Ninth Edition

HEALTH PROFESSIONAL and PATIENT INTERACTION

Amy Haddad, PhD, RN
Professor and the Dr. C.C.
and Mabel L.
Criss Endowed Chair in the Health Sciences,
Center for Health Policy and Ethics,
Creighton University, Omaha, Nebraska

Regina Doherty, OTD, OTR/L, FAOTA
Associate Professor and Program Director,
Department of Occupational Therapy,
School of Health and Rehabilitation Sciences,
MGH Institute of Health Professions, Boston, Massachusetts

Ruth Purtilo, PhD, FAPTA
Professor Emerita,
MGH Institute of Health Professions, Boston, Massachusetts

ELSEVIER

ELSEVIER

3251 Riverport Lane
St. Louis, Missouri 63043

HEALTH PROFESSIONAL AND PATIENT
INTERACTION   ISBN: 978-0-323-53362-1

Notices

Practitioners and researchers must always rely on their own experience and knowledge in evaluating and using any information, methods, compounds, or experiments described herein. Because of rapid advances in the medical sciences, in particular, independent verification of diagnoses and drug dosages should be made. To the fullest extent of the law, no responsibility is assumed by Elsevier, authors, editors, or contributors for any injury and/or damage to persons or property as a matter of products liability, negligence or otherwise, or from any use or operation of any methods, products, instructions, or ideas contained in the material herein.

Library of Congress Control Number: 2018951885

Content Strategist: Lauren Willis
Content Development Manager: Luke Held
Content Development Specialists: Laura Klein, Kelly Skelton
Publishing Services Manager: Deepthi Unni
Senior Project Manager: Manchu Mohan
Design Direction: Patrick Ferguson

Printed in the United States of America

Last digit is the print number: 9 8 7 6 5 4 3 2 1

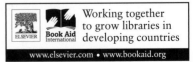

Working together to grow libraries in developing countries

www.elsevier.com • www.bookaid.org

With gratitude to the patients, professional colleagues, students, and friends whose stories and suggestions for content have enhanced the pages in this book—and enriched our lives.

Amy, Regina, and Ruth

There is a Chinese saying that a trip of a thousand miles begins with the first step. As this ninth edition of *Health Professional and Patient Interaction* goes to press, the authors are aware that opportunities in the health professions continue to expand and the level of education for participation in health care is evolving. This book is a companion for one of the first steps every person embarks on in a journey leading to a career in the health professions. Everyone must gain a basic understanding of the dynamics of the human relationships in a variety of care delivery settings. The core of these relationships consists of respectful interactions that shape and influence the success of all care and thus is the focus of this book.

Readers will have the opportunity to (1) engage in critical self-reflection; (2) clarify their roles in shaping the health professional and patient relationship; (3) explore effective models of interprofessional communication and collaboration for the delivery of quality, compassionate care; and (4) develop awareness of the larger health care and societal contexts in which each relationship takes place. Clarification of personal, professional, and societal values sets the stage for exploring the complexity of interactions and the unique perspective that a health professional and patient each brings to their relationship.

Respect is the thread that weaves together discussions regarding relationships in the health care environment. *Health Professional and Patient Interaction* includes evidence-based, respect-generating resources from the foundational disciplines of the social sciences, humanities, communications, ethics, medicine, and psychology.

The content is designed to apply to everyday clinical experiences across a variety of health professions, taking into account their specific disciplinary perspectives and the levels of formal education such preparation may involve, from two-year programs to doctoral-level preparation. Obviously, the autonomy and direct accountability for specific patient outcomes will differ, but the human-to-human encounter remains constant. Part of the function of this book, therefore, is to show the extent to which the different members of the interprofessional care team share common challenges, goals, and opportunities for service as they collaborate in the delivery of patient- and family-centered care.

In some instances, it is necessary to assign meaning to key terms. We mention four here: (1) *patient*—the recipient of and participant in a health care interaction, (2) *experiential learning*—the portion of formal education that takes place at the type of worksite where a person will practice, (3) *clinical experience*—the accumulation of actual experiences in one's chosen field, and (4) *interprofessional collaboration*—when multiple health professionals from different disciplines work together, interdependently, to deliver care.

The names of patients, families, health professionals, and other persons in the cases and other examples are fictitious. They represent a variety of clinical settings and disciplines to allow the reader to reflect on professional interactions across the life span and throughout the wide spectrum of care delivery settings.

When the last word of a manuscript has been written, its life has just begun. In sharing our ideas with you, the reader, we hope that in turn you will be stimulated to share yours with others, thus making us all more knowledgeable and skilled in respectful human interactions.

Amy Haddad

Regina Doherty

Ruth Purtilo

ACKNOWLEDGMENTS

One joy of preparing this ninth edition of *Health Professional and Patient Interaction* has been the opportunity for us to work together in its development.

Each of us also has discussed issues examined in the book with students and other readers, as well as clinicians and faculty members around the country and the world. We thank them for their insights. Several persons at Elsevier have been outstanding in their guidance and support. Finally, we extend our heartfelt thanks to our husbands, Steve, Dan, and Vard, who encourage us in all of our professional projects and enrich our lives, and to Regina's daughter, Olivia, who continues to be a source of inspiration as she charts her path in the world.

CONTENTS

Creating a Context of Respect

As you enter the pages of this book about your health professional and patient encounters, the first thing we bring to your attention are some key features of this special relationship. Understanding them will help ensure lifelong satisfaction in your career.

Chapter 1 introduces the concept of respect and the central function it plays in the professional role. Respect is essential to a good working relationship between health professionals and patients and is expressed in the everyday practice of the professions as specific conduct and attitudes. One indicator or expression of respect takes the form of the professional's sincere appreciation for the unique qualities of each person. Beyond that, respect is expressed through an acknowledgment that the other warrants the professional's considered attention. The ultimate expression of respect toward the other is found in the professional's genuine care for the patient.

Basic values—your own, those of the health professions, and society's—constitute a firm foundation for this respect to take root and grow into appropriate conduct and attitudes toward the people who become your patients.

Chapter 2 describes four benchmarks that are standards for measuring whether respect is at the center of a health professional and patient relationship. They include evidence that (1) the patient has grounds to trust that the professional is acting in that person's best interest, (2) the professional is addressing any deleterious effects of transference and countertransference that are influencing the relationship, (3) professional courtesy is being shown as part and parcel of the professional's duty, and (4) genuine human care is being exercised, guided by the expectations and contours of the health professionals' role in society, their specific scope of practice, and their commitment to providing optimum results in the interaction.

Chapter 3 continues to describe conduct and attitudes that express respect, this time in the form of a benchmark focused on professional constraints and sensitivities that honor the patient's dignity, privacy, and vulnerabilities. They include physical, psychological, and emotional boundaries that shape a healthful and satisfying relationship. These boundaries have their roots in the experience and wisdom of health professionals and other professions in society that contribute to the type of relationship that is acceptable to all parties involved.

The chapters in Section 1 are optimistic in tone and content, as are we, about your opportunity to honor and help foster respect in the health professions.

Respect in the Professional Role

The reader will be able to:
- Give a brief definition of respect and three indicators that respect is being expressed
- Describe why respect based on the idea of human dignity is so central to the success of the health professional and patient relationship
- Identify three spheres of values that constitute a person's value system
- Explain how one's value system influences the respect shown to others
- Name several criteria that describe a profession as a social role
- Discuss why the professions today have become concerned about professionalism
- List some "universal" values that are especially relevant in a health professional and patient relationship based on respect
- Cite the benefits of a fully integrated value system and reasons why a person may choose not to abide by that standard at times

Prelude

His way isn't the same as mine, nor mine as his. But we're both in search of our destinies, and I respect him for that.

PAULO COELHO[1]

Chances are you do not recall where you first encountered the idea of respect. For most it began with a parent or other authority rewarding you for your conduct or—if you were like most children—correcting you for attitudes or behaviors that implied you were doing something that was socially unacceptable. As you grew older, these teachings were reinforced until you realized that respect is a basic ingredient of getting along well in society. Respect involves treating others in ways that support a person's confidence or self-worth. Hopefully, over time you were guided to understand that respect is part and parcel of living a full life and that at the core, respect is relational.

Whether you are preparing to enter a profession for the first time or are continuing to seek excellence in it through further study, being able to show and receive respect is a key to the satisfaction you will be able to realize over the course of your career as a health professional. You might, in fact, think of respect as a linchpin that holds together your professional identity. Without respect for (and from) others, you will inevitably find the paths you are choosing in your professional life veering off course.

What Is Respect?

Respect comes from the Latin root *respicere*, which means "to look at closely." In common parlance, it has come to be interpreted as approaching an object, idea, person or group with regard or esteem.[2] This broad definition highlights that respect also applies to objects, situations, animals, and nature, but in your study of this book, we ask you to pay the most attention to its relevance for person-to-person interactions. In this context, respect for another conveys, "you matter," "you are worth the trouble." No matter how extreme our circumstances, we as humans hope above all that others will not discount our need to be somebody, that we will be sympathetically accompanied through the most difficult and unlikable or threatening aspects of our struggles. And when we rejoice, we hope others will join us in our celebration of happiness or accomplishment. In other words, we count on others' respect for who we are in a very fundamental sense, a recognition that we all are human. Many writers have tried to explain that this expectation arises because humans have basic worth. They agree that we share a common essence they term *dignity*. Even the ancients, in their myths, described this common essence, a theme also explored in virtually all the world's major religious traditions.[3] The essence is often referred to as the *inherent dignity* of persons to help emphasize that it resides beyond the physical, social, or psychological characteristics that distinguish us from each other.[4]

Inherent dignity is deeply ingrained in the idea of a profession. The assumption being that there is a common thread of humanity that warrants basic regard of a person as such. In your study of this book, we will help you look for specific evidence of this respect through such everyday actions as the tone of your voice when you address a patient, the adaptation of your pace and body language to meet the needs of a child versus an elderly patient, your trustworthy keeping of a patient confidence, your attention to cultural differences, your presence during a crisis, and your willingness to work together with a patient's support system, including family, significant others, and care providers.

Your skilled interventions can foster confidence that each patient is worthy to participate in health-related decisions that protect meaning in his or her life. Your communications can convey that you have the patients' back and that your intent is to protect them from exploitation or harm and advocate for them in ways that will be to their benefit.

Three Indicators of Respect

Three general indicators of respect will help you recognize a respectful health professional and patient relationship. The following indicators are described to take you a step further in helping you understand the deeper relational dynamics that take place in respectful conduct and communications within it.

1. *Appreciation.* Respect as appreciation means that you, a health professional, take notice of a person's unique character, manner, physical attributes, personality, and needs. This type of appreciation is not directed to a patient's superficial traits but serves as a tool to distinguish this individual from being one of a nameless crowd. In other words, you have not approached such an appraisal to make a positive or negative judgment about the person but rather to more fully "see" him or her as a unique individual. This expression of respect is illustrated in the comment by author Paulo Coelho at the beginning of this chapter. For the character in this novel just knowing that each is on a journey with a destiny in mind is basis enough for him to respect the other. More details of this aspect of respect based on our differences are emphasized in Chapter 5 and illustrated throughout this book.

2. *Attentiveness.* Respect as attentiveness means that you consciously turn your attention more fully to the person. Your stance comes from having taken note of the other as a unique individual, and this knowledge affects your encounter insofar as you move toward engaging him or her in a specific way consistent with the characteristics, needs, values, and conditions that have brought you to this point in your encounter. In Chapter 2 we take up the idea of becoming "patient-centered," which further highlights how respect conveyed as attentiveness is an essential indicator of a successful health professional and patient relationship.

3. *Care.* Respect as care—and its active form, caring—is the ultimate indicator of respect and goes to the heart of the professional relationship. It invites something of you that includes the appreciation of and attentiveness toward another, as discussed previously, but goes deeper. Now you commit yourself to providing appropriate measures demonstrating that you genuinely respect a person's worth as a human being. In other words, this indicator of respect involves a willingness to involve yourself as a human being in relationship with another. Care is conveyed not only by your actions but also by attitudes that reflect who you really are. For instance, in your professional role your negative feelings toward a person do not give you permission to limit your responsibility toward him or her but rather require you to find a means by which this person's reasonable goals can be met. Moreover, you must include but go beyond the sole application of the technical skills of your profession to consider the well-being of the whole person as your everyday standard of this care. For this reason, health professionals sometimes are referred to as *care providers*. There is no one set formula for this core aspect of the relationship, though basic characteristics of professional care are addressed later in this chapter and Chapters 2 and 3. An exploration of its many expressions are woven into every chapter of this book.

This introduction to respect and three indicators that one is being respectful (and respected) should emphasize some similarities between the function of respect in everyday life and help set the stage for you to further explore how respect factors into what is at stake in being a health professional.

REFLECTIONS

Think of a situation in your life when you felt you were not being treated respectfully.
- Of the three indicators of respect, which one or ones were not being honored?
- How did it make you feel?
- What could the other(s) have done to diminish your experience of being disrespected?

Respect and Your Values

To embrace and express respect for others, it is essential that you have insight into your own personal values and those of the subgroups and society in which you live. Moreover, there are some values that are especially vital to your role as a health professional. *Values* describe things one holds dear, and almost everyone can list many things that, on reflection, meet that criterion. We say that something is "of value" when we estimate it to have worth to us. One criterion of a "true" value is that it has become part of a pattern in one's life.

Values also provide the content to guide choices. They act as a compass to point where to put your attention and helps explain why you care what happens in regard to that object, idea, or person.

Taken together, your values constitute your *value system.* Some values in that system are highly specific to you as an individual. Some will be adopted through various subgroups to which you belong. Still others are shared by the majority of humans because of our common human condition. The unique value system for each person reflects a profile of his or her idea of how to survive and flourish. In Chapter 4 the authors focus more fully on how abiding by one's values becomes the fundamental basis of respect for oneself when challenging situations arise. Basic values find expression through the various roles one assumes—in your case, an important one being that of a health professional.

PERSONAL VALUES

Personal values are strictly one's own. Early values are absorbed from familial and social sources. These include parents, grandparents, relatives, childhood friends, caregivers, teachers, religious beliefs and traditions, and other sociocultural influences such as television and the Internet. Values are imparted, taught, reinforced, and internalized. We incorporate many of them into our lives as a personal value system. We exist in a complex world of bureaucracies and institutions that influence us, too. Our personal value system is dynamic. As we mature, our values may evolve with us to match our insights and experience.

Most people attach importance to more than one personal good, or value. History provides striking exceptions of persons whose lives seemingly were governed by one primary value that gave purpose to their everyday efforts. Examples are Joan of Arc, Mahatma Gandhi, Madame Marie Curie, Wolfgang Mozart, Sojourner Truth, and Babe Ruth. Most of us have many personal values, some more clearly defined than others, and go through life trying to realize or balance these personal values simultaneously.

The process of developing self-consciousness about one's values is the focus of values clarification exercises. Values clarification provides the means to discover the values one actually lives by day to day. An individual who can identify his or her own values is able to compare the worth of alternatives and make personally satisfying choices. Conversely, if unclear about your values or the connection between them and your choices, poor decision-making and dissatisfaction often result.[5]

REFLECTIONS

The following values clarification exercise is helpful in identifying personal values and how these values play out in real life.
- First, make a list of your 10 most important personal values in order of importance.
- Next, compare and contrast your own list of personal values with a peer's list.
- Then, compare the list of your own highest ranking values with your own behaviors.
- To what degree is your behavior consistent with your stated values?
- If there is an inconsistency, can you identify factors that keep you from integrating the two? Why?
- What can you do (if anything) to bring your stated values and behaviors into closer alignment?

Sometimes your personal values will conflict with each other. An example is Joe, a 35-year-old man with a diagnosis of severe obesity. Although there are many factors contributing to obesity, Joe reports to his care providers that he finds security in consuming vast amounts of food and identifies healthiness as being dependent on always having an ample supply of it. Unfortunately, his habitual eating now is causing increasingly poor health, and his care team tells him that he can expect a shortened life span with increasing debilitation. At this point, Joe's basic value of a healthful life is endangered by the competing personal value of feeling secure through food consumption. Because both values are essential to his good health, the goal is to help him derive security from aspects of life other than eating more food than his body needs to stay healthy. Similar examples of clashing values surround challenges related to other life-endangering practices, such as smoking, overwork, substance abuse, or lack of exercise or good sleeping habits.

REFLECTIONS

Your choice to make a career in the health professions has come from a desire to act on some of your most important personal values. Name some personal values that you recognize as consistent with your commitment to becoming and being a successful health professional.

When patients seek your services, their own personal values are almost always the motivation. They value staying healthy, getting well, or finding comfort during chronic or life-threatening illness. They want you to help them restore or maintain their value of health and optimize their functioning. Because health care is concerned primarily with personal values that are addressed through professional and patient relationships, your professional preparation gives you an opportunity to study and think about the challenges your own personal values may pose and to identify those that will facilitate your success. If, overall, you conclude that you share similar health-related values with patients it will help to more easily create a bond with them that reflects your genuine respect for their situation and its challenges. If your situation is so different from theirs that it is difficult to do so, your default during these times is your commitment to the fact that their dignity as a human being must be called on to guide you. A current helpful resource that addresses concrete steps professionals can take in such situations is the Dignity and Respect Campaign started in October 2008 by the University of Pittsburgh Medical Center. Under the heading "Dignity & Respect" it provides examples and incentives to its employees to encourage the inclusion of helpful pointers across the organization.[6]

PROFESSIONAL VALUES AND PROFESSIONALISM

Having chosen to become a health professional requires that you embrace values consistent with what being a professional means and professional practice entails. Fortunately, many of these values overlap with your personal values or at least do not conflict with them.

The word *professional* itself comes from the root "to profess" or declare something. When you adopt the values of your profession, as a professing-person you are publicly declaring something important to society about your place in it.

What is a Profession?

First and foremost a *profession* is a societal role with specific functions. Several criteria are the most often cited as describing a profession and how it is different from other societal roles. Among them are:

- Professions have an organized body of specialized knowledge and skills that require extensive training and are regarded by society.
- The knowledge and skills are designed to serve a basic human need.
- Basic need often renders the receiving person or group vulnerable in some way, so a profession promises to treat this vulnerability with due care.
- A profession has a code of ethics and code of conduct to which its members are expected to conform.
- Members of professions have privileges because of their societal role that other members of society do not have. For example, a health professional is licensed (literally given license by society) to touch, probe, and even invade a patient's body depending on his or her specialty, actions that would lead to arrest if performed by a citizen on the street. In turn a profession's code of ethics and various laws and other societal regulations detail the extent of and constraints on that privilege.

Many health professional organizations articulate basic values that undergird their specific identity. These values help explain the reasonable expectations that society can count on regarding all members of that profession. For example, the National Association of Social Workers lists the following core values, claiming them to be the foundation of social work's unique purpose and perspective: service, social justice, dignity and worth of the person, importance of human relationships, integrity, and competence.[7] Another example is the list of core values developed by the Education Section of the American Physical Therapy Association. It includes accountability, altruism, compassion and caring, excellence, integrity, professional duty, and social responsibility.[8] It is worth your effort to identify the values that your own professional organization has generated. You will readily see areas of overlap among the professions and begin to observe a general profile of professional values. For instance, several include ideals of selfless conduct, trustworthiness, and accountability.

WHAT IS PROFESSIONALISM?

In recent years, professional organizations have devoted growing attention to the idea of *professionalism*. The initiatives geared to professionalism share the common goal of identifying, protecting, and fostering the appropriate focus of the professional's role in society. The underlying concern is that forces outside of the professions themselves such as changes in the health care system and pressures from society to conform to its whims may place undue pressure on professionals.[9]

Professional responsibility is a dominant theme in professionalism. It emphasizes that the professions must be responsive to today's societal changes and demands. At the same time, in his probing analysis of the role of the professions in contemporary society, William Sullivan[10] advises professionals to be careful not to lose their own core values in their attempt to mold themselves to society's expectations. More than ever, he notes, they "have become responsible for key public values," and one such public value is personal health. It is this responsibility that sets off professionals from other workers and health professionals from other professional groups. Although professionals are engaged in generating or applying new ideas and technologies, each and all directly are pledged to an ethic of public service.

Of course, reflection by the professions on the values they uphold, and why, is by no means a novel phenomenon unique to the present age. Such reflection has been the focus of lively study and debate since the delineation of three traditional professions (law, medicine, and the clergy) during the Middle Ages. Today many still refer to a profession as a "calling" that requires total devotion, specialized knowledge, and extensive academic preparation. From these root terms and interpretations, the professions today are identified as groups whose members have responded to an opportunity to hold a special place in society, differentiated from those who hold other types of jobs. Their claims derive from society's values and society's beliefs. In other words, the task for you, the reader, is to incorporate appropriate values of professionalism into your value system. You may wonder why so much time is devoted to something like this that seems obvious in many regards, but the authors have found the preparation is well worth the effort because all health care providers will have conflicting claims placed on them and be involved in extremely complex situations. During such times the ability to ground yourself in your own and the profession's values, undergirded by your commitment to professional responsibility, creates a valuable foundation for informed, intentional movement forward.[11]

Care as a Professional Value

The basic idea of care as one key indicator of respect for another person was introduced earlier in this chapter. We view it here through the lens of professional values. The values of care and its active form, caregiving, are pivotal to realizing the goals of professional practice. Professionals are judged in part by whether they offer competent care appropriate to their area of expertise. In that regard, care expressed as a professional is different in some important aspects from caring in a relationship with a spouse, child, friend, or colleague. It is shaped by conscientiously applying clinical knowledge and skill along with abiding by ethical duties, rights, and character traits that describe the proper place of a professional in this relationship. Patients are drawn to the idea of care because the term conveys that a high-stakes human story is taking place, and for them it always is. Patients have a personal story that holds all their hopes, dreams, and fears. The health professional's caregiving must reflect that the story is heard and he or she is prepared to shape a care plan with the patient's values and goals an uppermost consideration.[12] A key question for a health professional, then, is, "Do I really value what is required of me in this type of human relationship to work toward fully expressing 'I care' for the wide variety of patients I will encounter?"[13] If a health professional, does not hold this value as essential in his or her own professional identity or a key to career satisfaction over time, professional service is not a good fit for this person. As this book unfolds, specific skills needed for effective care in different kinds of situations and many examples of care are explored in more detail.

SOCIETAL VALUES

A third set of values that make up your value system derive from the larger society. One well-recognized characteristic of the human condition is that we, as human beings, organize ourselves into complex interactions as groups of individuals called *societies*. You belong to many communities within the larger society already. Each subgroup has values that you are aware of and may accept, reject, or question how they support your attempt to lead a good life.

REFLECTIONS

Take a minute to name some of the societal subgroups you are most influenced by, such as your extended family, neighborhood, ethnic community, the part of the country where you live, school you attend, religious affiliation, and social or civic organizations to which you belong.

Can you name one or two values you have absorbed from your participation in each of these subgroups? If not, where did your values come from other than from these common sources?

The scope of societal values that influence value choices has expanded greatly in the past few decades. Millions have immediate access to societal values expressed through the Internet, social media, radio, and television. We can travel extensively or meet those who do. These broadening circles of access and influence have led some to conclude that we are all indeed members of a global society and to survive must come to grips with the common values that will help all lead a good life. As you will see in Chapter 10, the public has taken advantage of the Internet, television commercials, magazines, travel, and other means of data gathering to gain health care and clinical information not previously accessible to them.

In spite of the increasing exposure to new and ever-expanding sources of values, there continues to be a belief among many that some basic societal values are so fundamental that they can be deemed universal. Their argument is that human beings are fundamentally social beings and therefore rarely find satisfaction outside the social context of living in a society, so they agree to abide by basic values that apply to all.

REFLECTIONS

Consider whether you believe the following are universally held societal values and what supports your conclusion.
- Protection of human life
- Rights and liberties
- Having power and opportunities
- Financial security
- Adequate food and shelter
- Self-respect
- Health and vigor
- Intelligence and imagination
- Autonomy/Self-governance

What additional values would you add or substitute?

Some major sources of mainstream Western values are laws, philosophical inquiry, and shared experiences. For example, lawmakers in such societies rely on the principle that human life itself is a basic value and therefore ought to be protected and nourished.

Philosophers are an ongoing source of input as well. John Rawls, one of the most influential American philosophers near the end of the 20th century, argued that humans value several primary goods. *Social primary goods* include rights, liberties, powers, opportunities, income, wealth, and self-respect. (Self-respect is necessary for a person to feel assured his or her life plan is worth carrying out or capable of being fulfilled.) The realization of these goods is at least partially determined by the structure of society itself. *Natural primary goods,* also partly determined by societal structures but not directly under their control, include health, vigor, intelligence, and imagination.[14] Together, he says, these social and natural primary goods provide a sort of "index of welfare" for individuals in any society.

Other writers over the centuries have suggested character traits they propose produce a good life for the larger community; however, there is dispute over which character traits are the central ones. For instance, in ancient Greek society, the *cardinal virtues* of temperance, prudence, a desire to do justice, courage, and fortitude (or moral strength to do what is right) were considered central to being able to lead a good life. Early Christian thinkers argued that these alone were not sufficient for a good life and that faith in God, hope, and love were crucial. Other world religions and schools of philosophical thought have contributed their own lists.

Whether there are universally held societal values, they do have power to affect well-being positively or negatively on large groups of adherents. Whatever one's lot in life, most individuals need to be accepted within society and be able to embrace and live by its most basic values.

Respect, Values, and the Good Life

In this chapter, you have encountered examples of three spheres of values: personal, professional, and societal. Their differences have been highlighted, but in everyday life a person usually adopts a set of personal values that overlap in part and are harmonious with role-related values and the larger society's values. Fig. 1.1 shows a schematic representation of a person's integrated value system.

Motivation for this integration usually arises to reap personal and societal benefits that derive from doing so. It is possible to say of persons who live according to their value system, "That person has a good life." However, when a person's value system includes respect for values that help to uphold and further society as well, we say, "That person leads a good life."

Of course, not everyone adopts a set of personal values compatible with societal values or even with those of his or her own social or cultural subgroups. In the extreme form, this person has never integrated any societal or other cultural values into a value system or rejects them over time.

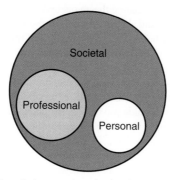

Fig. 1.1 Integrated personal, professional, and societal values.

Such a person likely believes there are no benefits to be derived from living in harmony with society's values. Some examples are the hermit, the outlaw, and the saint or martyr. The hermit and outlaw reject societal values and replace them with their own; the saint or martyr rejects societal values and replaces them with a "higher" set of values.

There are varying degrees to which persons periodically exempt or more permanently divorce themselves from societal values. For example, the woman who drives through a red light to make it to her tennis match on time is replacing a societal value of adherence to the traffic rules designed to protect all drivers with the personal value of reaching her tennis game. Or the conscientious objector who performs alternative service is refusing to accept the societal value of engaging in war to protect one's country on the basis of following the antiwar dictates of a higher law. Most people experience some such conflict from time to time, but often the default tendency is not to rock the boat, no matter how unsatisfactory the situation, until it is judged to be a crisis. And so it is jarring when something compels a person to reflect on his or her values and decide that they do not suffice. A powerful passage in the novel *Dead Man Walking* describes how Sister Prejean, the narrator of the book, understands suddenly after hearing a political activist speak that she is going to have to take a stand against capital punishment in response to data showing that this punishment is administered unfairly to rich and poor offenders. The speaker challenged audience members to reflect on their own values and action. Sister Prejean recalls, "She [the speaker] knew her facts and I found myself mentally pitting my arguments against her challenge—we were nuns, not social workers, not political. But it's as if she knew what I was thinking. She pointed out that to claim to be apolitical or neutral in the face of such injustices would be, in actuality, to uphold the status quo—a very political position to take, and on the side of the oppressors."[15]

For the health professional, a disconnect can occur when professional values that have been incorporated into legal and other institutional practices come into conflict with personal values or what the professional believes are appropriate societal values. Some current examples that arise in health care practices and policies today include an individual professional's personal values regarding legally and professionally sanctioned abortion, childhood vaccination, clinically assisted suicide and other end-of-life measures, or health care reimbursement mechanisms that the professional deems unfair to some groups. Any time a professional cannot conform in good conscience to practice and policy norms, it can become a source of discomfort for all but also an occasion for thoughtful reflection, discussion, and action.

Summary

Respect for others and reaping the benefits of it yourself are essential ingredients for a successful professional practice. Genuine respect involves both attitudes and conduct that acknowledge your regard for another person's dignity, no matter what his or her attributes and circumstances are. Indicators of respect can be found in appreciating the uniqueness of each individual, directing considered attention to their needs and values, and choosing action consistent with professional care. Our values constitute the content of what we hold dear and important and influence whether we will want and be able to express genuine respect for patients, their families, and other professionals. Some values arise from personal preferences, whereas others become internalized over time through the influences of our affiliations and societal forces. Professional values are transmitted through the educational, clinical, and research institutions of health care and are grounded in professional ethics. A professional identity based on respect will guide you back to the understanding that, in your relationships with patients, their assurance that they are being respected will depend on your ability to convey that you understand the stakes are high for them. They also will be reassured that you will devote your energy to addressing needs appropriate to your professional role. Your genuine care conveys your acknowledgment that respect requires action. Along the way you can make good progress on your road to respectful interaction by identifying your own values and developing a genuine interest in others.

References

1. Coelho P. *The Alchemist*. English translation by Alan R. Clark. Orig published in Portuguese, 1988. Eng trans 1993. New York: HarperCollins paperback edition, P 84.
2. *Shorter Oxford English Dictionary*. 5th ed. Vol. 2. Oxford, England: Oxford University Press; 2002:2250.
3. Purtilo RB. Chapter 1. New respect for respect in ethics education. In: Purtilo RB, Jensen GM, Royeen CB, eds. *Educating for Moral Action: A Sourcebook in Health and Rehabilitation Ethics*. Philadelphia: FA Davis; 2005:1–11.
4. Rolston III H. Chapter 6. Human uniqueness and human dignity: persons in nature and the nature of persons. In: Davis FD, ed. *Human Dignity and Bioethics: Essays Commissioned by The President's Council on Bioethics*. Washington, DC; 2008:129–154.
5. Hayhurst C. Measuring by value not productivity. *PT in Motion*. 2015;6(7):4–7.
6. Dignity and Respect Campaign. www.dignityandrespect.org.
7. National Association of Social Workers. In: *Preamble to the Code of Ethics*. Washington, DC: National Association of Social Workers; 2008.
8. American Physical Therapy Association. *Professionalism in Physical Therapy: Consensus Document*. Alexandria, VA: American Physical Therapy Association; 2003.
9. Tilbert JC, Sharp RR. Owning medical professionalism. *Am J Bioeth*. 2016;16(9):1–2.
10. Sullivan WM. *Work and Integrity, the Crisis and Promise of Professionalism in America*. 2nd ed. San Francisco: Jossey-Bass; 2005:4–9.
11. Doherty RF, Peterson EW. Responsible participation in a profession: fostering professionalism and leading for moral action. In: Braveman B, ed. *An Evidence-Based Approach to Leading & Managing Occupational Therapy Services*. 2nd ed. Philadelphia: FA Davis; 2016.
12. Purtilo RB. What interprofessional teamwork taught me about an ethics of care. *Phys Ther Rev*. 2012;17: 197–201.
13. Doherty RF, Purtilo RB. Chapter 2. The ethical goal of professional practice: a caring response. In: *Ethical Dimensions in the Health Professions*. 6th ed. St. Louis: Elsevier; 2016:27–50.
14. Rawls J. *A Theory of Justice*. 2nd ed. Cambridge, Massachusetts: Belknap Press of Harvard University; 1971.
15. Prejean H. *Dead Man Walking*. New York: Vintage Books; 1994:5–6.

Professional Relatedness Built on Respect

OBJECTIVES

The reader will be able to:

- Describe how trust and trustworthiness serve as a benchmark to gauge respect between patient and health professional
- Recognize professional competence and reassurance as supports in a trust-based connection between health professional and patient
- Explain how acknowledging and responding to the phenomenon of transference or countertransference in the health professional and patient relationship serves as a benchmark of respect
- Describe professional courteous behaviors and what is involved in meeting the benchmark of respect as the relationship develops
- Explain several examples of what is involved in meeting the respect benchmark of professional caring behaviors
- Distinguish the basic contractual foundation of the health professional and patient relationship from covenantal characteristics and the role of each in achieving the benefits of a professional career

Prelude

Of course the questions had to do only with illness. By the time he was through, this young man would know all about her years in the sanatorium, about her hysterectomy, and about her damaged lungs—and that is all he would know. Laura was amazed to discover that she was struggling to make a connection on another level. In a hospital one is reduced to being a body, one's history is the body's history, and perhaps that is why something deep inside a person reaches out, a little like a spider trying desperately to find a corner on which to begin to hang a web, a web of personal relation.

M. SARTON[1]

In this chapter, you have an opportunity to take the insights about respect you have gained from Chapter 1 and put them more specifically into the context of your relationship with patients. In May Sarton's reflection, above, you get a feel for her desire to make a fuller human connection with her young health professional—in her words, to find a "web of personal relation." She believes correctly that without their personal connection the professional cannot know who she is and cannot effectively express respect for her in her situation.

The health professional and patient relationship is determined by what you have subscribed to by becoming a professional and what the patient is experiencing that has brought this person to you instead of seeking out a friend, loved one, or business associate for help. Therefore, although respect is the foundation of any relationship, a good professional relationship has special respect considerations built into it because of your respective roles.

The phrase *patient-centered* is an apt example of terms and concepts that have evolved in the health professions literature to help keep an appropriate focus on this particular type of relationship.[2] Patient-centered does not mean that the patient has the right or prerogative to claim first place among all of the professional's personal priorities. It does, however, guide health professionals to decide among competing priorities when a conflict arises because of their professional role and its responsibilities. The goal of being patient-centered involves honoring the indicators of respect in its three forms—that is, appreciation of a patient's uniqueness among persons, attention to that person's health-related need, and commitment to conscientiously providing your professional knowledge and skills to address that need. In meeting this goal, health professionals and patients alike benefit from observable and measurable *benchmarks*. Benchmarks serve as standards and points of reference to assess whether an activity is in fact accomplishing its intended purpose. A respect benchmark measures observable actions that demonstrate that respect is operating at the core of a health professional and patient relationship.

Four important respect benchmarks include:

- evidence that the relationship is based on trust,
- conduct showing that health professionals acknowledge the realities of transference and countertransference and respond accordingly,
- expressions of professional courteous behavior toward patients and their support networks,
- markers confirming patient-centered care with the person's well-being the determinant of the specific shape it will take.

Build Trust by Being Trustworthy

Legally and ethically the health professional and patient relationship is based on trust. In the law, it is categorized as a *fiduciary relationship* in contrast to one that depends solely on the terms of a contract between two persons. The term *fiduciary* comes from the root *fides*, meaning "faith in someone or something." In this instance, it rests on an assumption that one of the two parties, the patient, cannot be expected to have all the relevant facts that would allow them to contract as equals.

Trust is the patient's sense of security that he or she is being respected by you, including confidence in your intent to provide your best professional services. The patient and others deem you *trustworthy*. In the traditional physician-patient relationship, trustworthiness was recognized by the patient's and others' blind faith in the physician. In almost all cases until the beginning of the 20th century, health care providers had few therapeutic interventions to offer except their presence and pain-relieving elixirs. At the same time the positive dimension of good doctoring of that era is that the provider was judged not only on mere physical presence but also that there was a personal connection with sufferers who were soothed by the professional's benevolence and compassion for the patient's and family's situation.

Modern interpretations of the role of trust in human relationships are molding the understanding of how it becomes recognizable in health professional and patient interactions. In the view of developmental psychologists, trust plays a central role in every person's developmental task of figuring out when and why to depend on others. Underlying this is the belief that no one else knows fully what is best for another individual and that to turn over that responsibility completely to someone else, even a professional, is not in a person's best interests. Therefore health professionals are considered trustworthy when a patient is helped to feel secure not only in the professionals' technical skills and decisions but also that he or she has been invited into fuller participation in decisions about personal well-being. The connection in the traditional relationship historically, nurtured by the professional's benevolence and compassion, continues to be vitally important, but choosing treatment alternatives together among possible courses of technical interventions shifts the focus.

Whereas "patient-centered" in more traditional understandings was interpreted to mean that the patient must submit trustingly to the professional's sole judgment, today it requires that the health professional also engage in more partnering with the patient, family, and other members of the interprofessional care team to plan a professional course of action based on what really matters most to the patient.[3] Only then can the patient feel confident that the professional's clinical decision is being guided by an underlying respect for that person's basic human dignity.

Other chapters in this book emphasize that trust and distrust do not arise solely in the one-on-one professional and patient interaction. Patients can trust or distrust the way the health care system itself is set up or the institutions or environments in which the services are offered. The important point here is that in almost all instances a health professional or professionals must be involved in assuming responsibility for building patient trust when any level of distrust occurs. This may be by reporting a problem to the appropriate authority, documenting abuses or injustices, working to change ineffective or unfair policies or practices, and in other ways participating in building a continuum of care respectful of patients' needs and preferences. For each area of trust experienced by the patient, the health professional has met the respect benchmark of helping to build a trust-based relationship.

PROFESSIONAL COMPETENCE AND TRUST

Trust building cannot be achieved fully without a patient's and others' confidence in your ability to apply skills specific to the unique modalities of your chosen profession.

Your *professional competence* includes:

- knowing what you know and are skilled to do within your specific area defined by your formal training and referred to in the literature and regulations as your "scope of practice,"
- a commitment to diligently stay current on the research and management of conditions within your scope of practice,
- awareness of your professional and personal shortcomings that could negatively affect optimum patient outcomes, and
- continual reflection and discussion with other professionals for self-improvement.

A patient's request for services in your scope of practice usually is generated by the presence of injury or illness resulting in a lack of ability to function, or some other disquieting physical, cognitive, or mental symptom. People also seek your counsel about how to stay healthy and prevent health-related difficulties. The patient counts on you and other members of an interprofessional care team, all strangers to the patient, to clinically assess the patient's problem, what it means for his or her everyday life, and what he or she needs to do to initiate and follow a clinical process leading to restoration or maintenance of the highest quality of life possible in the situation.

A trust-based professional relationship guided by the professionals' areas of competence builds over time, but that alone is not enough. Some challenges to trust result from the professionals' assumption that patients and others view the health care world just as they do. For instance, health professionals and institutions are so familiar with the professional setting that sometimes they become insensitive to unintended messages that get conveyed, causing patients and other laypeople to be wary of how patients are viewed. For example, one of the authors remembers overhearing a family anxiously discussing an ethics conference poster by an elevator near the intensive care unit (ICU) titled "Limiting Treatment in the ICU" and interpreted it to mean that professionals were looking for ways to transfer their loved ones out of the ICU prematurely. Fortunately, the surprised professional standing nearby was able to clarify that in fact it was a conference designed to further enhance this very effective treatment approach. Commonly used signs and terms such as the "bone clinic," the "allergy office," or "cardiac surgery," all can conjure patients' images of body parts or procedures rather than living, breathing human beings, leading one cartoonist to take this patient concern to the extreme (Fig. 2.1).

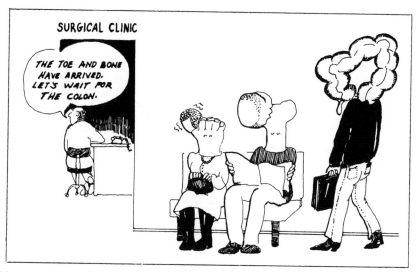

Fig. 2.1 At one extreme the patient may feel that the health professional is interested only in the body part or symptom. (*From the Swedish translation of Health Professional and Patient Interaction: Vård, Vårdare, Vårdad.*)

Some have called this phenomenon *thinging*. In it the patient fears being more valued for the "interesting thing" that he or she brings to the health professions setting than, above all, being a person with a human need. This is a serious challenge for health professionals because a necessary part of professional training is to look for the abstractive meaning of a condition: the chest sound, laboratory findings, x-ray films, the sight of the skin or tone of the muscle, and so forth. Common sense suggests that patients should not trust you if you seem more interested in their diagnosis or symptom than in what these mean to their well-being as persons. To the extent that you recognize the mistake of "thinging" and are sensitive to language that can be erroneously interpreted, you will have taken a giant step toward engendering a genuine bond of trust.

Clinically unattainable patient or family expectations also can be a barrier to trust. For example, consider the Case below regarding Mrs. Gleason, her family, and the team assigned to her care. This family's distrust rested on their inability or unwillingness to be reassured about the course of action being taken on behalf of Mrs. Gleason.

Case Study

Mrs. Amanda Gleason, a 70-year-old homemaker, has had amyotrophic lateral sclerosis (ALS) for just over a year. Mrs. Gleason and her family have gone on the Internet and learned that ALS, also known as *Lou Gehrig's disease,* is a progressive neurological condition affecting all voluntary muscles of her body. Most patients become weaker and weaker until they die, usually of respiratory arrest. Mrs. Gleason has only a small amount of movement left in her legs but can get around in a wheelchair. She is in the hospital for treatment of pneumonia that is probably due to weakness of her swallowing muscles, allowing aspiration of her throat contents into her lungs. Her weakness has accelerated since hospitalization, even though her pneumonia is responding to antibiotics. She is discouraged, knowing that the aspiration will continue and that in her present state it is unlikely she will go home. Her family realizes she is probably past the point of her ability to live independently. They feel unable to care for her in any of their own homes but are afraid of the terrible effect it will have on her when she learns this news. They ask several members of the interprofessional care team to do everything they can to reassure their mother that she will be OK.

Continued

Case Study—cont'd

Jaime Sills, the attending physician for Mrs. Gleason, meets with the interprofessional care team assigned to her, and they decide to conduct an evaluation by speech therapy and occupational therapy with the goal of determining the maximum swallowing function she has and any possible way she might be able to function well enough in her activities of daily living to manage in her own home with home health care assistance and the family's periodic help. Both therapists are extremely guarded in their conclusions, believing that her potential for a return home is limited.

Jaime Sills calls a family meeting with Mrs. Gleason, the children, the nurses primarily responsible for her care, the two therapists and a social worker. As the family feared, Mrs. Gleason is devastated, saying that she trusted them to help her and now they have let her down. The family, too, becomes assertive, telling this interprofessional care team that increasing her therapy at least would have given her some chance of a longer stay at home. No amount of reasoning about other alternatives seems to decrease their distrust and anger. Dr. Sills introduces the family to the social worker, Jake Sandersen, and says he will be glad to work with them to further explore their options. However, the family members by now have concluded that this meeting is further proof that their mother has been written off and stalk out of the meeting.

This situation was understandably uncomfortable for the health professionals who felt they had Mrs. Gleason's interests at heart but could not meet her and the family's expectations. Nothing the professionals said would convince or reassure them. When such situations arise the example of this team provides a process that, in the authors' opinion, should be of some comfort to professionals faced with similar situations. They all stayed with this family and took each concern and request seriously. At the same time, they were confident in their areas of professional competence and knew that genuine trustworthiness depends on exercising their best judgment accordingly.

Reality testing is a term often used to denote the health professional's attempts to keep the patient or others on track from setting unattainable goals, even though situations like the one of Mrs. Gleason occur at times. Communication and conduct based on professional judgment can help the patient and loved ones be realistic about their situation and therefore plan for unavoidable adjustments. How, when, and by whom unwelcome information is shared can help determine how it is received. Studies have found that most patients and their families or other supporters do want the truth about the patient's situation, which they can gain by being apprised of the professionals' best judgment at the outset and as the relationship progresses. But they also want to know that the professional is aware of the enormity of the information for the patient and family.[4] In other words, reality testing through compassionate and truthful conversations with the patient, family, and other spokespersons usually is welcomed as one characteristic of a trust-based relationship and facilitates planning for what lays ahead.

What are your resources for maintaining trust when you, the professional, are uncertain yourself about the best course for a patient? At one extreme the issue arises when there is consensus among professionals that their professional training and skills will be of no avail in achieving a positive result. There is a literature on *medical futility* that helps set professional guidelines for this circumstance and is worth the readers' further exploration. In these instances, the patient and loved ones need to know that the situation surpasses clinical knowledge at this point so as not to rest their trust on false hopes.[5] Other patients have complex conditions involving several bodily systems or symptoms that cause varying degrees of uncertainty among care providers. The uncertainty may be about the patient's actual diagnosis, the best plan of treatment, the likelihood of unanticipated complications, the expected timeline of results, or the eventual outcome (prognosis) even if all goes well.[6] The process of maintaining a trust-based relationship in these situations starts with offering any snippet of information that you can stand behind with certainty. Reassurance also may take the form of your willingness to respond compassionately to difficult questions about areas that are causing anxiety for patients or their families because abandonment is a common fear. Beyond that, though, are some challenges that are more difficult for many health professionals. For instance, many are very reticent to say "we don't know ourselves what to expect in your situation—it's not going as we hoped" because they worry that this admission will destroy the patient's hope. To the contrary, an honest admission usually does not have a lasting deleterious effect if this bad news is shared with compassion and deep respect for its significance to the patient and family.[7] One reassurance that can always be offered is, "You can count on us to continue to put our best effort forward on your behalf, and we will stand by you in the process."

REFLECTIONS

Think of a time in your life when someone tried to reassure you.
- What did the other person say or do that worked?
- Can you recount an example of when someone tried to reassure you but it did not work?
- Why did their attempts fail?

You can use these personal experiences to help guide you when you are faced with patients' or family's worries. Gentle probing may help uncover more specific causes for their concern and provide guidance for the direction your words and gestures should take. At the very least your assurance that you are trying your best to work on their behalf in this difficult time for them is always appropriate to help maintain their trust in your efforts. Your creativity about how to retain or regain their confidence in themselves and the relationship must be an intentional part of your work plan.

INTEGRITY IN WORDS AND CONDUCT

Integrity comes from the French root *integritas,* meaning "whole or undivided." The cultivation of integrity is your commitment to first and foremost know yourself thoroughly. A large part of this task is realized through living according to your value system as discussed in Chapter 1. Only then can you confidently demonstrate to others that your values and commitments are seamlessly aligned with your conduct so others experience a high level of consistency between what you say and what you do. We have been emphasizing examples of how trust does not build automatically in the health professional and patient relationship: It is the patients' judgment call as to whether they view you as trustworthy in declaring that you have their best interests at heart. Your integrity means that you project an authentic wholeness in your attitudes, words, and actions, providing evidence that they may confidently place their trust in you.[8]

The patient's reliance on the professional's integrity also extends to his or her experience with the interprofessional care team. Teams were designed to help coordinate care over time and across professional specialties so that the patient could experience a kind of collective integrity across the system. However, today sometimes the patient's encounter with multiple members of the care team breaks down confidence that there is a coordinated plan. In the absence of collaboration, interventions offered by team members, each representing differing perspectives on a patient's condition, can be confusing to the patient, leaving room for distrust to take root. We offer three general guidelines as preparation for your further study in Chapter 9 of interprofessional care teams to help patients see you as trustworthy.

- Be respectful of all team members' contributions, and decide among yourselves who will be the primary spokesperson in different situations that arise.
- Be an alert and active participant in team decisions. Provide your expertise, and listen to the perspectives and expertise of others.
- If a patient or family caregiver has a question that goes beyond your area of expertise, immediately convey this information to the appropriate team member, and let the patient know you are going to tap the expertise of others in response to their question.

In summary, trust and trustworthiness are central components of the success of any health professional and patient relationship. Having introduced you to several details of what is involved in meeting this important benchmark of respect, we turn now to another type of benchmark—namely, your acknowledgment of transference and countertransference in the professional relationship and your attention to its effects.

Tease Out Transference Issues

The psychotherapeutic notion of *transference* can help you understand certain kinds of behaviors some people exhibit toward you in your professional relationship with them. How you respond and use this insight serves as a respect benchmark. Transference has its root in the theories advanced by Sigmund Freud and further developed by other psychologists who employ this term to convey the process of shifting one's feeling about a person in the past to another person.[9] A young man, angry that his father brutally ruled with an iron hand, might conclude, "Here it comes again!" and respond aggressively to a male health professional as soon as something about the professional triggers a negative memory of his father. Or consider the example of Ray, a male nursing student who prepared extensively and carefully for his interaction with his first obstetrics-gynecology patient. Part of the clinical evaluation was to conduct a basic history and do a general physical examination. On entering the patient's room he said, "Good morning. I'm Ray Abrams, a student nurse who is going to be caring for you and examining you today." The patient took one look at this bearded, 6-foot-plus student and said, "Oh, no you're not! You look too much like my son, honey!" His supervisor, who had just stepped into the room, caught this woman's reaction and judged that to disregard the patient's discomfort would be a sign of disrespect, although she may have misunderstood what the student meant was not a gynecological examination. Instead the student's clinical instructor privately used the occasion as a teaching moment with the student, explaining that this type of transference sometimes happens. The instructor also informed the patient that in this case the examination simply included taking vital signs such as temperature, blood pressure, and pulse. Still, everyone was relieved when this patient was reassigned to a female student nurse.

Transference can be negative or positive. Examples of negative transference are the aggressiveness of the young man who "saw" his father in the professional and the discomfort stimulated by the similarity of the male nursing student to the woman's son. For reasons patients sometimes cannot identify or express, their comfort level is low and their guard is up. At the other end of the spectrum, positive transference, the good feelings a patient transfers to the health professional, usually can promote a well-working relationship.

It is not always easy to tell whether the transference will create a problem. A young occupational therapist caught a new male patient staring at her. Finally, he shook his head and said, "Man oh man, I could have sworn my first wife walked in when you came into the treatment area. Whew!" The man seemed a bit shaken, and of course this raised some questions for the therapist who responded by saying, "Well, is that a good or bad thing?" He said, "Both!" So, she was still in the woods on this one. She felt she had no choice in this moment but to continue with the patient, watching for further signs that this man's association seemed to be inappropriately affecting his responses and their relationship. (There were none, and the matter never came up again.)

The patient is not the only party in the relationship who experiences transference. *Countertransference,* a professional's tendency to respond to a patient with associations of others in his or her life, takes place every bit as often. A health professional may transfer feelings to the patient based on name, physical appearance, voice, age, or gestures that conjure up powerful associations of other people. It is up to you to be self-aware about such associations and adapt your conduct to correct for any negative or other troubling feelings and responses you think might be issuing from your mental association of the patient with someone in your past or present relationships.

At the same time, total neutrality is not required. If you have served on a jury, you know that the judge's concern is that the jurors' past experiences and associations do not in any discernible way adversely come into play to unduly sway the juror's judgment when the facts of the case and the identification of the defendant and plaintiff are made known. The basic concern is similar in the health professional and patient relationship. You can learn to listen for signs that such associations may be occurring. Fundamentally, what is necessary for maintaining respectful professional relationships with patients when this dynamic is taking place is to acknowledge transference or countertransference and try to respond to it in a way that honors it for the benchmark of respect that attending to it is. Your actions can range from simple awareness to providing for the patient to be referred to a colleague who is equally suited for the clinical challenges.

Distinguish Courtesy From Casualness

A third respect benchmark is based on the fact that basic politeness is an essential ingredient in every well-working relationship. You might think that everyday niceties such as "Hello, how are you today?" are such an obvious component of a respectful relationship that it need not be discussed. However, as important as a warm initial greeting is, the type of social exchange that is relevant as a benchmark of respect in a professional relationship is more akin to the idea of *courtesy*, which has a subtle level of formality to it. You can begin to see the difference in this simple dictionary definition of courtesy as ". . . elegance . . . of manners; graceful politeness or considerateness."[10] It includes but goes beyond minding your manners in the superficial sense that you were taught to do as a child. Professional courtesy requires doing so with words, attitudes, and gestures that convey your genuine acknowledgment of the other's dignity. Patients take their initial cues about whether they matter as people from the courtesy they receive when they first come through the door (or, in the case of home health care, when you pass through theirs). Although we must also strive to embed courteous conduct into the deeper understandings of care in the health professional and patient relationship, the patient's first, and often lasting, impression is connected to courtesies they receive (or do not receive) from you and others in the environment.

You cannot generate a welcoming, courteous environment on your own. In almost every instance you will be part of a group. Some will schedule patient appointments, keep patients informed, and collect fees. Others will work toward making a diagnosis or carrying out a treatment plan, and still others conduct discharge or follow-up activities. Another whole crew maintain a clean, tidy work environment. But you can and must also do your part, both personally and as a model for the others. For example, courtesies in an ambulatory care clinic, waiting room, or other common area that you can participate in maintaining include several signs of hospitality that anyone welcomes in a new environment:

- greeting a person warmly and by name, introducing yourself and your role;
- a safe place to hang a coat or umbrella;
- making sure that signage is present—that is, directions to bathrooms and dressing rooms, water fountains, extra seating, and clearly marked exits;
- offering assistance with mobility challenges and completing forms if it is requested of you or you notice that a person is struggling;
- keeping the patient (and family member) informed about delays or necessary changes;
- providing age-appropriate reading material, fresh water, and other calming distractions, including toys for small children.

The common denominator of this benchmark is that you show respect by initially directing your attention to each person's anxiety or questions and then structure your approach throughout the encounter so everyone can feel assured that you and your workplace colleagues' politeness is undergirded by attitudes and actions conveying genuine respect for that person's dignity from the get-go.

Take a minute to reflect on the last time you visited a physician, dentist, therapist, or other health professional. Picture the environment as you first entered.

- What did you find there that led you to feel confident you were welcomed and that the staff had given some thought to what would make you as comfortable as possible?
- How could the environment and conduct of the staff have been improved to make it a more commodious place?
- Now try to picture yourself being visited in your home by a home health care provider during your recovery from a serious accident. List some professional courtesies you would expect.

Today, many health care settings (as well as other public environments) try to create a feeling of casual relaxation as evidence of being consumer savvy. This can be effective to a certain degree, but for the most part a patient going to visit a health professional or to spend time in a health care institution is keenly aware that this journey is not like heading after work to the nearest bar or coffee shop or embarking on a vacation. In fact, this experience always involves some level of anxiety or uncertainty so that being approached in a very casual way may cause him or her to doubt that the professional cares. A good general rule is to be kind and forthright, trying to anticipate what the visit means to the individual patient. For instance, some are embarrassed to be in a place where their very presence suggests a weakness or malady. Others may cover their anxiety with loud laughter or conversely show excessive passivity (Fig. 2.2).

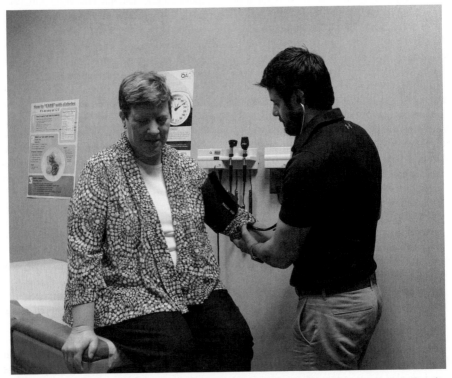

Fig. 2.2 The health care setting communicates that the patient and professional have different roles but share a common goal related to the patient's health. (*Courtesy Maren Haddad.*)

In summary, the onus is on the professional to attempt to meet the benchmark of respect through something as straightforward as genuine courtesy, a gracious acceptance of the other that takes the specific reason for their encounter into conscious account. From the patient's view professional courtesy is one visible sign that health professionals really care about him or her as a person.

Concentrate on Caring

As we introduced in Chapter 1, your role as a special kind of caregiver is so central to your purpose that your societal position is meaningless to others if you do not both profess and convincingly apply it. Your purpose in their life is to shape your relationship with each patient in light of their need for your professional expertise. The benchmark of respect in regard to this primary function is to go beyond competently applying the modalities of your profession alone to exhibit an approach that embodies care. This broader expression includes conduct based not only on your technical knowledge and skill sets but also on how your attitudes, experience, and reflection apply to an authentic human relationship with a particular individual.[11] What then are some markers that you and the patient can use to measure the success of meeting the respect benchmark of care? We offer several practical ones here, and others are woven throughout the pages of this book.

GAIN RESPECT FOR THE PATIENT'S UNIQUENESS

Referring back to the indicators of respect presented in Chapter 1 is a reminder that first you must infuse each relationship with convincing evidence that you see this patient as a unique individual. To be sure, most of the time your professional responses will fall within a general pattern of behaviors that apply to all patients similarly. In other words, the training defining the scope of your practice and a general template of appropriate professional attitudes and duties will guide you so that this person can perceive you as a trustworthy, competent provider of professional care. However, at times this process may take you down unexpected paths requiring creative responses to this individual and circumstance. The individualized aspect of care is illustrated by this excerpt about a surgeon's response to a dying patient. A woman named Caroline is dying of cancer, and when Caroline loses consciousness her friend Gail, who has been keeping vigil, panics and calls Caroline's surgeon:

> *I had found [Dr.] Herzog's home phone number and called him that evening from the hospital. He came into the room carrying a handful of lilies of the valley—he knew that whatever else had happened, Caroline would be able to smell and walked over to her and held them under her nose. It was a gesture that took my breath away with its exacting kindness. . . .*[12]

Dr. Herzog, a world-class surgeon, went beyond the essentials of his considerable technical expertise by paying attention to a small detail he knew about Caroline's and Gail's love of flowers, and that changed everything in terms of Gail's ability to cope. He also used his professional awareness of the senses still available to Caroline in her condition to "touch" her as a person when so many of their usual ways to relate were challenged. His unusual conduct was a sign that when the individual is seen as a unique person the professional soon learns that care cannot be bottled or reduced to a formula. Care has the malleability to be shaped to each circumstance.

Dr. Herzog's caring behaviors worked because he had been summoned in the first place to focus on the skillful application of the technical knowledge and skills that had brought him into the relationship with this patient and her friend. But that summons also gave him the opportunity to gain knowledge of Caroline as a person—which he did—and it resulted in an effective expression of personal care when his humanity called for it. His conduct demonstrates that paying attention to the *person* named Caroline is what resulted in a greater bandwidth of caring responses. This broader focus will not be accomplished without a deep respect for persons first and foremost.

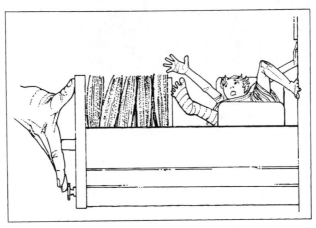

Fig. 2.3 Nothing is more upsetting to a patient than to feel you are treating her as a "case" to be filed before you go on to the next patient or commitment on your schedule.

STAY FOCUSED—ON THE PERSON

The undergirding of respect also operates on your behalf when you are faced with external challenges that threaten to deter you from your focused attention on what you have learned about the patient and how your professional care can best be expressed in your relationship. Recall from Chapter 1 that an indicator of respect is to be mindful that the unique person who has become your patient deserves your attention. At the same time, almost everyone struggles with effective time management in today's fast-paced health care and educational settings. Your commitment never to cut corners in patient care helps to keep you focused on fostering a relationship that goes beyond the mere minimum of caring behaviors. There is nothing more upsetting to a patient than feeling that you are seeing him or her simply as another case on the long list of cases, to be filed as "completed" at the end of the day (Fig. 2.3).

But even this commitment is sometimes difficult to keep. When you must take shortcuts, a patient is likely to maintain his or her assurance that you care if you explain why you are giving that person short shrift in this unfortunate exceptional circumstance, and then make it an unfortunate exceptional circumstance.

Your commitment to foster respectful care sometimes can be effective if at the outset you remind the patient of the amount of time you have to be with him or her and work together to discuss what you hope the two of you will accomplish in that time. Every health professional knows that on some days a particular patient needs extra time to work through a problem, which can wreak havoc on a schedule. Then there are patients who for good (or poor) reasons are late or need to linger, diverting your time and energy from other patients. Setting your daily schedule against a backdrop of differing patient needs will help to keep you on as clear a path as possible through the day. Although some patients you have kept waiting will become impatient, your focused attention on doing all that you are able to do for them when their turn comes will support their feeling that your behavior remains consistent with your respectful caring for them. Some waiting areas today list the professionals who are seeing patients, whether they are on schedule, and, if not, how long it appears it will be before the next patient can be seen. This can be effective to a point, especially if the professional apologizes for a delay and the waiting patient has an opportunity to learn something about the cause for delay when his or her turn comes.

Managing time with the goal of giving full attention to the patient can be aided by additional clues about how to conduct yourself with the patient during the time you actually are together.

- Remove the person from areas where distractions are likely to impinge on your time together.
- Sit down or in other ways convey your intent to give full attention to the person.
- Approach the person slowly and graciously, even though you may have had to run to get to your appointment.
- Look the person in the eye while conversing. A lack of direct eye contact communicates lack of interest.
- Place a clock at a place where you can be aware of the time without being obvious about it.
- Let others know you are engaged and should not be disturbed. For example, turn your cell phone to do not disturb mode and silence pagers.

This section on staying focused on the person who is a patient would not be complete without standing back from the individual patient to include a guideline for how you speak of a patient's condition more generally. The disability rights movement has taken leadership in drawing attention to the power of language in their emphasis on *person-first language:*

> *The language a society uses to refer to persons with disabilities shapes its beliefs and ideas about them. Words are powerful; old, inaccurate, and inappropriate descriptors perpetuate negative stereotypes and attitudinal barriers. When we describe people by their labels of medical diagnoses, we devalue and disrespect them as individuals. In contrast, using thoughtful terminology can foster positive attitudes about persons with disabilities.[13]*

An example is to use the phrase "a person with paralysis" instead of "a paralyzed person" or "a person who has Parkinson's disease " instead of "a Parkinson's patient." In Caroline's situation, Dr. Herzog would reinforce his caring conduct by speaking of, and to, her as "a person who has cancer." Although this may seem a subtle shift, reflection highlights that the latter does not equate the person Caroline with her diagnosis but communicates that this person has the diagnosis among many of her other traits and characteristics.

RESPECT FOR LITTLE THINGS

An important way to support a patient's feeling of self-worth and confidence in the caring relationship is to acknowledge little personal details that too often go unnoticed. The poet William Blake noted, "He who would do good to others must do it in minute particulars." A popular song heralds, "Little Things Mean a Lot!" If you think about your own life there are times when "little things" have counted as essential expressions of deep respect shown by another. Thoughtful little details take many shapes, but a few common ones are discussed here that apply to the health professional and patient relationship.

Personal Hygiene and Comfort Measures

When a patient has a straightforward hygienic need that can easily be relieved, your attention to it before any other activity or exchange will be deeply appreciated. It is surprising how embarrassed a person may be to admit that he needs to use the bathroom or needs a tissue to wipe a runny nose but cannot do it independently. A simple unsolicited act on your part makes the difference between an embarrassed or fidgety person and one ready to focus on the clinical issue at hand.

Comfort-enhancing details not only matter greatly to patients, but they also demonstrate respect for their dignity. A common error of omission that is extremely unnerving to a patient is to place cold clammy hands unexpectedly on his or her bare skin. But warming your hands and many other personal comfort measures can be taken. For instance, taking note to correct the temperature of a too cold room or too hot space where a patient is waiting to be seen or will be left as a part of your intervention always is appreciated. A patient sometimes experiences a certain amount of physical discomfort in a treatment, diagnostic, or other situation. It is easy to forget how often we humans automatically shift posture, scratch, blink, swipe at a tickle, or shrug to get comfortable, yet there are conditions or interventions that prevent a patient from performing these basic comfort functions. Watching for signs that such a need has arisen is a fundamental part of deepening your focus of attention on the patient. There are many ways a patient, even one with severe physical limitations, can be made more comfortable.

REFLECTIONS

- Have you been stuck in a situation where you could not get comfortable? Describe how it made you feel.
- What did you have to do to remedy the situation?

You can remember that situation as a starting point of your own responses when you are with patients. Asking "Are you comfortable?" or "Is there anything else I can do for you while I am with you to make you more comfortable?" expresses respect that will be interpreted as a genuine caring act.

Personal Interests and Landmark Events

Almost everyone has some area of interest, whether it be a hobby, job, family, or other focus. Showing interest in the person does not require probing unduly into his or her personal life. Some patients will want to chat about life outside of the moment, and others will not. At the same time, asking a hospitalized patient about the noon menu, complementing an ambulatory care patient on something he or she is wearing, reminding a teenager that her favorite rap artist has a special show on television that night, and spelling Mr. Schydlowski's name correctly on his appointment slip count as personalized care. Landmark events in the person's life often involve birthdays and anniversaries, and usually it is accepted as a sign of respect by this person if you mark it. For instance, if you think that he would enjoy the attention, on Mr. Arnold's birthday write "HAPPY BIRTHDAY, DICK ARNOLD" in bold letters on his lunch tray or let other staff know so that they can acknowledge it, too. You will think of other expressions of this type of respect to put into everyday action (Fig. 2.4).

In addition to personal events, most patients are very aware of holidays or even the passing of the seasons as holding special meaning they may or may not be able to acknowledge in ways they would like or remember doing. Asking them to share such memories can be interpreted as an expression of genuine care.

A special challenge arises for patients and residents who have been confined to a home, hospital, or other long-term care facility. You know how quickly one can lose touch with the rest of the world once schedules and everyday surroundings change. By sharing an incident observed on the way to work, reviewing a play seen the evening before, or taking the patient to a window to see a child and dog playing together, you can extend the patient's environment beyond the immediate setting, bringing him or her into contact with the outside world. The passing of the seasons can have significance for patients too. One of the authors once brought apple blossoms into a four-bed room in an assisted living facility only to have two of the residents burst into tears, saying they missed the sweet smells of spring more than anything else since being forced to make this their permanent home. This simple act opened the door to a discussion about springtime memories and was a reminder of how much such seemingly small things can be conducive to meeting the benchmark of care.

RESPECT FOR THE PATIENT'S AGENDA

Earlier in this chapter we introduced the notion of a patient-centered relationship and that in it the patient's say-so is essential for their his or her being. We pick up this theme again to underscore that a

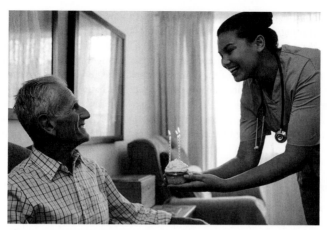

Fig. 2.4 A birthday is often an important opportunity to recognize a patient. © Wavebreakmedia/iStock/Thinkstock.com

patient's perception of the life challenges he or she is experiencing understandably can be quite different from that of the health professional's interpretation of the situation. This insight relies on the fact that patients are concerned primarily with what their clinical condition signifies in terms of their daily lives, loves, and activities. Hardly ever is the technical aspect of what is wrong the governing concern; rather it is "How does this affect the quality of my life?" The professional behaviors offered in this chapter provide clues to discovering the deeper personal meaning a patient assigns to his or her clinical condition. Chapter 7 describes how the patient's story (or stories) is the narrative he or she brings to the relationship that provides essential clues as to what this deeper personal meaning involves.

Because the professional's intent to partner with the patient will always involve blind spots, *humility* is one basic character trait a professional must cultivate. Humility acknowledges one's limits; thus respect for the patient partially is realized through humility in the form of acknowledgment of the patient's spheres of authority in the relationship. In the United States and many other countries, the mechanism of informed consent is a useful legal and ethical tool. *Informed consent* formally acknowledges a difference in power between the professional and the patient because of the professional's training. This difference places the onus of responsibility on the professional to level the playing field between them through a process of informing and being sure the patient understands and consents (or not) to a proposed course of action. This contract between you and the patient is just the beginning. Everything after that either reinforces or sets up barriers to the person's ability to participate confidently in details that give his or her life its content, texture, and meaning, many of them realized through mundane daily activities that the professional may think are not that important.

A patient who has lost control over many decisions in his or her life may still be able to take command of details such as what to wear that day or when to eat, thereby expressing his or her individuality. Sometimes the loss of so many areas of decision-making is taken as a signal to both parties that the patient should have everything done for him or her. It is easy for everyone, including family caregivers and friends, to fall into that mode out of a good faith attempt to help the patient. The health professional's efforts and modeling to counter unnecessary dependence can encourage everyone to do likewise. After a severe back injury, an active career woman in her 40s suddenly realized how passive and discouraged she had become about the need to remain bedridden for some time. This attitude was turned around by a close friend who sent a card with the following note:

NOBODY HAS EVER SAID THE
UNIVERSE CANNOT BE EXPLORED
FROM A RECUMBENT POSITION.

Obviously, this friend was tuned in to the patient's growing sense of despair and feeling of powerlessness resulting from her persistent back pain and fear of reinjury. A simple gesture was enough to give her a new perspective on her period of being bedfast! A patient who loses confidence in what he or she can still do often is at risk for becoming immobilized more by discouragement than by the clinical aspects of the condition itself. The good news is that in your role you can serve as a catalyst encouraging the patient to meet you halfway or more in working toward mutually arrived at and realistic goals. Patients and loved ones always will take this as a sign of care based on genuine respect for the person. When this dynamic is taking place a giant step toward the evidence needed to meet the benchmark of successful professional caregiving will have been realized.

Respect, Contract, and Covenant

Although a patient must successfully carry his or her share of responsibility for developing a flourishing relationship with you, the health professional must take leadership in the process of building a relationship that meets the benchmark of care based on respect. Toward realizing that result, ethicist William May proposes that thinking of ourselves as being bound by a *covenant* includes the contract elements of professional mechanisms such as informed consent and the items detailed in professional codes of ethics but goes further. Covenants place the parties in a situation of mutual benefit at the human level. Just as humility highlights areas of the professional not being all-knowing, covenants allow the professional to acknowledge benefits derived from health care practice and from the opportunity to be with a particular patient who arrives not only with signs or symptoms but also with talents, gifts, and histories. Therefore an element of *professional gratitude* enters the relationship, empowering patients to do their best and encouraging professionals to go beyond the bare minimum of expectations that are agreed upon in a strict contract approach.[14]

Summary

This chapter presents basic instruction for how to translate professional respect into specific everyday relational actions and offers four benchmarks of respect to assess the success of this goal. Through the remainder of the book the reader will delve more fully into these general forms of evidence that the health professional and patient relationship can help realize the well-being of each patient and be a welcome ingredient in fostering a flourishing society.

The benchmark of a trust-based relationship is met when both parties are free to move forward with confidence that the best possible course is being offered to the patient and that the professional's actions come from a place of integrity. The professional's acknowledgment of and considered response to the psychological dynamics of transference and countertransference is a second benchmark that allows the specific contours of a health professional and patient relationship to go forward true to its intended purposes. A third benchmark is manifested by courteous behaviors based on true respect for the human dignity of each individual and offered in everyday actions experienced by the patient and his or her support systems. Finally, the benchmark of professional caring behaviors is the ultimate measure of what the health professional and patient relationship should look like. The previously mentioned three benchmarks are instrumental in meeting this goal because each reflects an aspect of respectful care in action. Many expressions of professional care are possible, and even those that appear mundane at first glance are in fact essential considerations. Such expressions of care include everyday personal details that help give each patient hope for maintaining a meaningful quality of life. Taken together, these benchmarks of respect provide an overall measure of how health professionals and patients can effectively work together to achieve common goals. The test of the ideas presented in this chapter is the extent to which any of them supports genuine respect toward patients, their families, and the ideals of the health professions. Professional relatedness builds on basic human relational characteristics such as trust, sensitivity to the effects of psychological dynamics at play, behaviors assuring the patient that he or she is a person deserving of keen attention, and care offered in ways that embody and reflect genuine human respect for the patient.

References

1. Sarton M. *A Reckoning*. New York: Norton; 1978.
2. Stewart M, Brown JB, Weston WW, et al. *Patient-Centered Medicine, Transforming the Clinical Method.* 3rd ed. London: Radcliffe Publishers Ltd; 2013.
3. Interprofessional Education Collaborative. *Core Competencies for Interprofessional Collaborative Practice: 2016 Update*. Washington, DC: Interprofessional Education Collaborative; 2016. Accessed at: https://www.tamhsc.edu/ipe/research/ipec-2016-core-competencies.pdf.
4. Veatch R. *The Basics of Bioethics*. 3rd ed. Upper Saddle River, New Jersey: Pearson Education; 2012.
5. Jacobs BB, Taylor C. Medical futility in the natural attitude. *Adv Nurs Sci*. 2005;28(4):288–305.
6. Robinson E, Hamel-Norduzzi M, Purtilo R, et al. Complexities in decision making for persons with disabilities near end of life. *Top Stroke Rehabil*. 2006;13(4):54–67.
7. McGuigan D. Communicating bad news to patients: a reflective approach. *Nurs Stand*. 2009;23(31):51–56.
8. Hardingham LB. Integrity and moral residue: nurses as participants in a moral community. *Nurs Philos*. 2004;5(2):127–134.
9. Freud S. *The Ego and the Mechanisms of Defense*. New York: International Universities Press; 1966.
10. *The Shorter Oxford English Dictionary*. 5th ed. Vol. 1 (*A-O*). Oxford, England: Oxford University Press; 2002.
11. Doherty R, Purtilo R. *Ethical Dimensions in the Health Professions*. 6th ed. St. Louis, Missouri: Elsevier; 2016:61.
12. Caldwell G. *Let's Take the Long Way Home: A Memoir of Friendship*. New York: Random House; 2010.
13. Arc The. What is people first language. http://www.thearc.org/who-we-are/media-center/people-first-language.
14. May WF. Code and covenant or philanthropy and contract? *Hastings Cent Rep*. 1975;5:29–35.

CHAPTER 3

Professional Boundaries Guided by Respect

OBJECTIVES

The reader will be able to:

- Describe the idea of a professional boundary as a benchmark of respect
- Distinguish a respectful, professional approach from one based on objectivity and efficiency alone
- Identify and discuss appropriate physical boundaries, compared with inappropriate or unconsented touching
- Describe three types of situations in which setting and maintaining emotional boundaries are crucial to avoiding enmeshment
- Identify clues that may alert you that your sympathy is becoming pity
- Define overidentification and describe its negative effects
- Describe what it means to care too much
- Explain some ways that honoring professional boundaries serves the positive goals of the health professional and patient relationship

Prelude

I remember the wintry day she called from a phone booth not too far from the office, barely hanging on. I got somebody to take me out to find her and bring her back to the office. I remember the moment when I realized that the absurd choice before me was to do grief work or find insulin. After a frustrating morning on the phone trying to find some public or private source of help—a struggle she was in no shape at the moment to handle—I took her to a drug store and bought the insulin myself. I was feeling a bit of shame. There's an emphasis in our field now on maintaining proper boundaries, with the implication that those who do not are overfunctioning, codependent, and other compound words even more dreadful. Emotional disengagement was expected. Technically—though no one forbade it—it was not part of my job to go find people in phone booths or pay for their medicine. I was aware of stretching the limits of what I usually do.

B. JESSING[1]

The health professional in the quote is struggling with the appropriate professional limits of involvement with a patient who is homeless. She is experienced and knows she could go beyond behaviors that are appropriate in their relationship and in so doing may cause more harm than good in the long run. Still, almost everyone can sympathize with her attempt to be respectful of her patient's desperate situation. As her hesitance suggests, her challenge is not only to show respect by acting to meet the positive benchmarks of the relationship but also to consider the wisdom of understanding its limits.

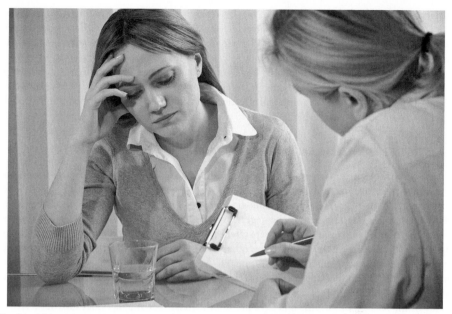

Fig. 3.1 Maintaining professional boundaries helps put the goal of facilitating a patient's well-being at the forefront of the professional and patient relationship. (© *Alex Raths/iStock/Thinkstock.com.*)

What Is a Professional Boundary?

Professional boundary is a term developed in the professional literature and professional practice guidelines to provide guidance regarding appropriate, prudent physical and emotional constraints to intimacy. Although most benchmarks of respect involve positive action, this one calls for understanding where and when to exercise constraint. The general rule is that the physical and emotional boundaries between you and patients must always be guided by the goal of facilitating a patient's well-being and maintaining profound and caring respect in the interaction (Fig. 3.1). But knowing the general rule will not necessarily always help you with the complex human stories you face in the line of work you have chosen. For one thing, relationships are dynamic, and there are changes in them with every encounter. Boundary issues may arise from physical or psychological/emotional sources. An extreme example sometimes is reported of health professionals losing their licenses or in other ways being sanctioned for engaging in sexual intercourse with patients. We discuss this type of breach in a section that broadly describes physical boundaries. Guidelines regarding emotional boundaries are designed to prevent psychological dynamics that are harmful to the patient or to you during the relationship. We discuss these, too. It is easy to see that breaches may involve aspects of both. Some boundary guidelines have arisen from external considerations (e.g., the time you spend in the encounter), whereas others are internal (i.e., characteristics you and the patient bring to it).

Guidelines for physical and psychological or emotional boundaries are derived from several sources. Some come from professional codes of ethics. These draw on a long history of differentiating the role of the professional from that of a citizen. Others come from institutional codes of conduct, laws, and regulations that have grown out of the experience of health professionals and patients and serve to regulate conduct and protect the public trust.

Sometimes guidelines change based on insights from psychology regarding tensions that may arise from human needs for privacy, intimacy, and acceptance. Today, studies of power differentials among the respective roles of persons within institutions and relationships add another component of understanding.[2]

One way the wisdom of maintaining boundaries has been dramatized in the past is through advancing the erroneous idea that being professional requires one to be aloof, objective, and efficient at the price of personal warmth and affectionate conduct. But to suggest that respect entails aloofness is a distortion of the highest goals to which professionals aspire.[3]

RECOGNIZING A "MEANINGFUL DISTANCE"

In everyday life, we seldom are consciously aware of the distance between oneself and the other; rather, we automatically position ourselves among others to maintain our comfort zone. However, in human interactions, psychological and physical distances have societal and often personal meanings determined by the degree of intimacy it represents for both parties. At one pole, there may be a complete sense of separateness such as accidentally being physically pressed against each other in a crowd, and at the other there is a realm of togetherness that is highly personal, informal, and familiar (i.e., intimate). At any point along this continuum, certain messages and expectations are put into play, whereas others remain in the background. The nuances with which the appropriate boundaries of respect must be maintained are the impetus for many of the reflections on this topic. We present the most fundamental ones for your learning and reflection.

Physical Boundaries

As a rule, mainstream Western societies do not condone much touching, especially among strangers. You may find a clerk in a store who physically touches the palm of your hand in returning change. You may be jostled in a crowd. You may shake a stranger's hand in meeting. Among some a formalized form of kiss or buss on the cheek is expected. Strangers may impulsively hug the man or woman next to them during an important sports event. However, the occasions when touching among strangers is socially sanctioned can probably be counted on one hand. At the same time, many tasks in the health professions environment require caregivers to be in close physical contact with strangers who are their patients and to do so respectfully. In addition, displays of affection expressed by a pat on the shoulder, a gentle hug, or other signs of support are behaviors you may be comfortable engaging in as a part of your interaction if you feel confident that the patient is welcoming it.

> **REFLECTIONS**
>
> Think of a time in the past couple days that you and a stranger came into physical contact.
> • Was it comfortable? If so, what made it so?
> • If not, what happened that you had a brush with discomfort?

All cultures and subcultures have socially constructed rules about when and between whom touching (or even visual access) is condoned. Such rules often extend to the acceptable conduct between health professionals and patients. For example, in some a male caregiver may not touch or even look at a woman's bare body. At the same time, when taken seriously, appropriate touch can be an effective means of establishing rapport or showing reassurance—and may be required for diagnostic or treatment regimens. In short, acceptable contours of physical contact between health professional and patient require considered attention.

UNCONSENTED TOUCHING

Informed consent, mentioned in Chapter 2, is one of the most basic societal acknowledgments that professional contact may permissibly depart dramatically from general accepted social norms of physical contact. Informed consent arose in part from the concept of battery. *Battery* is a legal term acknowledging society's deep prohibition against unconsented touching. By giving informed consent the patient is saying, in effect, I give you—and others involved in my care—consent to hold, stroke, rub, poke, or even puncture or cut me, depending on the scope of practice in your professional role. Obviously, the permission to make physical contact already puts the health professional and patient relationship into a special category in which usual socially acceptable distances are breached on a regular basis.

Your right to make physical contact does not give you permission to impose on a patient's sensitivities or dislikes regarding physical contact. Cultural, social, and personal factors come together to create a patient's comfort zone regarding physical contact, and the health professional must be guided by a sensitivity to these individual differences.

Inappropriate Touching

Some types of physical contact are deemed unacceptable in the health professional and patient relationship under any conditions, even with the consent of the patient or client. Under law you cannot make contact with a patient with an intent to harm him or her physically or psychologically. If you do, you will be charged with abuse.

The type of inappropriate touching that has received the most attention is physical contact delivered with an intent to excite or arouse the patient sexually. Although sexual intercourse is the most prohibited of inappropriate touching between a health professional and patient, the prohibitions are not limited to it. For example, the American Medical Association's 2016 *Code of Medical Ethics: Current Opinions with Annotations* addresses the broader notion of sexual misconduct, including "'romantic involvement" as one factor.[4] In another example the American Physical Therapy Association states explicitly, "Physical therapists shall not engage in any sexual relationship with any of their patients/clients, supervisees, or students."[5] In this case the boundary is tied to the value of maintaining professional integrity. You might wonder why it is forbidden if a competent, adult patient consents to or even seems to invite sexual contact. The strongest argument against this type of contact is that it betrays the reasonable expectations built into the essence of the health professional and patient relationship. Patients have a right to receive the best care possible without having to satisfy the professional's needs. The reasoning is that sexual activity is never free from other types of claims on the other person, so both patient and health professional may begin to alter the conditions of the relationship considering the power of its sexual dimensions rather than the conditions under which a patient sought professional care in the first place. In short, it is never considered fair that the patient would have to meet your need for sexual pleasure, sexual intimacy, sexual fulfillment, dominance in a relationship, or any other gain, no matter what either you or the patient believes would be gained.

SEXUAL HARASSMENT

The importance of the idea that sexual boundaries must be maintained in public settings is being aired today in the notion of *sexual harassment*. The U.S. Equal Employment Opportunity Commission (EEOC) defines harassment as unwelcome sexual advances, requests for sexual favors, and other verbal or physical conduct and includes activity that creates a hostile or unwelcome work environment for the person who feels "harassed." A more specific description follows:

> *Sexual harassment is a form of sex discrimination that violates Title VII of the Civil Rights Act of 1964. Unwelcome sexual advances, requests for sexual favors, and other verbal or physical conduct of a sexual nature constitute sexual harassment when this conduct explicitly or implicitly affects an*

individual's employment; unreasonably interferes with an individual's work performance; or creates an intimidating, hostile, or offensive work environment. Sexual harassment can occur in a variety of circumstances, including but not limited to the following: The victim and harasser may be a woman or a man. The victim does not have to be of the opposite sex. The victim does not have to be the person harassed but could be anyone affected by the offensive conduct. The harasser's conduct must be unwelcome. It is helpful for the victim to inform the harasser directly that the conduct is unwelcome and must stop.[6]

Although harassment was developed within the context of employer-employee and related situations, most state licensing acts governing the professions have similar provisions prohibiting such behavior by professionals toward patients or others, and many institutions include prohibitions in their policies. You will have ample opportunity to learn more about the particulars of the legal and regulatory issues involved in this evolving area of professional practice, and it is in your best interest to do so. An important aspect of sexual harassment that has not been explored deeply enough involves sexual advances that issue from patients or their family members toward professionals. Many professionals can recall such an incident and often do not know how to respond. No one in the workplace needs to be a victim of harassment, and most institutions will have protections in place to support health professionals who experience this type of conduct from those they are there to serve in a professional capacity.

What About Dual Relationships?

Dual relationships are defined as those in which "[a] professional . . . assumes a second role with a client, becoming . . . friend, employer, teacher, business associate, family member, or sexual partner."[7] In the past the typical belief has been that once a health professional and patient relationship formally ended, two consenting, competent adults ought to be free to do whatever they please. This makes good sense on the face of it. However, Baca[8] notes that dual relationships exist when there are other personal or professional demands, stresses, or considerations in the relationship in addition to the provider-patient relationship.[8] This behavior may begin before, during, or after the professional relationship. Dual relationships in the professions for the most part involve health professionals who often rationalize their behavior, arguing that the situation is unique.

Friendships initiated after the termination of a professional relationship can be injurious to a former patient should the professional relationship have to be reinstated. Other relationships, such as business partnerships, can interfere dramatically with the professional's ability to be sensitive while remaining appropriately objective in the professional and patient relationship.[8] At one end of the continuum is a long-held general precaution or prohibition against treating members of one's own family.

Current thinking about dual relationships is not conclusive, and more research in this general area is necessary. Not all major health profession guidelines include a caution against it, especially once the formal therapeutic relationship has ended. To take seriously the potential for harm to a patient or former patient is to weigh in on the side of better judgment. Although a rare exception may present itself, a good rule that remains is to honor physical and emotional boundaries with great thoughtfulness and care, referring to the professional and patient relationship contours of care as the primary consideration.

We turn, now, to three types of situations in which maintaining emotional boundaries become markers of a respect benchmark in the health professional and patient relationship.

Psychological and Emotional Boundaries

The previous two chapters have outlined strengths that result when the health professional follows the benchmarks of respect, going beyond applying the minimum technical tasks required for a patient-centered relationship. At the same time, there are some specific ways the emotional responses and psychological attachments of the health professional or patient can interfere with respect for the patient and do damage to the relationship. Taken together these feelings and conduct can be summarized in the term *enmeshment:*

> *The nurse who has become enmeshed often develops an emotional connection with or an emotional availability to the client that may be impossible to maintain over the life span of the client. This can ultimately lead to client feelings of anger or emotional pain and to a sense of abandonment. The process of enmeshment may also complicate provision of adequate care at a later time. This can occur if the patient sees the other care team members as not caring sufficiently or as providing inadequate care, in comparison with the nurse who is enmeshed.*[9]

In these situations, a self-conscious attentiveness to what is happening when the relationship is tending toward enmeshment will help each person gain (or regain) perspective on the appropriate nature of the relationship and the reasonable expectations of each. Challenges include the health professional's tendency for sympathy to slip into pity, for overidentification with the patient's plight, or misjudgments regarding the scope and type of respectful caring you should exhibit toward the patient.

THE SLIP FROM SYMPATHY TO PITY

Some patients' clinical conditions or social circumstances may be so appalling to you that you shrink from imagining how terrible it would be to be in their place. Emotional constraint may have to be exercised in this circumstance because your usual attitude of sympathy can slip into pity. Psychologically speaking, observing something one finds horrible may lead to self-protective feelings of withdrawal from or contempt for the situation as likely as ignite the desire to relieve the other's suffering. For example, one can view the plight of starving people in another part of the world and feel immense pity toward them, but that does not necessarily move one to want to relieve their suffering. Once pity is conveyed by your words or conduct in the health professional and patient relationship, it becomes impossible for the patient to trust that you really have that person's interest at the heart of your encounter. Most health professionals can name at least one type of illness or injury that profoundly affects them emotionally and therefore is an area in which the slide into pity is most likely to occur.

REFLECTIONS

- Can you name one type of physical or psychological trauma that would be horrendous if it were to befall you?
- What symptoms or other aspects of that condition would be the most difficult to accept?
- Would you want people to have pity for your plight? Why or why not?
- What kind of response would you hope for in this unwelcome situation?

Looking inward at your own strong reactions can provide insight into a block you may feel when faced with treating certain conditions. Recognizing that such a block exists does not mean you are unfit for practice in your field. Sometimes discussing your reaction with a supervisor or trusted colleague can help you find a way through your initial pushback. There are also mechanisms within most health care environments such as referring such a person to another colleague who can relieve you of your responsibility of caring for this person. One of the best approaches is to be proactive by seeking employment where your sensitivities will not regularly be challenged in this way.

At the same time, it is not at all unnatural for you to periodically become so involved in a patient's tragic situation that you take his or her problems home with you. Almost any health professional can recall the time he or she had trouble falling asleep or was moved to tears or laughter by a sudden tragic or joyful announcement touching a patient's life. There is, however, a significant difference between this depth of professional caring, which stimulates a purely human response, and fruitless or destructive enmeshment occasioned by a persistent feeling of pity. The difference can be illustrated with this case study.

Case Study

Michael Bodenheimer was admitted to the psychiatric ward of City Hospital after the police brought him there from the streets. The police found him unconscious in a doorway of a downtown office building. Mr. Bodenheimer is a 64-year-old veteran with posttraumatic stress disorder and a substance use disorder. He has held down a variety of part-time jobs and has lived in various boarding houses until evicted for his drunken behavior or failure to pay his rent. His mother died when he was 15 years old, and he left home shortly after that. When he was in his early twenties his father died of a heart attack while Michael was serving active duty in Iraq. Craig Hopkins, who works on the psychiatric ward at City Hospital, is a little younger than Michael but only by 4 years. However, his similarity to Michael Bodenheimer ends there. Craig Hopkins grew up in an upper-middle-class home and served as an officer in the Marines before entering professional school when he retired from the military at age 57. Some of the officers in the military certainly had alcohol dependencies, but being a teetotaler himself he tended not to hang out with them much. He tells his wife that he is fascinated with Michael. He finds Michael very warm and human, and they enjoy sharing what they call "war stories." Michael is admitted to the detoxification unit on the ward, where he will spend some weeks. Craig asks to remain one of his caregivers, and the supervisor initially is happy to comply. The two men chat when Craig has a few minutes, and, over the next few days, Craig arrives at the conclusion that Michael has had more than his share of misfortune.

One day when Craig goes into Michael's room, he finds Michael doubled up, writhing in agony. With a trembling voice, Michael tells him that the doctor has not given him anything to "take the edge off" his withdrawal from alcohol. To Craig's surprise, Michael grabs him by the wrist and pleads, "Please, please, I can't stand this agony. If you will just get me something to drink, just enough to make it over the hump, I swear I'll never touch another drop. If I can't get a little relief, I will kill myself. The doctor is a sadist."

Craig Hopkins tears himself away and leaves the room. He knows he should report this exchange in the medical record but rationalizes that it could cause Michael more suffering by reporting this outburst. That night he cannot sleep. He is haunted by the picture of this man who has survived the death of his parents, claims to have been divorced three times, and has "some kids somewhere who don't want anything to do with their old dad." He has been on the front lines as an enlisted man "with a few notches" in his belt and has succumbed to the bottle. Craig sees clearly the beads of sweat that clung to Michael's forehead as he spoke, thinks that Michael is clearly all alone in the world, and realizes he is irrationally angry at Michael's physician for not making detoxification a little easier for Michael.

The next morning the unit supervisor motions to Craig to step into a quiet area of the unit. She says that Michael is in a restless sleep and experiencing some visual hallucinations. She adds, "I see you are spending quite a bit of time with him. I don't know how much experience you have in this area but you've got to watch these alcoholics. They're all liars. They'll do anything to manipulate the staff so be on your guard."

Craig remembers Michael's pleading eyes the day before and is overcome with a desire to make a sharp retort to the supervisor's statements. He goes instead to Michael's room and deftly slips a half pint of whiskey he bought the night before into the drawer of the bedside stand and makes enough noise so that Michael stirs from his tortured sleep and sees what he is doing. As Craig leaves he suddenly thinks, "*What am I thinking?!*" But he continues hurriedly out of the room.

We can see that Craig has reached the point where he is responding impulsively out of pity rather than with genuine caring conduct. Because pity distorts what he should not do so as to maintain the appropriate boundaries of this relationship, his enmeshment leads him to err. In fact, we may include him among the patient's many problems, as well as jeopardizing his own position with this unethical behavior.

REFLECTIONS

- What details of this story do you think contributed to Craig's sympathy turning to pity?
- What else could Craig have done to help alleviate the patient's suffering?
- Was it his professional duty to admit his wrongdoing? Why or why not?

You cannot solve the type of problem arising from pity simply by enmeshing yourself more deeply into the patient's personal life, as Craig did. Of course, your pity is in response to a genuinely felt need of a patient. Michael Bodenheimer may be manipulative, but Craig saw the depth of his suffering. What was called for was sympathetic acknowledgment of the person's problem but also clarity that Craig's professional role required him to put boundaries on what he could do to intervene constructively in Michael's plight.

Many patients who become objects of pity are suffering and do not know how or when to limit personal revelations when they find a professional person with a sympathetic ear. Health professionals in general are in no position to solve most of the patient's often life-long personal problems. As one colleague commented, "Overall, we are just a flash in the pan of a patient's life!" He is right. Craig went beyond his best considered judgment to try to become more than his professional role warranted.

Pity is a powerful emotion. It can be communicated to the patient in one meeting and over a period of time. Facial expression can instantly convey one's feelings. Quick nervous movements, coupled with a sudden departure, are sometimes correctly interpreted as expressions of pity. The desire not to talk about the patient's problem and trite comments such as, "It'll be *fine*, I'm sure," also can be interpreted to mean, "Poor, poor you." Often, patients abhor pity, even if it serves some small immediate purpose. Pity is destructive and belittling to the patient, who will eventually recoil from it.

We can assume that Craig, with a life as an officer in the military, had encountered other difficult situations, but something about Michael hit him deeply. We do not know for sure what it was.

Checking one's feelings with trusted other professionals in such situations can be helpful. Craig bristled when the supervisor confronted him and responded antagonistically. However, if he had listened to what she said, he might at least have taken it as a signal to back off a little and discuss his feelings with someone else on the ward. This might have given him a clearer insight into this patient, into others like him, and into himself, providing a chance to reset his own professional compass.

OVERIDENTIFICATION WITH THE PATIENT'S PREDICAMENT

Maintaining appropriate emotional boundaries and psychological distance can become a challenge when you have had an experience so like the patient's that you believe your experiences to be identical. Such a reaction of *overidentification* is a little different from transference as discussed in Chapter 2. Transference highlights an association you have of that person with someone else you know or have known. Overidentification puts you personally into very close alignment with the other and is another variety of enmeshment.

At first it seems a mistaken idea that having had similar experiences may actually hinder the effectiveness of a respect-based health professional and patient relationship. But everyone has had the experience of beginning to relate a traumatic (or exciting) event only to have the other person interrupt with "Oh! I know *exactly* what you mean!" and then go on to describe his or her own story. One feels cheated at such times, thinking, "No, that's not what I meant, but you are more interested in telling me about yourself than in listening to me!" The way such overidentification works within the health professions can be illustrated in the following Case Study.

Case Study

Mrs. Rita Garcia, an elementary school teacher, became interested in teaching language skills to hearing-impaired children after her third child, Lucia, who was born deaf, successfully learned to communicate by attending special classes for those with hearing impairment. Mrs. Garcia enrolled in a health professions course directed toward training teachers of hearing-impaired persons.

In her first position, she was surprised and alarmed that some of the mothers requested that she not be assigned to their children. Finally, she approached one of the mothers whose child she had been working with and with whom she felt comfortable. "What's wrong?" she asked. "Do they think I'm incompetent because I was older when I went back to school or am new in my field? Is it my personality or the fact that I have a Spanish accent? I want so much to help these children, and I can't understand what I'm doing wrong." The embarrassed mother replied, "Well, since you asked, I'll give you a direct answer. I don't feel this way, but some of the mothers think that you don't understand their children's unique challenges because every time they start to tell you something about their child, you immediately interrupt with an experience you have had with your daughter."

Unfortunately, Rita Garcia's intent was a good one, but her effectiveness as a teacher was hindered by her own intense experiences and, likely, her need to share what she had been through. She would benefit from recognizing that the tendency to overidentify is bound to be present because of her own situation. It also will be helpful to remind herself periodically that attempts to relate to the patient (or in this case the parent of the patient) by pointing out superficial similarities between her own experience and theirs may be interpreted as her desire to talk about her own problem. Overidentification, once it becomes a part of the caregiver's thinking, cannot be easily erased. But giving the other an opportunity to fully describe his or her unique experience and express the feelings attached to it before superimposing any similarities can help convey respect for the other's unique situation and decrease the deleterious effect on the relationship. Co-workers also can be valuable when a health professional's close relationship with the patient prevents him or her from seeing the patient's situation clearly. They may see what is happening and thus provide insight into the challenge occasioned by one's own similar, intense experience.

REFLECTIONS

- How might Mrs. Garcia have become better prepared to overcome her tendency to use her own child as a reference point to secure a bond between her and the parents of her clients?
- As you think about your own situation, what types of patients or families in your care might pose a challenge for you to not overidentify with them?

The task for all professionals who encounter a patient's situation that lends itself to overidentification is to be on the lookout for and honor the unique details and differences as well, thereby meeting the benchmark of respect.

CARING TOO MUCH

A third situation addresses the awkwardness that ensues when a relationship that began with appropriate expressions of professional care, including adherence to its limitations, evolves into a situation signaling that a new set of boundaries must be established. This type of occurrence often is precipitated by genuine affection many people in health professional and patient relationships learn to feel for each other. This situation leads to what can be characterized as caring too much; that is, the professional becomes sensitively drawn into the other's whole life situation, not just those aspects that lend themselves to being helped by the health professional's area of expertise. One study suggested that professionals who have been brought up to view themselves as "caregivers" in their own family may be the most susceptible to overstepping the professional contours of the relationship than others because they become sensitively drawn into circumstances of the other's life and are more likely to feel responsible to help "fix" problems.[10] Signs that affection, a positive component of the relationship, has spilled over into enmeshment lend themselves to some general suggestions about what can be done to rectify the tendency to care inappropriately. Obviously, in most cases such enmeshment is more likely to develop in health care settings in which longer term professional relationships exist. An example of how a problematic dynamic can arise is illustrated in this Case Study.

Case Study

Jack Simms has been an ambulatory patient at University Rehabilitation for 6 months. His affable, optimistic spirit has made him popular with the staff. At 23 years of age, he was involved in a car accident in which his fiancée was killed and he suffered a traumatic brain injury. Some health professionals have long suspected that Jack's optimism is a veneer for the deep grief and frustration resulting from this sudden, dramatic change in his life. However, attempts to encourage him to visit with the staff psychiatrist have been largely unsuccessful, a problem exacerbated by the fact that his insurance plan covers only 6 hours of psychiatric evaluation and treatment anyway. One day he tearfully tells Karen Morgan, a health profession student who has been treating him, that he is bored and desperately lonely. Up to this point, their interaction has been full of banter, and they have felt quite comfortable with each other. Karen does not divulge to the rest of the staff Jack's expression of boredom and loneliness, but that night on the way home, she stops by a local coffee shop where he has invited her to "come by and have a coffee" after work.

In the following weeks, she begins to visit him more often. She finds him attractive, they share common interests, and he is obviously happy in her company. During this time, however, Karen also leads her own private life, going on dates or out with friends and interacting with a world of other people. However, Jack hangs around the clinic before and after treatments, and he counts the minutes until she arrives at the coffee shop.

During her holiday vacation Karen visits old friends in a distant city and has a marvelous time. In fact, her original plan to spend the last few days back home is revised so that she can extend her time away. When she returns, bursting with enthusiasm and eager to share her stories, she finds Jack sullen and angry at her for staying away from him for so long. He has arranged for her to receive a present from him, which he plops angrily on the clinic desk. He says, "That's for you. Take it if you want." Then he stomps out of the clinic. A colleague who has witnessed this exchange exclaims, "Well! What was *that* about!"

Karen did not pity Jack or overidentify with his situation. Still, Jack's reaction indicates that he feels Karen has betrayed something important about their growing relationship. He has now reached the point at which someone he thought was a friend has rejected him. Karen, who acted in good faith on her feelings of warmth and affection for Jack, has thus unwittingly fostered a dependence on her that is detrimental to his well-being. Subsequent attempts to explain her sudden cutting back of the social aspects of their relationship may have profound, lasting negative effects on Jack. Instead of being a friend and confidante—maybe eventually a lover—as he had hoped, she will become just another of a long line of losses he has experienced. He has relied on her for more than she had intended or could manage.

As you may know from your own professional or personal experience, it is easy to get more involved with a person than you intended at the outset or miss clues that the other is becoming more attached than you.
- In Karen's situation, in retrospect were there any junctures that would have served as a warning sign to her that Jack's expectations were growing in a direction different from hers?
- What might she have done then?
- What can she do now to help ensure that the professional goals appropriate for him are met optimally?

In retrospect, Karen paid too much personal attention to Jack, meeting with him in an environment that invited more involvement than she apparently realized would result. With rare exceptions, it is always wise for the health professional to refrain from visiting the patient in a social setting until certain that the patient's feelings and life situation are such that an injury to the patient's feelings and dignity will not result.

Often an effective way to maintain respectful emotional boundaries is to remind the patient of the real situation between them. A young man, for instance, should know that the health professional he adores is engaged to someone else. A lonely older woman can bring small appropriate gifts of appreciation but be kept to the time frame and clinical environment of the relationship so if she expects more than a genuine acknowledgment for her generosity, you can contain the involvement. By discreetly sharing personal incidents from your everyday life you will introduce reality testing for the patient to consider if the fantasy of a different relationship is building. It is the health professional's responsibility to give and receive pertinent personal information in such a way that it allows both parties to maintain respectful limits in the relationship.

There are no hard and fast rules about how to proceed when genuine affection and enjoyment of the other is present in the professional relationship. Many of the caveats regarding dual relationships discussed earlier in this chapter can be useful if a relationship seems to be becoming sufficiently intense to cause you to question. Periodic reexamination of your own motives and conduct or others' assessment of your relationship is essential. For example, when the awkward situation occurred after the holiday break and another colleague witnessed it, this could have been an opportunity for Karen to share what she believed was behind Jack's behavior. Although it is important to maintain a professional demeanor, you will best be served by showing genuine warmth and affection but also tempering that with awareness that the other person's needs and wishes may exceed or differ from your own. In fact, a powerful antidote to enmeshment of this type is the health professional's strong professional identity, knowing that one can rely on the duties, rights, and values of the professions to help steer a respectful response of care when it seems to be veering off course.[11]

Maintaining Boundaries for Goodness' Sake

The examples of physical and emotional boundaries described in this chapter illustrate that exercising respectful constraint will serve everyone's interests well. The good news is that although an emphasis on boundaries taken alone sometimes leaves one feeling hemmed in, the reverse is true when it is understood that respect for basic limitations simply are instruments for everyone being able to fully flourish within the unique goals of a health professional and patient relationship.

People who seek your services to remain well or who become ill or injured are thrust into a new, unique relationship when they begin their encounter with you. The starting point for a flourishing relationship is to once again acknowledge the difference between your two roles. Most patients probably do not fully understand their feelings toward you; they may be expressed as awe or deference, as vague admiration, as infatuation, or as resistance and hostility. Some patients may not have a good idea of how to act in their role as a patient or how to honor yours. For many the whole environment is new or strange, sometimes influenced by popular television shows or other misleading depictions of the health care environment. To a large extent, you can alter the patient's attitude and expectations by learning about the basis of their feelings and by consciously keeping your own focus on your societal role as a health professional.

This understanding about the terms of involvement is usually easily established at the first meeting with refinements along the course of the interaction. If the relationship is more sustained, rough spots may have to be navigated, aware that adherence to the appropriate goals must continue to inform attitudes and conduct toward each other. When necessary limitations in this type of relationship are understood by both, there is not good cause for a patient's fear or anger. At the core of the relationship lies a paradox. The people who respect each other find that in their closeness they can provide each other freedom and mutual benefit as it applies to the health professional and patient relationship. What occurs is the knowledge (though not always spoken) that health professionals find satisfaction in applying professional skills optimally for each person, and the patient discovers satisfaction by benefiting from the services of skilled, caring professionals.

Their involvement is personal to a degree and not merely a business transaction; they express to each other those feelings and opinions that can be shared within the limited professional setting. When the patient no longer requires the services of the health professional, there will be no regret about ending their relationship because each one has benefited from it, whether it lasted for 10 minutes or 10 months. This is how goodness itself is served in the work we are privileged to do.

Summary

This chapter promotes respectful interaction through your becoming aware of and willingly acting within the physical, emotional, and psychological boundaries that serve as a benchmark of respect appropriate in professional relationships. We have shown that maintaining professional boundaries is not achieved by employing a cold or impersonal approach because such an approach may increase patients' conviction that you are being disrespectful of them and their situation. At the same time, the line between behaviors and expectations in your personal versus your professional relationships can be stretched thin in some situations. Your physical conduct, emotional responses of pity or overidentification, and actions that lead a patient to believe you care in ways that go beyond your professional relationship may present themselves as challenges to person-centered care. You are faced with the opportunity to respectfully structure the individual situation to uphold the dignity of both the patient and yourself through the guidelines offered in this chapter.

References

1. Jessing B. Back to square one. In: Haddad A, Brown K, eds. *The Arduous Touch: Women's Voices in Health Care.* West Lafayette, IN: Purdue University Press; 1999.
2. Lantos J, Matlock AM, Wendler D. Clinician integrity and limits to patient autonomy. *J Am Med Assoc.* 2011;305(5):495–499.
3. Swisher LL, Page CG. *Professionalism in Physical Therapy Practice.* Philadelphia: Saunders; 2005.
4. American Medical Association. Section 9:1.1 romantic or sexual relationships with patients. *AMA Code of Medical Ethics with Current Opinions.* Chicago: American Medical Association; 2016.
5. American Physical Therapy Association. *Principle #4.E American Physical Therapy Association Code of Ethics.* Fairfax, VA: American Physical Therapy Association; 2012.
6. Equal Employment Opportunity Commission. *EEOC-FS/E4: Facts about Sexual Harassment: EEOC Guidelines On Sexual Harassment.* 29 CFR 1604 11a. 93.

7. Kagle JD, Giebelhausen KB. Dual relationships and professional boundaries. *Soc Work*. 1994;39(2): 213–220.
8. Baca M. Professional boundaries and dual relationships in clinical practice. *J Nurse Pract*. 2011;7(3): 195–200.
9. Rich RA, Hecht MK. Staffing considerations. In: Haddad A, ed. *High Tech Home Care: A Practical Guide*. Rockville, MD: Aspen; 1987.
10. Farber NJ, Novack DH, O'Brien MK. Love, boundaries and the patient-physician relationship. *Arch Intern Med*. 1997;157:2291–2294.
11. Beauchamp TL, Childress JF. *Professional-Patient Relationships. Principles of Biomedical Ethics*. 7th ed. New York: Oxford University Press; 2012:288–331.

Respectful Interactions in the Delivery of Care

Section 2 begins with a focus on you as an individual because a key to all respectful human interaction lies in respecting yourself. When you and your colleagues enter the health professions, you bring with you your own unique combination of abilities, needs, values, and dreams. Understandably, as you transition into your professional role, you expect to incorporate these into the work positions you assume that are embedded in the health care system and society.

Chapter 4 focuses on developing self-respect in your role in the health professions. The tools to take care of oneself include benchmark conduct and attitudes, including building resiliency, relying on professional competencies, and finding balance in life and work. Of prime importance for your well-being is to take to heart the suggestions for how to use and contribute to your support communities—family, friends, and colleagues—and what to look for in the setting where you choose to work.

Chapter 5 offers a broader view of respect for oneself and others encountered in a variety of health settings, with a special focus on the challenge of looking below the surface at the differences that affect interactions with patients and devise strategies to overcome barriers and facilitate communication. This chapter explores commonly encountered differences such as cultural, geographical, socioeconomic, gender and sexual identity, and ethnic variations and the negative impact of bias and prejudice on health professional and patient and relationships.

Chapter 6 examines the environment in which care is delivered and its impact on respectful interactions with patients and others. Although not all health professions place people in the role of direct patient contact, some of the most challenging aspects of this work are in a health care delivery system. Attitudes toward and understanding of the clinical setting and the types of relationships that are appropriate influence the effectiveness of interaction with patients.

The role of being one of a whole matrix of persons caring for a patient is examined, with attention to the importance of interprofessional care teams and being able to decide when and why to refer a patient to someone else. By the end of Section 2, you should be better able to view yourself as respectfully as others will in your several roles in the health professions in the increasingly diverse world of health care.

CHAPTER 4

Respect for Self in the Professional Role

OBJECTIVES

The reader will be able to:

- List some positive goals related to self-respect that can be realized by attending to one's own needs and healthful habits
- Describe some reasons why striking a balance between socializing and solitude is important for a lifetime of professional vitality
- Explain what competence involves as a criterion for maintaining self-respect as a qualified practitioner
- Identify four professional practice skills that serve to sustain self-respect
- Understand the need to balance personal and professional life, including the need to put family and friends high on one's priorities list
- Name two types of bonds that can develop among work colleagues to help create a network of support and mutual respect
- Describe guidelines to assess how supportive an employer and future colleagues are likely to be
- Distinguish intimate from personal relationships and therapeutic from social relationships
- Identify the benefits of mindfulness as it relates to self-care and the health professional and patient interaction
- Evaluate why addressing one's anxieties and accepting responsibility for one's actions are essential to maintaining self-respect and realizing professional satisfaction

Prelude

Dignity can be considered as two values: other-regarding by respecting the dignity of others, and self-regarding by respecting one's own dignity or self-respect.

ANN GALLAGHER[1]

In this chapter, we stand back from some specific aspects of your professional role and identity formation to examine the fundamental question of how you can care for yourself and make physical and psychological space for optimal professional functioning.

Sustaining Self-Respect Through Nurturing Yourself

Nurturing comes from root words meaning "feeding," "taking loving care of," and "bringing into full bloom." In Chapter 1 you were introduced to the idea that a professional life guided by respect depends in part on the ability to identify and shape your own life according to your personal values and those that help to build a stronger community. The basic question we ask for your reflection in this chapter is, "What kinds of activities and attitudes can you cultivate to stay authentically you—healthy, happy, satisfied with your job, and able to integrate your professional and personal values and goals?"

There is the issue of who is responsible for your well-being. Today the consensus is that individuals ultimately are responsible for their own health. Do you agree and, if not totally, what are some exceptions? It certainly is the case that people feel better, look better, and can function more fully when nurturing their own sense of well-being, seeking balance in their lives, and mapping a life course that has opportunity for changing priorities.

None of these goals comes easily for most! The positive results of keeping life-affirming habits, practices, and goals in the forefront of your life plan as new situations arise seem obvious. However, if you are among the millions who make New Year's resolutions each year, you know that acknowledging the benefits of staying healthy physically, mentally, and spiritually and being successful in doing so are not the same. Consider with us some insights and suggestions to help you succeed in staying happy and healthy through enjoying self-respect in your professional role.

Self-Respect and Self-Care

You were introduced to care in previous chapters as an essential benchmark of respect in professional practice. You will recognize some themes about professional care in the following paragraph

Everyone talks about care as a positive feature of human relationships. It is. But care has a much more serious function in sustaining them than often we acknowledge. It is the link we make with another human being in distress, taking their suffering and well-being into account. At its core, care is not limited to the warm sentimentality so often expressed on the inside of greeting cards. True caring requires us to choose among our priorities and may become a challenge or even a burden. Caring always requires involved concern about the specific barriers to the other person's well-being and the action required to relieve them.

What do you notice about this statement? It is about care of *others*. This is not surprising, because professionals' reason for being is to determine and provide a caring response to a patient's plight. At the same time, this emphasis on caring for others points to a deeper issue. The emphasis on caring for others is so deeply rooted in professional identity that the care of oneself can easily get left out of the equation. In fact, many health professionals are so attuned to being caregivers or care *providers* that they perceive themselves as immune to needing care themselves.

The illusion that in caring for others one need not or cannot afford to pay attention to one's own needs and life-affirming instincts can lead to deep wounds over time, distorting what it means to place the patient first. For instance, to override feelings of deep distress, the need for relaxation or other healthy activities may set up a pattern that engenders inappropriate guilt or resentment toward patients. Medical historians tell us that the famous 18th-century physician Galen suffered nightmares for the rest of his life because of his feelings of guilt after he fled his inevitably dying patients during the plague of Rome to protect his own life and that of his family. A friend of one of the authors who was serving her time as a medical intern and had been on call for more than 24 hours, when this practice was still allowed, confessed, "By 4 a.m. I had no compassion at all for the patients coming into the emergency department, whatever their circumstance. All I could think of was getting them out of there so I could get some sleep." This person went on to be an outstanding physician who shared her story with students to urge them to be aware of the deleterious effects that resulted from abuse of their body and mind. The health professions have been slow to incorporate policies that respect the importance of self-care even though a professional obviously is in a better position to serve others well when acting from a position of personal strength gained through self-respecting habits and activities. In the words of Eleanor Brownn, a contemporary self-care workshop leader, "Rest and self-care are so important. When you take time to replenish your spirit, it allows you to serve others from the overflow. You cannot serve from an empty vessel."[2]

REFLECTIONS

The benefit that can come from respecting your own limits seems to be a blind spot in most discussions guiding professionals. Find and review the code of ethics in your field.
- Does it include this important aspect of professional life?
- If so, what is the wording that encourages you to remain true to your own healthful habits and needs?
- If not, write a statement that does include it.

You can get a fuller picture of what is at stake by looking at the quote about care on the previous page but this time thinking of it in terms of self-care:

Everyone talks about care as a positive feature of human relationships. It is. But self-care has a much more serious function in sustaining me than often I acknowledge. It is the link each of us makes with our own inner selves in distress, taking suffering and well-being into account. Often it is not limited to the warm sentimentality so often expressed on the inside of greeting cards. True caring requires me to choose among my priorities and may become a challenge or even a burden. Caring for myself always requires involved concern about the specific barriers to my well-being and the action required to relieve them.

Note that none of this attention to the self deflects from the realization that being in a professional relationship with patients means putting their specific health-related needs at the center of your professional decisions. At the same time, self-care gives you a measuring rod of qualities that allows you to fully engage in a person-centered approach with patients without being in a constant state of alert self-protection. The gift of this effort is a feeling of well-being.

REFLECTIONS

- In a few words describe a couple of things that give you a feeling of personal happiness and well-being.
- Why do you think this is the case?

Noting these is a great start because in declaring them you are taking a conscious step toward the self-respect that results from seeing yourself worthy of care. However, we also reminded you earlier in this chapter that most good ideas remain in the realm of "resolutions" that fall away. Starting with right now, take a few minutes to follow up on what you have just listed as some things that will help you experience well-being as a normal state.

REFLECTIONS

- Given how pressed I am for time and in light of my other priorities, when push comes to shove one thing I will do during the coming 6 months to enhance my personal well-being is:
- My strengths and most promising resources for keeping this resolve are:

Self-respect requires self-care. One must consciously identify what is important to oneself and find ways to follow it through into everyday choices, exercising the discipline to remain true to it over time.

Striking a Balance Between Socializing and Solitude

One step in following through on choices that demonstrate self-care is to recognize the importance of setting a balance between being with others and having time to yourself for spacious self-reflection. To fail to strike such a balance undermines the self-respect that you assiduously have honored in making choices that show you care about yourself.

Socializing yields both professional and important personal benefits. Of the former, the language often used in the description of what happens in the process of becoming and being professional is that the person becomes *socialized* into this identity. It goes almost without saying that personal benefits gained from informal socializing as leisure and relaxation activities are for most readers an essential component of their self-care.

Why, then, be concerned with the importance of striking a balance between constant interactions of socializing and reflective aloneness as a criterion of self-care? One compelling reason is that the professions are a *reflective practice,* not just direct application of material you have absorbed. Benner[3] and others have shown that the process of going from being a *clinical novice* to becoming a *clinical expert* is a self-reflective dimension of learning. In self-reflection, you fly solo and need time and open space to do so without continuously charging ahead to the next activity or responding to who or what calls for your immediate attention.

A second reason is that personalities differ in their need for internal "quiet time" to grasp and integrate material and feelings.[4] Even the most extroverted person needs some solitude. Some of you will need it to survive, others can practice it for their own self-enrichment as well as not always imposing on others one's extroverted need to be connected.

What is solitude and why is it important? *Solitude* is a time to *be with yourself only,* not responding to others, and to engage in reflections and restorative activities. Some people are active in their solitude, finding walking, jogging, biking, reading, or other solitary activities a time for honoring oneself. Others prefer the stillness of meditation, yoga, or just sitting quietly as a positive, active state of being. The experience of solitude is not identical to happiness and may even be "bittersweet" (accompanied by sorrow or anger) because it reveals parts of ourselves to ourselves that we otherwise may never recognize even though they are influencing our health. It is a form of self-respect realized by embracing the necessity of not always responding to other people whenever they need or want it and not reacting to every circumstance that comes one's way. As one health professional commented when he began to turn off his cell phone for an hour each day, "I realized over time that I had been acting like a service organization by always interrupting what I needed to do to link up with someone else!" Unlike loneliness, which is a form of suffering, solitude is a life affirming and self-respect–supporting activity.

REFLECTIONS

- List here the things you most like to do by yourself.
- If you do not currently make or have enough time for some of these activities, make two columns, one listing the reasons why you do not do them and the other making some suggestions about how you might make more opportunities to enjoy them.

Some ideas to help you make time for yourself include:

- Set a time and place, and rigorously try to adhere to it.
- Become bold in identifying to others what you are doing.

- Breathe, think, breathe again.
- Take notes on your reflections or keep a log of your solitary activities.

Remind yourself often that a basic minimum requirement for many other health-supporting activities is to take time and make space to be with yourself. In addition, you can help others have their own time alone by learning to recognize this need in others and encouraging it.

With this backdrop of self-care and some aspects of your environment to help realize it, we turn to other issues that incur self-respect and offer suggestions for ways to support and enrich it.

Self-Respect and the Motivation to Contribute

Most readers know that they would like to be able to contribute to others in society. It is a motivator for applying to an education program in the health professions, and this choice in itself is a good example of acting out of self-respect. Many psychologists, philosophers, and others have demonstrated that a life of satisfaction for most adults includes making a contribution that has benefit to others, whether to one's children, partner, or spouse, as a volunteer, or in the public workplace. Often, though not always, the choice of a professional career also arises from an individual's experience of illness or injury and how he or she or a friend or family member was helped by a professional, a friend, or loved one. Sometimes the desire to become a professional is based on a student's recognition that he or she has a talent for being a good listener or a capacity for helping friends when they are in trouble.

The desire to help others is not always the primary or only motivation that leads people to choose a career in the health professions. Love of science, the desire to be in a "people-oriented" line of work, the desire for status, and a career that promises to provide a good salary and high personal satisfaction are other important and understandable motivators. However, above all, the desire to make a significant contribution in life is paramount in helping you stay true to your initial intent when the going gets rough.

CONTRIBUTIONS THROUGH PROFESSIONAL COMPETENCE

Fortunately, health profession education is designed to prepare you to competently carry out your commitment to make a worthwhile contribution to society while realizing a certain type of lifestyle. You have already learned that your identity as a health professional carries with it expectations on the part of society, privileges, and responsibilities. You will be considered an expert in your field. You will be looked upon as a person whose special knowledge, skills, and attitudes can make the world a better place and improve individuals' lives. Thus, in choosing to be a health professional, you are accepting that self-respect requires professional competence. This involves not only what you will do but also what kind of person you will be in your own eyes and in the eyes of patients and others.

Knowledge

What knowledge do you need to become and remain a competent health professional?

- The physical and clinical sciences provide a foundation for understanding the body and the natural forces acting on it.
- The behavioral and social sciences of psychology, sociology, and anthropology provide understanding of people's needs and behaviors and how they affect healthfulness.
- The liberal arts expose you to the great political, religious, literary, and philosophical ideas and establish your own and your patients' link with history.

- Economic and legal concepts prepare you to understand how delivery of health care is financed today and some basic guidelines governing the activities of health care institutions.
- Statistics and information technology furnish baseline knowledge for research design, data analysis, and communication functions.
- Policy and administration courses help you understand the links between practice and the larger social context in which you work.

Depending on the level of your professional preparation, you will be exposed to all or most of these areas.

Skills

At the time you entered your professional curriculum, it is highly likely you had been more accustomed to classroom learning than to laboratory and clinical learning. The acquisition of skill often requires long, tedious hours of hands-on practice.

The frustration that often accompanies mastering a skill was illustrated when one of the authors decided to learn to fly fish. She read several books, watched a video, and studied the types of flies and equipment; then she hired a guide to take her to a trout stream in northern Maine.

The first half-day was spent far from the water, in a field, learning to cast out the fly. At least half the time the fly caught in trees, bushes, and other obstructions. After lunch, finally in the water, she learned that the coordination required to lay the line flat and cast the fly out far enough from her hook to attract anything other than shoreline weeds was a far cry from the pictures in the video. That night, nursing a sore shoulder and wrist, she remembered her instructor's encouragement to rest up and "with practice you'll see yourself improving day by day." She wondered. Hundreds of casts later it still was not perfect, but the fly more often landed in the stream where she was trying to set it.

Several basic skill sets are needed for acquiring and maintaining professional competence in a health profession. Each receives much attention in professional preparation.

Technical Skill

Technical skill is the ability to safely and effectively apply technology, often using highly specialized techniques of your field to secure a diagnosis, conduct an evaluation, or provide a treatment intervention.

Clinical Reasoning Skill

It follows that a key component of professional competence is creativity and problem-solving arrived at through your clinical reasoning and related critical thinking, leading to the exercise of sound informed judgment. Clinical reasoning requires that you consider the situation; gather relevant information; interpret, predict, and synthesize information; select a course of action; evaluate the outcomes of your actions; and reflect on your actions.[5] Reflection is a key component of clinical reasoning. It allows the health professional to extract meaning from clinical experiences and engage in life-long learning. Thinking about one's own thinking is critical to professional development and models best practice across a variety of care delivery settings.

Skill in Interpersonal Relationships and Communication

Most health professionals interact with a wide variety of people during a day: other members of the interprofessional care team and support personnel, patients and their families, students, visitors, administrators, and business contacts such as equipment salespersons. This activity demands that you understand appropriate conduct in different types of relationships. It means being able to accept responsibility as a supervisor and constructive criticism when supervised. It involves tact, diplomacy, consistency, and forthrightness. Many areas of this book describe means whereby professionals express respect toward others and thereby also maintain the self-respect that comes from competence in communications.

Teaching and Administrative Skill

Education of individual patients or clients, including families and significant others, and the larger public is essential in every health field. This may involve patients, families, students, other professionals, support personnel, and the public. You will be required to assess an individual's readiness to learn, determine any barriers to learning, and provide teaching in keeping with the patient's ideal learning mode or style. Administrative skills allow you to organize and implement workable solutions to potential problems; set reasonable short- and long-term goals in your workplace; engage in fair, objective evaluation of yourself and others; and do your share to maintain a cost-effective operation.

ATTITUDES AND CHARACTER

Your attitudes toward caring for others, responses to persons who may be different from yourself, and the qualities you believe make life worth living all are part of how your feelings of self-respect are either supported or diminished by challenges in the health profession environment. In most instances, your intuitive responses are a great resource. Attitudes that seem to keep you at a distance from being able to engage wholeheartedly in your professional tasks warrant deep reflection.

Some basic attitudes and character traits needed for successful professional practice were outlined as core professional values in Chapter 1. Almost all of them are other-directed as resources for care of others. They apply to self-care as well. In addition, a career in the professions requires lifelong learning, and so it follows that one important attitude to cultivate at the outset is a love of learning and discerning what matters most for your own sustenance and growth at any period of your career. Keeping abreast of key opportunities to enhance your expertise is rewarded with the self-respect that comes with professional competence.[6]

Self-Respect and Acceptance of Support

We turn now to several additional considerations; among the most important is the necessity of being willing to graciously accept support when you need it and set priorities that keep the most important people in your close circle of caring. Family and friends are at the top of the list. Professional colleagues are close behind.

BALANCE PERSONAL AND PROFESSIONAL LIFE

Because professional life can be so involving, family and friends outside of your work environment are at risk for being left out of your life in important ways unless you make conscious efforts to include them. Still, there is much evidence that the support of family and friends is key to thriving in almost all walks of life. Often, they are taken for granted and may get the leftover part of your days, the majority of the best hours having been spent in workplace activities.

In the circle on the next page write the name of the most important person (or persons) to you in the center. Add those who are in a second tier. Finally, add those around the periphery but still in the mix.

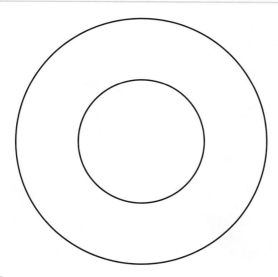

Your challenge is to establish priorities and conduct that will reflect the rhythms needed for your family members and friends to be able to support you when you need it. A young lawyer has this comment as he recounted the choices he began to exercise when he felt himself being consumed by his work:

> There were a few things that helped to restore my sense of equilibrium. The first was to make a conscious effort to spend time with my wife. In the beginning, I resisted when my wife would plead, cajole, and sometimes push me out the door of our apartment so that we could spend a few hours watching a movie or going to dinner. Eventually, I realized how important this time was. It strengthened our relationship by keeping the lines of communication open between us. Not only that, it also made me a better worker by giving my anxious mind a much-needed rest.
>
> A second source of balance came from getting together with other people who were facing similar pressures at work. Two or three times a month I would meet with a few friends from law school who were working in other firms around town. Our get-togethers were combination lunches and b.s. sessions. These meetings did wonders for my perspective. I found myself becoming less anxious and self-absorbed as I discovered that my friends were dealing with the same worries and concerns I was facing. We helped ourselves by helping each other.[7]

In short, this young professional used the resources of family, friends, and his own form of solitude for spiritual reflection to create the balance he felt slipping away from him. In the process, he created a support network that not only benefited his work but also helped him maintain a balance that showed respect for himself and those closest to him. He also mentions his professional colleagues as a resource. This is so important that we now examine it in more detail.

HONOR BONDS WITH COLLEAGUES

One source of support is that persons working in a health care setting have several common bonds, all of which help establish rapport and support among them. Of special importance and sometimes easy to overlook in the hubbub of everyday tasks are the professional colleagues in one's immediate workplace.

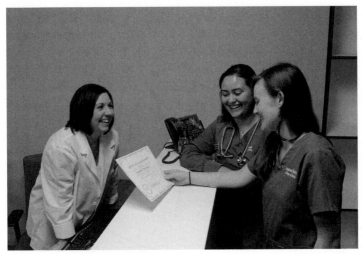

Fig. 4.1 Sharing good news such as professional accomplishments with colleagues at work helps build strong working relationships. (*Courtesy Maren Haddad.*)

Bond of Shared Concerns

At your worksite, self-care that buttresses self-respect can be realized through having a place to air common concerns about a particular patient's clinical problems, about the department, about what is happening in one's field, and about health services in general. This can be achieved while respecting confidentiality regarding specific patients or others and refraining from gossip. As health professionals, we voluntarily place ourselves in the mainstream of human suffering. No one commits us to this role. We choose to be there because we care enough about human well-being to want to effect certain changes using our professional skills. But this life you chose makes intense demands on you, and an essential resource is to know there is a trusted group with whom to share your common worries, uncertainties, and questions.

Bond of Shared Care and Gratitude

In the crush of everyday work, colleagues take less time telling one another directly that they appreciate and care about them than they do sharing their concerns. Creating a generous atmosphere of such expression helps transform a workplace from a work site only to a true community. Gratitude, too, is expressed too seldom by persons working together. A simple word of thanks can create more goodwill than months of competent work together during which neither person tries to express appreciation for the other. There are many ways to say "thank you" or "you are appreciated."

REFLECTIONS

- What are some ways in previous jobs you have held or currently hold that you and your colleagues have shown appreciation for each other's contributions?
- What ideas do you have for helping to create a happy and supportive workplace for yourself and your colleagues?

Many things are quite simple to implement. Remembering when colleagues complete a milestone in their professional studies such as passing a board examination or attaining certification in their discipline is one example. Performing other "random acts of kindness" creates a general environment of congeniality in which the language of mutual respect for the efforts and gifts of one another's skills and presence can flourish (Fig. 4.1).

SEEK SUPPORTIVE INSTITUTIONAL ENVIRONMENTS

The bonds of shared concern, caring, and gratitude work together to encourage the realization of mutually shared goals and values. However, it is not enough for individuals alone to desire to create a respectful environment—respect also must be reflected in the structure and values of those who have policy authority. One group of health care administrators suggest the following for the design of organizational structures that meet the requirement: "Optimally there is full alignment among (1) the moral identity of individuals, which informs and shapes their behavior as they work in an organization; (2) the implicit values of the organization as embodied in the organizational culture and stated and unstated practices; and (3) the organization's explicit social purpose and stated mission."[8]

It is a good idea, then, when considering a position to seek at least one person who appears to be a potential source of support when problems arise that could challenge your self-respect in your position. You should be bold in asking questions that will allow you to gain some understanding of how support is expressed within the department and larger institution. To make an assessment, the following guidelines may be useful:

- Inquire of your future employer whether there are meetings or other sessions in which problems associated with the everyday workplace stresses of health care delivery are discussed.
- Ask potential colleagues what they think the sources of the most intense stress in that environment are and how the group typically handles them.
- Make a mental note of those who appear to be potential sources of support or if no one appears to be. If everyone denies that problems exist or become defensive about such questions when they are tactfully posed, this probably signals a setting in which stresses are dealt with alone, without the support of one's colleagues or the institution.[9]

Fortunately, only in rare situations are no support mechanisms available. In fact, being a support to others is often the key to finding support from them when it is needed. The adage "To have a friend is to be one" almost always holds true in the workplace.

PLAY: ENJOY ONE ANOTHER'S COMPANY

No one can—or should—keep he or she self-respect if he or she unnecessarily puts up with or contributes to an atmosphere of doom and gloom. Persons in the health professions are fortunate to be in a line of work in which they know they are usually making a positive difference in patients' lives. That in itself is reason to enjoy their work.

But there's more. Shortchanging the joy that can come from remembering to put some levity and fun into the environment is doing yourself a disfavor. It does not take much—a cartoon, a good joke, a lighthearted story that a colleague or patient is trying to tell, or some other type of pleasure can do the job. One author, himself a health professional, observes:

> Joy is only possible for persons who are attentive to the present. One cannot be happy if one is continually ruminating about what might have been or fretting over whether wishes will come to pass. Americans have a tough time with real joy. Americans are oriented toward outcomes, expectations, and the future; toward ever more competition in proving that they deliver the best results, and anxiously pondering how things might have turned out if only they had chosen differently. This makes it hard to be happy. In health care, these tendencies are exaggerated. Worries about what will happen next to the patient and worries about their own future careers blot out the possibility of joy for many health care professionals. Joy is a present tense phenomenon. It is possible only if one attends to the moment.[10]

Attending to the moment is a key component of *mindful practice*. Mindfulness is setting an intention to "pay attention systematically and nonjudgmentally to the present moment for

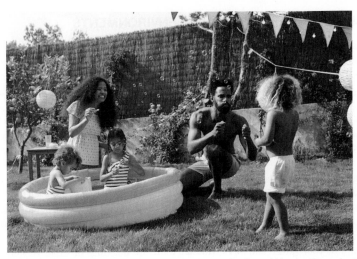

Fig. 4.2   Health professionals should remember to make time for family and friends. (© *monkeybusinessimages/iStock/Thinkstock.com.*)

whatever arises."[11] Mindful practices such as mind-body awareness, purposeful pauses, breathing exercises, body scans, and informal and formal meditation have been correlated with resilience in the health professions.[12-14] Sometimes mindful activities such as yoga outside of work hours enhance the ability for co-workers to enjoy one another in a more relaxed environment as well as enhance the time spent with family and friends (Fig. 4.2).

Activities do not have to stop with an informal afternoon coffee, holiday party, or sports team. For instance, two of the authors were part of a writing group some time ago. We met regularly with several other health profession colleagues after work. We wrote about our work experiences in the form of fictionalized short stories, poetry, and essays. At first all of us were too shy to share anything, thinking it would not be good enough. However, as we became more comfortable with one another, we started looking forward to hearing one another's stories. In addition to writing about some serious problems, we found our gathering to be a great vehicle for laughing at ourselves and good-naturedly at one another, as well as an "excuse" to get to know one another better. One delightful outcome was that we could publish some of our work for others to share, too.

Obviously the professional or interprofessional care team who substitutes a good time for good work is not one who will, or should, last long in a position. However, finding and helping to further create a positive work environment can do much to generate an enriched, respectful environment for everyone involved and, not the least important, for you.

Refining Your Capacity to Provide Care Professionally

The development of basic professional competencies discussed earlier in this chapter is not only a requirement for self-respect but also a splendid opportunity for your continued growth and flourishing. The chapters in Section 1 are basic building blocks of professional identity and benchmarks of respect and boundary setting that help give further shape to the professional role. We return here with some additional refinements to those basic foundations. Consider with us some distinctions between intimate and personal modes of caregiving and important differences between strictly social and therapeutic relationships. The former focuses on the depth of a relationship and the latter on the avenues of expression.

INTIMATE VERSUS PERSONAL RELATIONSHIPS

Acts of caregiving, both intimate and personal, depend on the depth of involvement in which the persons engage in each other's lives. *Intimate care* is what you offer to someone you love or for whom you care deeply. Most often that inner circle of intimate relationships is limited to a few such as family members or beloved friends. One test is that the offer of intimate forms of assistance in its most extreme form means that you would be willing to risk personal danger to yourself for this person. In contrast, *personal care* is what you are willing to offer colleagues, friends, acquaintances, or strangers whose human needs you see you can respond to without getting more deeply entwined in their lives. It takes many forms in everyday interactions from giving directions, assisting a person physically, or donating money to a good cause. Random acts of kindness express care of this sort. Both types of relationships demand an investment in the well-being of others, and the boundaries are not always hard and fast between the two. For example, in a group of acquaintances you may over time become closer to one and find yourselves increasingly more engaged in each other's lives.

Professional caring belongs to the category of personal rather than intimate relationships. Maintaining the respectful conduct that characterizes personal helping in health professional and patient interaction is the primary focus of this book.

REFLECTIONS

Reflect on the past couple days of your encounters with family, friends, and others with whom you have come into contact.
- Which of the encounters would you say were intimate?
- Which ones met the general criteria of personal caring conduct toward the other(s)?
- Why?

SOCIAL VERSUS THERAPEUTIC RELATIONSHIPS

A related way to view your relationships as a care provider emphasizes the types of activities rather than degree of involvement with the other person. Any care you provide in which your resources are not prescribed by specific, well-defined professional skills that maintain boundaries specific to the professional-patient relationship are examples of *social relationships*. Social caregiving takes many forms because the numbers of resources you can use are as numerous as your imagination and your willingness to extend yourself for someone else's benefit. One helps a child cross the street, lessens an old man's loneliness by paying him a visit, or lends $5 to a neighbor in need. On the face of it, this example of caring could stem from wanting to benefit someone else while feeling the benefit of self-respect as well, and in most cases this is true. But offers of the social help variety are not always welcomed by the recipient and in fact may not be interpreted as showing genuine care at all. A study by several scientists interested in altruism concluded this is especially true if the recipient perceives the offer as being motivated primarily by the person supposedly offering care but needing only to fulfill his or her own needs.[15] Persons with disabilities are often victims of this displaced motive. Consider this experience recounted by a health professions student.

Case Study

On weekends, the student cared for a 13-year-old boy with paraplegia who mobilized with the help of a wheelchair. One Saturday, the student and boy were shopping in a large department store and paused at a vending machine for a Coke. First the student bought a soft drink for his young friend and then turned to buy one for himself. The boy had just taken the first sip and was resting the can on the arm of his wheelchair when a woman laden with bundles rushed up and dropped a dollar in his lap. She patted the astonished boy on the head and exclaimed, "Poor, poor boy. I hope that helps you get better." She then gathered up her packages and scurried away.

REFLECTIONS

- What seems not to be caring behavior in this woman's actions?
- Supposing her motives were indeed to show personal care toward this young man, what should she have done that would have made a difference?

In short, the carer in the social relationship may use any available means to offer assistance rather than depending on specialized skills, but how the offer of care is perceived by the recipient will be determined in part by what the motive seems to be and how sensitive the caregiver is to the effects of the offer. There is another kind of care available and when put into the relational context is recognized as a therapeutic relationship.

A *therapeutic relationship* develops when the professional caregiver performs professionally competent acts designed to benefit the person who needs his or her services. Therapeutic caring is personal but not intimate. At times, this is a difficult difference to grasp because often there are aspects of the therapeutic relationship that involve the patient's sharing of deeply intimate details of his or her life and that impinge on the usual physical boundaries of propriety. The prosthetist may massage the stump of a patient's bare thigh in order to be sure the muscles are relaxed sufficiently for a prosthesis mold to fit accurately; a dietitian may interview a patient about deeply personal eating habits to evaluate nutritional status and plan the dietary regimen; nurses, assistants of all kinds, therapists, and others regularly touch, probe, hold, and stroke patients. Some ways in which close physical contact requires attention were addressed in Chapter 3 regarding how to understand and honor professional boundaries. The common denominator is that your unique professional role determines what is permitted for truly therapeutic care to be provided. The differences between care as a social relationship and a therapeutic relationship are summarized in Box 4.1.

REFLECTIONS

- Name some unique therapeutic activities you might engage in during your interactions with patients that would not be considered appropriate in other societal environments.
- Name some that are not necessarily unique to your field but fall within the broader scope of a therapeutic relationship.

BOX 4.1 ■ Comparison Between Caring in a Social and Therapeutic Relationship

Caring in a Social Relationship
- May be an intimate or personal act
- Helper uses a wide variety of resources

Caring in a Therapeutic Relationship
- Is a personal but not an intimate act
- Helper primarily uses well-defined, specialized professional skills

---

Self-Respect, Anxiety, and Accountability

This chapter has focused on several tools and some key insights that can help you maintain your self-respect. Still, as authors, we know from experience that some stresses are inevitable because nothing that presents worthwhile challenges comes without its burdens. *Anxiety* is a psychological response to a stress that is calling for attention. *Accountability* is a means of remaining true to your core values when they are threatened. Both can be seen as resources when you care enough about yourself to take the time to both pay attention to them and act accordingly.

RESPONDING TO ANXIETY

Anxiety is the result of unresolved stresses, some of which can lend themselves to resolution but, if not attended to, may gnaw at one's confidence, happiness, and most important, self-respect. Anxiety arising from deep uncertainty or unresolvable situations is more difficult to bring to a full resting place but does not have to remain destructive to one's well-being.

Anxiety may arise from situations in your workplace ranging from feeling unprepared for some of the challenges facing you with particular types of patient situations to feeling frustrated with institutional conditions that are not allowing you a sense of satisfaction. At another level, the troublesome feeling may be pointing to something deeper in yourself. For example, one of the most difficult things to admit is that you find you are not cut out for the type of work you are preparing—or have prepared—to do. If you take the time for solitude and reflection, you may hear that inner voice saying, "You do not want to be—or stay—in this type of work." Not everyone is cut out for what the health professions demand. Maintaining self-respect must not hinge on trying to do the impossible for whatever reason or deceiving oneself into believing that because you began a career, or were encouraged to do so, you made the right choice. Not everyone can just change careers midstream, but dropping out prematurely would be a tragedy if the source of unease is temporary and there is a way through an unsettling period characterized by anxiety.

Anxieties arising from personal issues can engender disabling effects too. An impending divorce, either one's own or that of one's parents or child, a serious illness, an unexpected or unwanted pregnancy, the news that a loved one is seriously ill, sudden changes in financial viability—these and many other personal, family, and other relational problems can threaten a person's feeling of well-being and affect workplace performance.

Age-related concerns can combine with one or more of the previously listed sources of anxiety. Pressures on young people to decide what they are going to be have led some to choose a career path early in life only to wonder if it was a wise choice. A growing number of professionals come into their field having raised children or spent many years in another career. Common anxieties expressed by this group spring from the belief that they are acting on their last chance to realize a dream when other hopes have not panned out or have gone into debt to desperately retool to stay afloat financially when another line of work has dried up or that they are not giving enough time to other obligations of midlife. Under these pressures it is understandable that any doubts are open season for anxiety.

If anxiety persists, it should be addressed. Following are three suggestions on how to respond constructively out of your commitment to well-deserved self-care.

- *Identify the source:* One of the most important steps in dissipating the destructive tension associated with anxiety is to identify its source if you can do so on your own. Is it directly work related? Is there some other obvious reason that anxiety has descended on you, or is the source too diffuse to identify? Are there times when you are free from it and, if so, when? What activities seem to help allay it?

- *Share feelings with a trustworthy friend or family member:* The sting of anxiety is that it can alienate you from others who know that something is wrong but do not know what or why. Keeping the source to yourself can baffle them when they observe your change in conduct or become aware of your self-deceit that obviously is covering a deeper problem (Fig. 4.3). They may even think it is something they have done. In sharing your anxiety with a trusted person, you have overcome the isolation of the experience and in most cases have gained an ally who can help you address it. An unintended but encouraging side effect of this process is that you may find out how common your feelings are. By knowing that others, too, are feeling stressed, you feel less "out of joint" with the rest of the world.

- *Seek professional help:* When talking with a trusted friend or family member is not adequate, you deserve the benefit of help from a professional. In such cases, an instructor or counselor

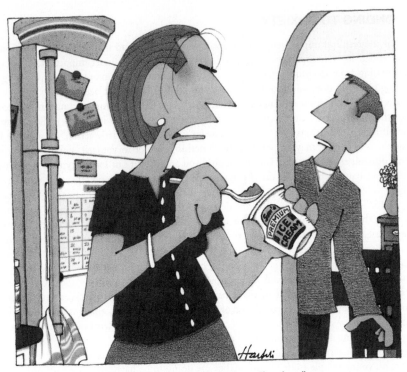

"I'm not eating. I'm self-medicating."

Fig. 4.3 "I'm not eating. I'm self-medicating." (© *The New Yorker Collection 2001. William Haefeli from* cartoonbank.com. *All rights reserved.*)

can help you discover why you feel anxious. Many workplaces today provide such services, knowing that anxiety affects the productivity of their employees. The treatment for stress may require an extended course of intervention over weeks or months. Your well-being is at stake, and this is an area of caring for yourself that, when acted on, will help bolster your self-respect for what you took the time to do.

ACCOUNTABILITY

In Chapter 1 you were introduced to the basic ideas of knowing and remaining true to your values and those that are expected of you as a professional. The reward for doing so is that you will be sustained over a lifetime of challenges to your personal and professional integrity. In a word, you can remain whole in the presence of destabilizing situations and forces that threaten your very core of being.

Accountability means taking responsibility for one's actions and is the key to maintaining your integrity. A professional is viewed as an *agent*—that is, one who has the specialized knowledge, skills, and other authority to be held legally and ethically responsible for his or her professional judgment and actions taken on behalf of patients. This includes the pleasure of taking credit for a job well done but also readily admitting mistakes or errors in judgment. Fortunately, almost all institutions and your professional codes of ethics have guidelines for how clinical or other errors in the professional role must be reported and steps taken. In addition, your professional educational experiences teach you in more detail how to honor this requirement.

One of the most unwelcome but important aspects of modern health care is the legal and ethical responsibility of professionals to report unethical, unsafe, or impaired conduct observed among one's peers. This type of accountability signals the trust that society places in the health professions to police themselves when wrongdoing is observed and is taken up in more detail in Chapter 6, in which institutional policies within care delivery systems are emphasized. Strict procedures to protect all involved during the process of discovering, reporting, and following through on such allegations have been developed in the very structures of health care to emphasize the weight society places on the professionals' expanded role as protectors of the cherished value of health.

REFLECTIONS

- What does the Code of Ethics of your profession say about your professional responsibility and accountability toward patients? About reporting suspected wrongdoing or impairment among peers?
- Does it give you adequate guidance for you to feel confident about these requirements?

Participating in Goodness

This chapter focusing on respect for yourself in your professional capacity understandably includes ways that you can be supported sufficiently to provide a foundation for patients to have confidence in you (Fig. 4.4).

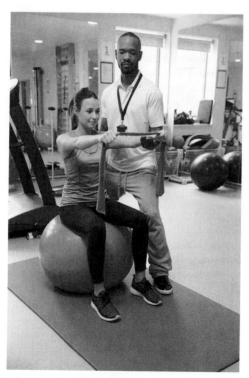

Fig. 4.4 One expression of mutual respect is participation in shared goals that are valued by each. (© monkeybusinessimages/iStock/Thinkstock.com.)

Attention to these suggestions will allow you to shift from being a caregiver following the must do's and must not do's to the joy of experiencing the goodness that your role allows you to share with others in the everyday practice of your profession.

What is goodness? Everyone's experience of it will vary somewhat, but we think a common denominator is that professionals who include self-respect in all its forms in their daily practice are the most prepared to think they are participating in something wonderful that goes beyond the everyday routine of their particular tasks.[16]

Although we do not often think of being in love with our work or experiencing and sharing goodness through our daily conduct, there is the potential for that type of richness. Physical and emotional healthfulness is a cherished value in every culture. We participate in promoting that goodness as caregivers in health profession settings, including our own. Continuing to find work satisfaction year after year requires striving for the most value one can be in the professional role and the most value one can contribute and receive.

Summary

This chapter highlights how to realize self-respect for your choice of profession and implement self-care throughout your career. All along the trajectory from student to experienced professional, self-respect and the caring it generates are cherished resources to be used. A balance between socializing and taking time for reflection and solitude is essential. Taking seriously the emphasis on professional competence through the acquisition and life-long updating of essential knowledge, skills, and ennobling attitudes should help you remain focused on the self-satisfactions such a career offers.

Showing respect toward and accepting support from family, friends, and the people you work with daily also are invaluable resources. Their support of you is essential to break your fall should you ever feel like you are losing your footing. The appropriate nature of your relationships with patients is basically personal and therapeutic, not intimate and social, providing additional guidance for respect to be honored all around. Addressing understandable bouts of anxiety and embracing areas of professional accountability will help keep you focused on the necessity of including care of yourself while expressing professional care toward patients and society. Remember to enjoy the benefits of this type of work, including the opportunity to participate in a basic type of goodness as its own reward!

References

1. Gallagher A. Dignity and respect for dignity—two key health professional values: implications for nursing practice. *Nurs Ethics.* 2004;11(6):587–599.
2. Brownn E. © Eleanor Brownn. https://www.goodreads.com/author/quotes/10614034.Eleanor_Brownn (accessed April 9, 2017).
3. Benner P. *From Novice to Expert: Excellence and Power in Clinical Nursing Practice.* Commemorative edition. Upper Saddle River, NJ: Prentice-Hall; 2005.
4. Cain S. Quiet. *The Power of Introverts in a World That Can't Stop Talking.* New York: Random House; 2012.
5. Jensen G. 42nd Mary McMillan Lecture. Learning what matters most. *Phys Ther.* 2011;91:1674–1679.
6. Doherty RF, Purtilo RB. *Ethical Dimensions in the Health Professions.* 6th ed. St. Louis: Saunders; 2016:78.
7. Loving Your Job, Finding Your Passion: Work and the Spiritual Life, by Joseph G. Allegretti. Copyright © 2000 by Joseph G. Allegretti. Paulist Press, Inc., New York/Mahwah, NJ. Reprinted by permission of Paulist Press, Inc. http://www.paulistpress.com.
8. Rambur R, Vallett C, Cohen JA, et al. The moral cascade: distress, eustress, and the virtuous organization. *J Org Moral Psych.* 2010;1(1):41–54, with permission from Nova Science Publishers, Inc.
9. Doherty RF, Purtilo RB. *Ethical Dimensions in the Health Professions.* 6th ed. St. Louis: Elsevier; 2016.
10. Sulmasy DP. *The Healer's Calling: A Spirituality for Physicians and Other Health Care Professionals.* Mahwah, NJ: Paulist Press; 1997.

11. Kabat-Zinn J. *Full Catastrophe Living: Using the Wisdom of Your Body and Mind to Face Stress, Pain, and Illness*. New York: Dell Publishing; 1990.
12. Olson K, Kemper KJ. Factors associated with well-being and confidence in providing compassionate care. *J Evid Based Complement Altern Med*. 2014;19:292–296.
13. Foureur M, Besley K, Burton G, et al. Enhancing the resilience of nurses and midwives: pilot of a mindfulness-based program for increased health, sense of coherence and decreased depression, anxiety and stress. *Contemp Nurse*. 2013;45:114–125.
14. Pidgeon AM, Ford L, Klaassen F. Evaluating the effectiveness of enhancing resilience in human service professionals using a retreat-based Mindfulness with Metta Training Program: a randomised control trial. *Psychol Health Med*. 2014;1:355–364.
15. Dugatkin LA. *The Altruism Equation: Seven Scientists Search for the Meaning of Altruism*. Princeton, NJ: Princeton University Press; 2007.
16. Purtilo R. New respect for respect in ethics education. In: Purtilo R, Jensen G, Royeen CB, eds. *Educating for Moral Action: A Sourcebook in Health and Rehabilitation Ethics*. Philadelphia: FA Davis; 2005.

Respect in a Diverse Society

The reader will be able to:

- Provide a working definition of culture and its relevance to the health professional and patient relationship
- Define cultural bias, personal bias, and unconscious bias
- Define prejudice and how it relates to discrimination and health disparities
- Describe how discrimination of all types affects patients and health professionals and some ways you can counter its disrespectful dimensions
- Recognize primary and secondary characteristics of culture
- Examine the various types of diversity in health care settings and society at large
- Explore ways that the label of "race" is problematic
- Describe the dimensions of culturally appropriate care
- Define cultural humility, and describe the process of viewing the health professional and patient relationship in this manner

Prelude

Ultimately, the immigrant must find himself in an American environment, must attach himself to American institutions, must contribute his gifts to their support and to their further development. As a means toward establishing such Americanizing contacts, the immigrant must at least be able to communicate with his English-speaking neighbor in the language of America, and to appreciate in an elementary way the things which Americans hold dear.

H.H. GOLDBERGER[1]

Section 1 of this book focused on creating a context of respect in one's professional role. Respect also involves sensitivity to individual and group differences in the interactions that are part of the delivery of health care. Thus you may discover that, even with deep understanding of your personal values and clarity about building relationships and setting boundaries, respectful interaction still does not result. And even with experience, you may sometimes fail to appreciate significant differences in others with whom you interact. It is a continual challenge to look below the surface at the differences that affect interactions with patients and devise strategies to overcome barriers and facilitate communication. Many such differences have come to be viewed collectively as being characteristics of a person's *culture*. However, just exactly what culture is or how the concept is to be used in health care interactions is open to a variety of interpretations. For our purposes, an apt working definition of culture is:

… the totality of socially transmitted behavioral patterns, arts, beliefs, values, customs, lifeways, and all other products of human work and thought characteristics of a population of people that guide their world view and decision making.[2]

It follows that yet to be considered in your examination of the health professional and patient relationship is the fact that each person interprets another's actions, facial expressions, choice of words, and other characteristics according to his or her cultural conditioning and past experience, social context, and other factors that shape how ultimately he or she views the world. From the perspective of culture, our interactions take place within a society that, at least within the United States, has long been described as a "melting pot" in which all the various cultures blend together. The melting pot metaphor has its origins in the days of vast numbers of immigrants entering the United States at the turn of the 19th century to help explain the relationship between the dominant culture and the new arrivals in America. However, this metaphor hides the negative side effects of such a view of US society that forces assimilation, which strips immigrants and refugees of long-standing cultural traditions and practices and requires adoption of the cultural practices of the mainstream culture. Some still hold to the melting pot description of the United States, and you can hear this view when people say something like, "At least they (the immigrant population in question) could learn to speak English." This view is reflected in the introductory comment at the beginning of this chapter. The quote is from a manual for teaching English to "foreigners" that was written in 1921. Although that was more than 100 years ago the sentiment sounds disturbingly contemporary.

Others claim it is no longer accurate or appropriate to expect newcomers to a society to lose all connection to their cultural traditions or ethnic identity, so they describe contemporary America as a "chunky stew" or a salad savored both for the character of the individual ingredients (ethnically derived differences) and for the delicious melding of flavors (social integration).[3] Other countries, such as Canada, have traditionally likened society to a "vertical mosaic," with each person comprising an integral part of a complex but comprehensive picture, or, similarly, a jar of jelly beans, with each color contributing to the diversity of the contents of the jar (an organization or society at large).[4,5]

Furthermore, members of cultural groups can individually or collectively adapt traditions or borrow traits from other cultures, which is quite common when members of diverse cultures are in prolonged contact.[6] The phenomenon of merging cultures is called *acculturation*. In this chapter, we examine the diversity you will encounter in clinical practice and the barriers (e.g., personal and cultural biases, prejudices, discrimination, or ignorance) that get in the way of appreciating differences and inhibit respectful interaction.

Bias, Prejudice, and Discrimination

A *cultural bias* is a tendency to interpret a word or action according to culturally derived meaning assigned to it. Cultural bias derives from cultural variation, discussed later in this chapter. For example, some cultures view smiles as a deeply personal sign of happiness that is only shared with intimates. Others view smiles as an indication of general friendliness to be shared with all. It is quite possible that another can interpret a friendly smile on the part of one person as disingenuous or inappropriate. Regarding health care, attitudes toward pain, methods of conveyance of bad news, management of chronic illness and disability, beliefs about the seriousness and causes of illness, and death-related issues vary among different cultures. These different kinds of beliefs about disease and illness have an impact on health care–seeking behavior and acceptance of the advice, status, and intervention of health professionals. Understanding a patient's concept of health and illness is critical to the development of interaction strategies that are clinically sound and acceptable to the patient.

A *personal bias* is a tendency to interpret a word or action in terms of a personal significance assigned to it. Personal bias can derive from culturally defined interpretations but also can originate from other sources grounded in personal experience. The individual internalizes the cultural attitudes until he or she believes them to be entirely personal. Put another way, a personal bias is an individual's feeling about a particular person or thing that colors his or her interpretation of it. The bias can lead to more favorable or less favorable judgments than are warranted. This process is similar to internalizing societal values described in Chapter 1.

Understanding the way personal biases influence us and their effect on our attitudes and conduct are important to the health professional. Whenever bias is present, it affects the type of communication possible between the persons involved and therefore must be recognized as one determining factor in respectful interaction. In some cases, personal bias may produce a positive bias, or "halo effect," on certain individuals; that is, a single characteristic or trait leads to positive global judgments about a person. For example, a patient who is pleasant and cooperative during office visits also could be thought by the health professional to be compliant with therapy because of the halo effect even though the opposite could be true. Although showing favoritism on the basis of personal bias alone is not permissible in the patient and health professional relationship, common interests can, of course, have legitimate positive effects on the relationship between two persons working together and thus improve the health professional and patient relationship.

Personal biases can lead to discrimination. *Discrimination* is negative, different treatment of a person or group. Usually it is derived from prejudice. Gordon Allport, in his definitive work, *The Nature of Prejudice* (which, although written over 50 years ago, is still widely considered an authoritative study), describes *prejudice* as "an aversive or hostile attitude toward a person who belongs to a group, simply because he belongs to that group, and is therefore assumed to have objectionable qualities ascribed to that group."[7] In this way we see how prejudicial attitudes of health professionals tend to manifest in discriminatory behavior that can have concrete implications for patients regarding the care they receive.

In short, every exchange between a patient and health professional undoubtedly will be influenced by cultural differences and other sources of personal bias. Sometimes these feelings will create an attitude of prejudice and a desire to discriminate. However, despite legal restrictions to eliminate discrimination in the health care environment, it occurs craftily and evasively. You must watch for it in yourself and others because both parties involved are inevitably injured by the interaction. Allport warns, "It is a serious error to ascribe prejudice and discrimination to any single taproot, reaching into economic exploitation, social structure, the mores, fear, aggression, sex conflict, or any other favored soil. Prejudice and discrimination may draw nourishment from all these conditions and many others."[7] At the same time, treating people differently because of race, religion, ethnicity, gender, or other attributes does not necessarily imply prejudice and discrimination. Respect for differences includes understanding when those differences should count to benefit patients, how they inform the responses of people, and the process of providing patient-centered, culturally informed care.

What can you learn from the previous pages? One thing you can discern is that the cultivation of respectful attitudes and conduct begins with self-examination and consideration of what cultural and other differences mean to you. As you learned in Chapter 1, getting to know yourself and the values supporting your positions is essential. Still, this is not as easy as it may seem at first glance. It requires that you enter into a "difficult dialogue" (i.e., you are asked to reconsider long-held assumptions about individuals and groups that raise questions about your values and beliefs). Engagement in this type of activity may lead to feelings of discomfort and uneasiness.[8] These uncomfortable feelings result from the limited experience most of us have in interacting and talking with individuals different from ourselves.

We explore here a variety of differences, both obvious and subtle, that exist among people, such as differences in language, one of the most basic reasons for miscommunication—why, for example, even when we speak the same language, we may hear what a patient says but not understand its true meaning. Once you become aware of your often *unconscious biases*, you can more easily avoid being controlled by them in your interactions with others. Unconscious biases influence our interpretation of what we hear and see to conform with previously established beliefs.

Furthermore, by becoming aware of your hidden biases, you will be less likely to form inappropriate judgments about patients, colleagues, and others and more likely to remain sensitive and open to differences that influence your interactions with them.

Respecting Differences

A cursory look around almost any community in the United States or most other countries would indicate that we live in multicultural societies. Some assert that we are all "multicultural beings—living in worlds of multiple cultural identities. We are born into one world, and perhaps as adults live in another world where we move between cultural references of family, work, and community."[9] Sensitivity to cultural differences today has increased owing to the various underrepresented minority rights movements over the past several decades, the recent increase in displaced persons from war-torn countries, and the ever-growing percentage of ethnic minorities in the United States. In fact, in 2011 for the first time in US history, babies born to ethnic minorities outnumbered the number of white toddlers.[10] The US Census is the official count of the US population and is completed every 20 years. According to the 2010 US Census, the national population was approximately 308,745,538; of this total, 16.3% self-identified as Hispanic or Latino; 12.6% as black or African American; 4.8% as Asian; and about 1% as American Indian, Alaskan native, Hawaiian native, or Pacific Islander.[10]

Clearly there is growing diversity on a national basis, but this change in composition is also felt on the local level within large urban and even smaller communities. Perhaps the shift in the makeup of the population is felt even more strongly in rural areas in which the arrival of refugees and other immigrants seeking a better life has dramatically changed the homogeneous nature of and long-held assumptions about their communities. This growing diversity also has strong implications for the provision of health care. Although the patient population is growing more diverse, today the composition of health professionals remains overwhelmingly white with Northern Hemisphere cultural and ethnic roots. The significant underrepresentation of minorities in the health professions contributes to the disparity in the health status of minority groups. For example, in 2015, approximately 19.5% of employed registered nurses in the United States were racial or ethnic minorities, which is much lower than the almost 40% of ethnic minorities in the US population.[11] The challenge in nursing and other health professions is to bridge from a predominantly white perspective to meet the needs of a racially and culturally diverse population. Additionally, efforts should be made to increase the number of minority groups in the health professions not only to offer culturally informed care but also to serve as role models for young people to enter such professions. Seeing health professional role models who are African American, black, Hispanic, or from other underrepresented groups will be especially important for students entering college in the future, because it is predicted that in 2027, approximately 49% of high school seniors will be students of color.[12] Adding to the challenge are the historical data that show students of color are less likely than white students to enter and complete a college education.

Depending on where you live, you may be aware of the percentage of persons from backgrounds that are significantly different from your own who are living in your community. One way to identify the variety of diverse groups in your area is to use data from the US Census Bureau, which are organized by state, county, and towns with populations greater than 5000 people. You can access the most recent information by going to the home page of the US Census Bureau (https://www.census.gov/quickfacts/fact/table/US/PST045217). There you can find the cultures represented, the languages spoken, and other information about the people who live in your community and where you work. If you are interested in additional information about other countries in terms of population, geography, etc., an excellent resource is the US Central Intelligence Agency's *World Factbook* to give you an idea of the background of patients from different countries (https://www.cia.gov/library/publications/the-world-factbook/geos/us.html).

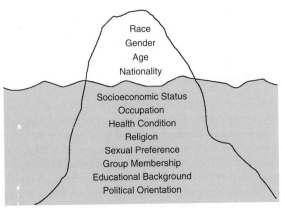

Fig. 5.1 Iceberg model of multicultural influences on communication. (*From Krepp GL. Effective Communication in Multicultural Health Care Settings. New York, NY: Sage Publications; 1994. © 1994. Reprinted by permission of Sage Publications.*)

In almost every health care setting, you will interact with patients of backgrounds different from your own. Certain differences are obvious, and others are hidden. The iceberg model (Fig. 5.1) illustrates how much remains below the surface at various levels that others cannot see or discern. For example, we may notice that a new patient, a woman, is wearing a scarf that completely covers her hair and quickly conclude that she is Muslim. The head covering or burka is "above the waterline" in that we can see that symbol. When we look at her, we might be able to tell if she is a young or old woman but not be able to accurately arrive at her age. When we speak to her, we might be able to tell if English is her first language. However, we cannot know without further inquiry what values or beliefs lie below what we see and hear or how it could affect health care decisions. We may not be as accurate as we think in determining exactly who the person sitting in front of us is. With limited information about potential differences, a professional can take steps in the right direction to adjust communication patterns and approaches accordingly. However, it is more difficult to assess hidden differences that can have as profound an effect on a patient's health beliefs or behavior. Differences that are hidden may create more stress than those that can be more readily identified. These considerations are what has led sociologists and others to develop the notion of culture to better grasp our variations and their importance.

Culture can be viewed in terms of primary characteristics such as race, ethnicity, gender, sexual orientation, or age and secondary characteristics such as place of residence, education, or socioeconomic status. All are part of the web of social interactions in daily life. Cultural practices and beliefs can have a significant effect on the following health-related issues: diet, family rituals, healing beliefs, understanding of illness symptoms and causation, communication process and style, death rituals, spirituality, values, art, and history. The National Center for Cultural Competence notes the following reasons why cultural competence is so critical in contemporary health care: to respond to the aforementioned demographic changes in the United States, improve the quality of health outcomes, and comply with the growing number of regulatory and professional mandates including accreditation standards.[13]

We turn your attention to specific primary and secondary cultural characteristics beginning with a difference that is the root of numerous, deep-seated conflicts among social groups—race.

RACE

Race is one characteristic of culture almost always mentioned in discussions about cultural differences and is the characteristic or descriptor most fraught with controversy. However, even the distinctions used by the US Census Bureau constitute a system based on outmoded concepts and dubious assumptions about genetic difference. The 1999 Institute of Medicine Report edited by Haynes and Smedley[14] stated that in all instances race is a social and cultural construct based on perceived differences in biology, physical appearance, and behavior. An editorial in *Nature Genetics* flatly stated, "Scientists have long been saying that at a genetic level there is more variation between two individuals in the same population than between populations and that there is no biological basis for race."[15] If the biological understanding of race seems to have been settled, that is not the case. Postgenomic science has revived the idea of racial categories as proxies for biological differences and with it a revival of controversy and new opportunities for racial hierarchies and discrimination.[16] At a minimum the present idea of race clearly has social meaning because it is a socially constructed way of grouping people. It assigns status, limits opportunities, and influences interactions between health professionals and patients.[17] Take a moment to reflect on the race categories listed in Box 5.1 that are presently being used to classify people by the US Census Bureau, and consider the questions in the following Reflections box.

REFLECTIONS

- What does the speaker mean by the following quote: "The fact that we know what 'race' we are says more about our society than it does about biology."[18]
- What is society's role in the determination of racial categories?
- Would someone meeting you for the first time place you in the same racial category or categories you chose for yourself? Why or why not?

The same difficulty with racial identification can occur in your relationship with patients as well. Although it is generally thought that patient treatment and counseling are more effective when obtained from members who apparently are of one's self-identified racial group, it does not mean that patients must always be treated by members of the same race to receive quality care. First, this would not be possible because there are so few health professionals who are

---

BOX 5.1 ■ How Are the Race Categories Used in Census 2010 Defined?

The standards have five categories for data on race: American Indian or Alaska Native, Asian, Black or African American, Native Hawaiian or Other Pacific Islander, and White. The concept of race is separate from the concept of Hispanic origin.

Racial Categories and Definitions

American Indian or Alaska Native. A person having origins in any of the original peoples of North and South America (including Central America) and who maintains tribal affiliation or community attachment.

Asian. A person having origins in any of the original peoples of the Far East, Southeast Asia, or the Indian subcontinent including, for example, Cambodia, China, India, Japan, Korea, Malaysia, Pakistan, the Philippine Islands, Thailand, and Vietnam.

Black or African American. A person having origins in any of the Black racial groups of Africa. It includes people who indicate their race as "Black, African American, or Negro."

Native Hawaiian or Other Pacific Islander. A person having origins in any of the original peoples of Hawaii, Guam, Samoa, or other Pacific Islands.

White. A person having origins in any of the original peoples of Europe, the Middle East, or North Africa.

Two or more races. People may have chosen to provide two or more races either by checking two or more race response check boxes.

From U.S. Office of Management and Budget, http://www.whitehouse.gov/imb/fedreg/1997standards.html. Accessed November 16, 2016.

underrepresented minorities. Second, it is essential for all health professionals to learn how to work effectively with patients different from one's own racial and ethnic backgrounds through sensitivity, knowledge, and skills in cross-cultural communication, especially when informed by the virtue of humility.

There are other barriers to be overcome between patients and health professionals that are, unfortunately, deeply tied to notions of race. In a national study conducted by the Institutes of Medicine on disparities in health care, evidence indicated that stereotyping, biases, and uncertainty on the part of health care providers can all contribute to unequal treatment.[19] Additionally, there are ample historical reasons for members of minority populations to mistrust the health care system. For example, in the not-too-distant past, black and African American patients were refused treatment at "white-only" hospitals. Some were undertreated and deceived in the infamous Tuskegee syphilis study. Mistrust in the health care system on the part of African Americans and others who identify with the treatment of black Americans continues to this day because of these historical events and continuing discriminatory events in health care.[20] Gaining the trust of patients whose racial identity is different from one's own can sometimes be a challenge but is not an insurmountable one if health professionals show that they are trustworthy through dignity, respect, and providing optimal care, while working to eliminate racial disparities and health inequities.

GENDER

Gender alludes to characteristics designed to designate a person as masculine or feminine. Gender issues interact with other primary and secondary characteristics of culture to shape a person's identity. There are many implications for assessment and treatment of patients based on differences in gender. Gender has traditionally been viewed as binary in mainstream American society in the sense that a human being is either male or female, man or woman. However, some people do not fall into these discrete socially constructed categories. *Transgender* "is an umbrella term for the broad spectrum that includes all individuals who have gender identities or expressions that are at odds with the sex they were assigned at birth."[21] Providing respectful care to all patients requires a recognition of the complexity of gender identity and education about how people self-identify according to gender-related distinctions.

Gender inequities in health status, access, and treatment exist worldwide and are strongly related to other social determinants of health such as education and economic status. For example, women in developing countries often lack access to basic health care and suffer from domestic violence and murder at a higher rate than their counterparts in countries with more education and economic resources.[22] Even in the relatively affluent United States, women have a history of unequal access to sources of economic and political power that has an impact on access to health care resources.[23] This is especially true for women of color or older women who experience the combined impact of race, gender, and age discrimination.

Transgender individuals also experience discrimination. including social sanctions such as ostracizing or even violence for not conforming to the social identity of the sex ascribed to them at birth.[24] Consider the recent uproar about transgender people's use of public restrooms in schools and attempts to legally restrict such usage because of alleged safety risks to others as an indicator of how strongly some people react to those who are transgender. Gender inequities in health care are inexcusable but often subtle and unfortunately widespread. At the same time, it is also important to simultaneously acknowledge differences that should be taken into consideration and accommodated in planning and delivering optimum care.

Let us take as an example the preferences of patients regarding the gender of their physician. Numerous studies have documented the fact that 20% to 56% of women explicitly prefer a female physician for women's health problems.[25,26] Because many women feel uncomfortable and perhaps embarrassed during a gynecological examination, they may prefer female physicians because the latter are familiar with the female body and have firsthand experience with the examination. It follows that if women are more comfortable with the examination, then they will be more likely to follow through with checkups and follow the recommendations of the physician. A recent study shows that outside of the specialty of obstetrics and gynecology, communication skills was the most important factor for women patients regarding their interaction with a physician,[27] although women physicians are still rated lower in communication skills than their male counterparts.[28] The take-away lesson here is that all health professionals need to adopt behaviors and communication styles to compensate for any differences from their patients.

A patient's preference for a health professional of the same gender also may be culturally or religiously grounded. Many cultural groups are concerned about modesty and may require that only a female health professional examine a female patient's breasts and genitalia or be present when the patient is undressed. Gender differences regarding modesty can have direct implications for diagnosis and treatment, as is evident in the following case study.

Case Study

> Two of the three places I have had mammograms over the years have been great for women. One of them, however, had no privacy. I was required to change clothes in a booth with a curtain that couldn't quite close, while other patients, including men, sat facing the booths less than 5 feet away. It was also necessary to walk by this row of men while clutching my purse and trying to keep the skimpy paper top I was wearing from flopping open.[29]

The importance of modesty can have its origins in culture, religion, or personal preferences and is especially important to consider in the health care environment in which patients are often subjected to being unnecessarily exposed. Regardless of the reason for modesty, inattention to respecting a patient's modesty can lead to poor follow-through with preventive procedures such as the mammogram mentioned in the case or follow-through with agreed-upon treatment or therapy.

AGE AND INTERGENERATIONAL DIVERSITY

Stigma associated with being old is related to the prejudices of an ageist society. The word *ageism* was coined to designate the discriminatory treatment of older people. Older adults living in mainstream Western societies are constantly confronted with ageist conduct in their day-to-day interactions with others. Unfortunately, ageist conduct occurs in the health care environment as well. Older patients often receive less attention or are denied services on the basis of age alone. Physical and psychological problems may not be addressed because health professionals assume that they are normal for an older person. Additionally, older patients are highly complex regarding the numbers and types of health problems they possess, so more time is necessary when diagnosing and treating them. Older patients are prime targets for overmedication and frequently experience the effects of poorly coordinated care. Regardless of his or her state of health or physical ability, an elderly patient is commonly met with a patronizing attitude. Ways in which you can overcome the tendencies to engage in ageist behavior are discussed in more detail in Chapter 14.

Intergenerational diversity is another aspect of patient care that is different from discriminatory behavior on the part of the health professional based on age. In fact, working across the generations is a very common occurrence between young health professionals and older patients that can cause a great deal of misunderstanding for both. Adjustments in communication tactics and exploration of differences in values or meanings express respect in contrast to responding to older patients with negative stereotypes, such as assuming hearing loss or diminished mental capacity, that results in the health professional's use of inappropriately loud or oversimplified language.

ETHNICITY

Ethnicity refers to a person's sense of belonging to a group of people sharing a common origin, history, and set of social beliefs. Ethnicity also may refer to an individual's place of geographical or national origin. For example, the US Census Bureau states that Hispanics may be of any race.[9]

It used to be easy to identify an ethnicity-based cultural variation because one could readily distinguish among the various ways of doing things in different parts of the world. Frequently, early explorers were stunned by the practices they encountered as norms in cultures, and all too often they used the occasion to demean or diminish the importance of the cultural practices of other societies. The world often seems small today with the accessibility of media of all types and movement of large groups of people due to war and famine. Health professionals who encounter these displaced refugees in their own communities may be unfamiliar with the beliefs, traditions, and values of these newcomers, as is the case in this excerpt from Anne Fadiman's comprehensive work on the Hmong refugees who immigrated to Merced County, California, in *The Spirit Catches You and You Fall Down:*

> *When refugees from Laos started settling in Merced County in the early 1980s, none of the doctors at MCMC [Merced County Medical Center] had ever heard of the word "Hmong," and they had no idea what to make of their new patients. They wore strange clothes—often children's clothes, which were approximately the right size—acquired at the Goodwill. When they undressed for examination, the women were sometimes wearing Jockey shorts and the men were sometimes wearing bikini underpants with little pink butterflies. They wore amulets around their necks and cotton strings around their wrists (the sicker the patient, the more numerous the strings). They smelled of camphor, mentholatum, Tiger Balm, and herbs. When they were admitted to the hospital, they brought their own food and herbs.[30]*

Today, in most parts of the world, a large variety of external influences such as Internet access, telecommunications, the ease of global travel, and the presence of foreign visitors affect what used to be isolated, homogeneous cultures. Although the United States has a history of immigration from various parts of the world, "Never before has the United States received immigrants from so many countries, from such different social and economic backgrounds, and for so many reasons."[31] As for refugees, the United Nations Refugee Agency asserts that "we are now witnessing the highest levels of displacement on record," largely from Somalia, Afghanistan, and Syria.[32] A result of the influx of immigrants and refugees is that it is often more challenging to sort out and identify specific cultural differences that modify behavior in various ethnic groups.

Sometimes as a health professional you may have a difficult time remembering that members of an ethnic group are not homogeneous. Their ethnicity is only one characteristic of the culture or cultures they bring to their present experience. At times, each of us becomes aware of cultural beliefs held by an individual that, on the surface, seem to be incongruent. For example, a Chinese American may be highly assimilated into the majority culture and seek mainstream health care for a gastrointestinal disorder yet also seek care from a traditional Chinese healer who might prescribe herbs, teas, or other forms of therapies appropriate for his culture. Because we can identify with individual variations in our own cultural beliefs and the blending of seemingly opposite beliefs that can occur within us as individuals, we must appreciate the profound variability that can exist within cultural groups.

One of the widest cultural gaps you will encounter in your role as a health professional is that created by the "ethnocentrism" of health professionals. (Although separate professions often are not thought of as cultures in themselves, they are.) *Ethnocentrism* is the belief that one's own cultural ways are superior. Health professionals often believe that their way is best and so are guilty of medical ethnocentrism. In fact, while you are a student you are learning and adopting the culture of your chosen health profession. The culture of a health professional encompasses the interrelationships of professional values, beliefs, customs, habits, and symbols. You are learning the cultural meaning that your profession gives to concepts such as pain, disability, independence, disease, and illness. You will find that even within the culture of the health professions, there are different meanings and understandings of identical phenomena. Thus, as an individual, you may share the same ethnic origin, race, and gender as the patient you are working with and yet not hold the same beliefs and perspectives about some important values related to what his or her health care or treatment should involve. The alignment of patient-centered values and evidence is called *values-based practice.* In this practice model, the unique preferences and expectations of patients are integrated into clinical decisions based on evidence-based care.[33]

SOCIOECONOMIC STATUS

As was mentioned previously in this chapter, a vast majority of US and Canadian health professionals are white, with average incomes that are in the upper-middle to high economic range when considered globally. The income level and accompanying higher social status of health professionals tend to create barriers in their relationships with many patients. "Ethnic minority groups and economically disadvantaged individuals may have particular difficulty feeling in control within a setting dominated by well-educated professionals."[34] The difference in socioeconomic status may hinder patients from asking you important questions, hinder you from empathizing with patients, and limit your knowledge of the practical everyday obstacles that prevent or facilitate the ability of patients to pursue, and adhere to, medication or treatment regimens.[35] The following example highlights the challenges some patients face just getting to a medical appointment.

Case Study

A young mother and her two small children, a toddler and a 3-month-old, leave their apartment at 7:00 a.m. for a 9:00 a.m. clinic visit. In the rush to leave the apartment to get to their appointment, the mother forgot her cell phone. With the baby in a stroller and the toddler at his mother's side, they head for the bus stop that is four blocks from their home. The first bus is late because of icy conditions. She must transfer three times to get to the clinic and walk two blocks to the clinic building. She arrives at the clinic 45 minutes late for her 9:00 a.m. appointment. The medical assistant at the intake desk looks at the clock as the mother signs in and says, "Couldn't you have called if you were going to be late?"

We will address different interpretations of time in Chapter 10, but in this case, there is no disagreement between the clinic staff and the patient about what "on time" is. The medical assistant does not understand the complications that arise from having to be dependent on public transportation or the hassle of finding a pay phone today. The fact that this patient made it to the clinic at all is a testament to her desire to receive care. Yet this fact becomes lost in complaints about the patient's tardiness and lack of consideration for the clinic staff. Health professionals may take for granted owning a car or carrying a cell phone, items that could be completely beyond the financial means of some patients.

The differences in social class and economic status also affect the type and frequency of interaction between patient and health professional outside the health care setting. The informal networks that exist in neighborhoods and communities provide opportunities to establish cooperation, exchange information, and determine appropriate behavior. Health professionals who have mainly been socialized in largely white, urban middle-class values see underrepresented minority patients as "noncompliant" when such patients are actually following a different set of rules and culturally appropriate principles.[36] For example, a patient may be told to increase his exercise and go on daily walks, which sounds easy for someone who lives in a safe neighborhood. But in a crime-ridden area, a walk around the block could be seen as foolhardy and dangerous.

Outsiders can make unintentional errors in judgment because they underestimate the effects of ethnicity, age, or class on insiders' responses or actions—that is, the responses and actions of individuals born or socialized into membership of the group. Outsiders must work to "get in," to earn, build, and maintain trust with a group.[37] Even gaining enough trust to adequately treat a patient is not sufficient to understand what goes into staying afloat on a minimum-wage salary or holding down two or three part-time jobs to make ends meet.

Level of education is another difference between health professionals and patients related to socioeconomic status. Although patients may respect education in the abstract, they may also be suspicious that you will use your education to take advantage of them rather than to assist them. Patients also may be too intimidated to admit when they do not understand something. For fear that they will be seen as ignorant or superstitious, patients may neglect to mention that they are also seeking alternative methods of care or providers. Even when patients are well educated, they may not speak the dominant language well enough to adequately express themselves. You may understand what it means if you have struggled to make yourself understood across a language barrier. It is important to remember that the "language" of health care is often foreign to patients as well. In Chapter 10 we discuss in more detail how language, vocabulary, and health literacy can facilitate or block what patients perceive as respect from you.

OCCUPATION AND PLACE OF RESIDENCE

One of the first questions we often ask a new acquaintance in a social setting is, "What do you do?" We deeply identify with our occupations in mainstream American culture. Some would go so far as to say that their occupation defines who they are more than their ethnicity or other primary characteristics. Occupations shape how people see the world and what they value. The importance of a person's occupation is sometimes seen more clearly when illness, injury, disease, disability, or retirement forces a change in occupation. How patients occupy themselves, whether they spend their time in the formal workforce or not, can give important cultural clues that have an impact on health care beliefs and decisions.

We do not often think of place of residence as a cultural variable in our interactions with patients, yet there is increasing evidence that place of residence has an impact on how patients think about health. For example, certain health beliefs and practices sometimes differ between urban and rural patients. People who live in rural areas, because of their environment, must often travel a considerable distance to see a health professional. Thus rural patients are often more independent regarding the use of health care services than their urban counterparts. Another significant difference between rural and urban dwellers is the way health needs are viewed. Rural dwellers, both male and female, from a variety of locations, tend to determine health needs primarily in relation to work activities.[38] Thus it is important to consider not only where someone lives but also the other cultural values they bring to their place of residence. A striking example of the impact values held by rural dwellers can have on health decisions is evident in the following case.

Case Study

The O'Mara family has ranched in the Sweetwater Valley since the 1850s. "It's what my grandfather left us," says Sam, "and I don't plan to let him down." There's nothing easy about this life—too much snow in the winter, not enough rain in the summer. On eight sections of land, Sam and his sons graze their cattle, grow hay, and, if they're lucky and get the moisture, harvest some wheat. "In a good year, we make a buck, and in a bad year, lose two, but we're here and we're not going anywhere else," says Sam. The little hilltop cemetery on the edge of his property quietly underscores Sam's statement. Fenced with barbed wire, it's the resting place for Sam's grandparents, parents, uncles, and others who worked this land during the past one hundred years.

When Dr. Olsen moved to this ranching community about 5 years ago, Sam was one of the first people he met. Since then, Dr. Olsen has provided medical care to Sam, his wife, and sons. He attended the festivities at the ranch when Sam's son was married, and just last year he delivered Sam's first grandchild.

When Sam arrived for his recent appointment, he admitted to "being a little slow this spring." But it was a cold spring, he explained, and there were long hours spent protecting the new calves. He'd be grateful, though, if he could get something for his chest pain and his shortness of breath. The "funny, sick feeling" he's had for the past few weeks doesn't seem to be passing.

Dr. Olsen examines Sam and is frankly concerned. He suspects coronary artery disease and explains to Sam the need for more tests. "You need to go to the city," says Dr. Olsen. He carefully explains the tests that will be conducted and the procedures that might be done. "I've heard of those bypasses," says Sam. "And I know Pete, my neighbor, had an angioplasty; that was the beginning of his troubles. He died anyway but not before he had more surgery and a lot more bills." Sam says he'll go home and think about the whole situation. He and his wife have bare bones health insurance, and there's nothing they can sell right now to pay for a lot of medical care.

"The boys can take care of the ranch," he says. "And they'll take care of their mother and she'll have a home. My grandson can grow up knowing he has a place. But if I ransom this place to pay for a heart, well there won't be much left for anyone to live for."

"I expect that we can keep this between us," says Sam. "The wife is just glad I made the appointment. I'm not going to have her choose between life for me or life for her boys." Sam does not indicate exactly what he will tell his wife, their sons, and his friends. Dr. Olsen suspects Sam will just attribute his difficulties to hard work—and nothing that a little rest can't cure.[39]

From University of Montana. The National Rural Bioethics Project. http://www.umt.edu/bioethics/healthcare/resources/educational/casestudies/ruralfocus/decisions.aspx.

- Consider Mr. O'Mara's choice of words when he says he doesn't want to "ransom the place," to pay for his treatment. What does this tell you about his values and priorities?
- Do you think Mr. O'Mara is making a foolish, courageous, short-sighted, loving, or another kind of decision about his health?
- How might Mr. O'Mara's values and beliefs contrast with yours? Would any differences affect your ability to care for him? If so, how would you work through these value conflicts?

Sam O'Mara no doubt shares many attitudes and beliefs about health status and health care with his urban counterparts, but his place of residence introduces additional cultural variables. Rural residents tend to value self-reliance more than urban residents. Rural residents, particularly farmers and ranchers, often are required to maintain a higher level of physical fitness as they take care of their land, tend animals, manage the maintenance of and use heavy machinery, etc. Their ability to accomplish these tasks is tied to their self-identity and self-worth.[40]

Whether a patient lives on a farm, in the inner city, or in the suburbs, you will show respect when you are mindful of the impact place of residence can have on your interactions with patients and their health-related routines. This is especially true when the patient does not have a permanent place of residence or is homeless. The challenges of working with patients whose only home is the streets include major issues such as ensuring the safety and basic well-being of the patient but also practical considerations unique to this environment such as the need for access to a bathroom, warmth and dry clothing, or a source of clean drinking water. Persons who live on the street either by choice or necessity are part of a subculture that is often hidden from view and requires openness and understanding from health professionals.

RELIGION

Religious beliefs are another feature of culture that influences your relationship with patients. Religion gives meaning to illness, pain, and suffering. Religious beliefs are often most apparent when a patient is seriously injured, critically ill, or dying. For example, the Christian faith, with its valuing of human life and belief in eternal life, states that whereas a struggle for health can be meaningful, a struggle against death at all costs to the point that the effort becomes a torment, may be antithetical to their beliefs.[41] The Christian cultural view of the dying process and death itself influences treatment decisions and may promote requests for symbolically meaningful activities such as receiving rituals in the form of sacraments.

A different view of illness is evident with believers in Islam. "The word *Islam* means to submit; that is, to submit their lives to the will of God (Allah). A fatalistic worldview is common whereby the person attributes the incidence and outcome of a health condition to "inshallah" or, to put another way, to leave it in God's hands. This belief may make preventive health behaviors or self-care programs difficult to institute. Because God is perceived to be in control of the outcome, what can humans do?[42] However, what may appear to be "fatalistic" could also be shaped by another Muslim duty regarding stewardship of one's body and health. This duty prescribes clear responsibility for one's health. Thus, once again, there is more to culture and beliefs than appears on the surface.

Christian, Jewish, and Muslim beliefs are widespread established religions in Western societies and relatively well known; therefore health professionals may not find much difficulty in recognizing them even if they don't know a lot about underlying beliefs and rituals. Religious beliefs that are further removed from these three mainstream religions are present in many patient populations today and may challenge health care professionals' understanding, tolerance, and willingness to make accommodations.

SEXUAL IDENTITY AND ORIENTATION

In modern society, sexual self-identity or orientation is yet another characteristic of culture that may elicit biased responses to a person. Lesbian, gay, bisexual, transgender, questioning, and other (LGBTQ+) patients are often treated differently because of their gender identities or sexual orientation. One commonality among gay men and lesbian women is that they may hide this aspect of their life for fear of prejudicial attitudes and discrimination. Thus the sexual orientation of patients may be somewhat invisible. However, given the number of men and women who report being homosexual (and that number is probably an underestimate of the actual total), it is highly likely that most health professionals are assigned to provide care to individuals without knowledge of their sexual orientations.

In addition to the negative attitudes expressed by health professionals toward patients with a sexual orientation different from their own, gay, lesbian, transgender, and bisexual patients find themselves in a health care system that is built on heterosexual assumptions. Common examples include women seeking gynecological or obstetrical care who may not even be asked about their sexual history and lesbian and gay patients' partners not being formally acknowledged in family education or care planning. Providing sensitive, culturally appropriate care requires taking the patient's sexual orientation fully into account and ensuring that the information is used to optimize his or her quality of care.

Cultural Sensitivity, Competence, and Humility

The overall lesson to be gleaned from the brief preceding descriptions of various primary and secondary cultural characteristics is that the atmosphere in health care must rest on fully appreciating what each culture brings to the richness of our society and on acceptance rather than on fear and misunderstanding.

What is needed is an approach to each patient, client, and colleague that takes into account cultural differences, and that begins with cultural sensitivity (i.e., appreciating that you are a multicultural being, as are others). *Cultural sensitivity* is a necessary foundation for becoming culturally competent. *Cultural competence* is "an ongoing process in which the health care professional continually strives to achieve the ability and availability to work effectively within the cultural context of the patient (individual, family, and community)."[43] An important component of becoming culturally competent is the ability to conduct a cultural assessment when interacting with patients. Among numerous cultural assessment tools in the literature, one set of questions developed by Kleinman stands out because the questions focus on the patient's perspective regarding illness, as follows:

- What do you call your problem? What name does it have?
- What do you think has caused your problem? Why do you think it started when it did?
- What do you think your sickness does to you? How does it work?
- How severe is it? Will it have a short or long course?
- What do you fear the most about your sickness?
- What are the chief problems your sickness has caused for you?
- What kind of treatment do you think you should receive? What are the most important results you hope to receive from this treatment?[44]

Regardless of the patient's cultural background, the preceding questions are a logical and respectful place to start in trying to understand what brought the patient to the health care encounter. Additionally, beyond individual patient encounters, health professionals should consider solutions that let go of traditional approaches to patients in general that focus only on problem identification and methods to bridge divides. Put simply, the traditional approach looks at patients, particularly patients from diverse cultural backgrounds, and asks, "What does this patient need, and how is she or he different so I know what to do to compensate for these differences in providing care?" It is important to acknowledge that a focus on good communication and culturally informed care can shore up these deficits or problems that present barriers to quality care. Use honest questions to open conversations with patients such as, "Many of my patients experience racism/ageism/sexism in their health care. Are there any experiences you would like to share with me?"[45] From an equity-minded standpoint, health professionals would assume diversity and approach all patients to create an environment in which everyone will receive the best care.[46] From this perspective, health professionals would ask, "Why are our practices failing to produce successful outcomes for all patients, and what do we need to change?" This perspective shifts the focus to factors within the health professionals' control.

Along these same lines, *cultural humility* should be factored into an understanding of culturally appropriate care and requires more than knowledge about cultural practices. Cultural humility requires commitment to ongoing self-reflection and self-critique, particularly identifying and examining one's own patterns of unintentional and intentional prejudices and negative attitudes and practices.[47] In Chapter 1, you were charged with approaching each patient respectfully. This means, among other things, consciously avoiding unfair judgments about other people's traditions, values, and beliefs. We are much more likely to respect a patient's decision or action if we understand its rationale. Misunderstandings can result in harm to the patient in that he or she may hesitate to seek medical attention or follow the advice of someone so out of touch with his or her beliefs.

One common barrier to respectful interaction is the tendency for health professionals to adopt stereotypes and expect certain behaviors from patients from a certain culture simply because they are from that culture. Avoid scripted remarks such as "Syrian refugees all believe . . ." or "All Chinese patients practice . . ." because it is impossible to generalize from one patient to an entire culture. "Although some behaviors may appear similar within an identified cultural group, the astute health provider must assess for differences both within and among groups to plan appropriate care."[48] You may think that you do not hold any of these limiting beliefs about ethnic or cultural differences, but we all have implicit biases. These learned biases are unconscious and can operate automatically with clinically based decisions or actions despite our intensions.

In the face of cultural differences, you will need basic negotiation skills. This means finding a place where you can feel confident in the exercise of your professional judgment yet incorporate the beliefs and values of patients into their treatment plan to achieve mutually desirable outcomes. The goal of cultural humility is to provide care characterized by respect. Such care is meaningful and fits with cultural beliefs and ways of life for those involved. Because diversity in society is likely to increase rather than decrease in the coming years, access to the most current statistics regarding demography and tools to assist in providing culturally appropriate care is vitally important. Table 5.1 provides a sampling of web resources to assist you in obtaining the most current information.

TABLE 5.1 ■ Web Resources That Support Delivery of Culturally Appropriate Care

Organization	Web Address
National Center for Cultural Competence	https://nccc.georgetown.edu/
U.S. Administration on Community Living.	http://www.aoa.gov
Stanford Geriatric Education Center	http://sgec.stanford.edu
American Society on Aging	http://www.asaging.org
Center for Applied Linguistics	http://www.cal.org
ALTA Language Services	http://www.altalang.com
The Cross Cultural Health Program	http://www.xculture.org
Culture Clues	http://depts.washington.edu/pfes/CultureClues.htm
Culture, Language and Health Literacy	http://www.hrsa.gov/culturalcompetence/index.html
Ethnogeriatrics and Cultural Competence for Nursing Practice	https://consultgeri.org/topics/ethnogeriatrics_and_cultural_competence_for_nursing_practice/want_to_know_more
Institute for Health Care Improvement	http://www.ihi.org
Project Implicit	https://www.projectimplicit.net

Summary

The issues relevant to showing respect for diversity must continually be examined and be a topic for reflection. The concept of culture provides an appropriate starting point for health professionals to become aware and learn to honor different characteristics among groups, remaining cognizant that individuals may not always fit a predictable cultural pattern. Making every effort to avoid prejudice, discrimination, unconscious bias, and other negative attitudes and conduct based on difference is part and parcel of being a health professional. The only constructive approach to evaluating human differences with the goal of providing patient-centered care is to take each experience as an opportunity to learn more about the rich diversity of the human condition and to take what one learns as a gift that will help achieve the goals of the health professional and patient relationship, as well as enrich one's own life.

References

1. Goldberger HH. *Second Book in English for Coming Citizens*. New York: Charles Scribner Sons; 1921:5.
2. Purnell LD. Transcultural diversity and health care. In: Purnell LD, ed: *Transcultural Health Care: A Culturally Competent Approach*, 4th ed, Philadelphia; F.A. Davis; 6.
3. Spencer M, Markstrom-Adams C. Identity processes among racial and ethnic minority children in America. *Child Dev*. 1990;61:290–310.
4. Porter J. *Vertical Mosaic: An Analysis of Social Class and Power in Canada*. Toronto: University of Toronto Press; 1965.
5. Thomas Jr RR. From affirmative action to affirming diversity. *Harv Bus Rev*. 1991. Retrieved from https://hbr.org/1990/03/from-affirmative-action-to-affirming-diversity.
6. *National Health Service Corps: Bridging the Cultural Divide in Health Care Settings: The Essential Role of Cultural Broker Programs*. Rockville, MD: U.S. Department of Health and Human Services; 2004.
7. Allport G. *The Nature of Prejudice*. Reading, MA: Addison-Wesley; 1954.
8. Baldwin D, Nelms T. Difficult dialogues: impact on nursing education curricula. *J Prof Nurs*. 1993;9(6):343–346.
9. Marshall P, Koenig B. Accounting for culture in a globalized society. *J Law Med Ethics*. 2004;32:252–266.
10. U.S. Department of Commerce. *U.S. Census Bureau*. Washington, D.C.: 2010. Retrieved at http://www.census.gov.
11. The 2014 National Nursing Workforce Survey. *J Nurs Regulation*. 2015;7(1):S4–S6. Retrieved at: https://www.ncsbn.org/workforce.htm.
12. Witham K, Malcom-Piqueux L, Dowd A. *America's Unmet Promise: The Imperative for Equity in Higher Education*. Washington, D.C.: Association of American Colleges and Universities; 2015.
13. Goode TD, Dunne C. *Policy Brief 1: Rationale for Cultural Competence in Primary Care*. Washington, D.C.: National Center for Cultural Competence, Georgetown University Center for Child and Human Development; 2003. Retrieved from https://nccc.georgetown.edu/documents/Policy_Brief_1_2003.pdf.
14. Haynes MA, Smedley BD, eds. *The Unequal Burden of Cancer: An Assessment of NIH Research and Programs for Ethnic Minorities and the Medically Underserved*. Washington, D.C.: Institute of Medicine. National Academies Press; 1999.
15. Editorial: Genes, drugs and race. *Nature Genet*. 2001;29:239–240.
16. Fitzgerald KJ. The continuing significance of race: Racial genomics in a post-racial era. *Humanity and Soc*. 2014;38(1):49–66.
17. Pinderhughes E: *Understanding Race, Ethnicity, and Power*. New York: Free Press.
18. Kreiger N, Bassett M. The health of black folk: disease, class and ideology in science. *Mon Rev*. 1986;38:74–85.
19. Smedley B, Stith A, Nelson A. *Committee on Understanding and Eliminating Racial and Ethnic Disparities in Health Care, Institutes of Medicine, Unequal Treatment: Confronting Racial and Ethnic Disparities in Healthcare*. Washington, D.C.: The National Academies Press; 2003:1.
20. Scharf DP, Matthews KJ, Jackson P, et al. More than Tuskegee: understanding mistrust about research participation. *J Health Care Poor Underserved*. 2010;21(3):879–897.
21. Carabez RM, Eliason MJ, Martinson MM. Nurses' knowledge about transgender patient care: a qualitative study. *Adv Nur Sci*. 2016;39(3). 257–217.

22. Diaz-Granados N, Pitzul KB, Dorado LM, et al. Monitoring gender equity in health using gender sensitive indicators: a cross national study. *J Womens Health*. 2011;20(1):145–153.

23. Conway-Turner K. Older women of color: a feminist exploration of the intersections of personal, familial and community life. *J Women Aging*. 1999;11(2/3):115–130.

24. Konsenko K, Rintamaki L, Raney S, et al. Transgender patient perceptions of stigma in health care contexts. *Med Care*. 2013;51(9):819–822.

25. Kerssens JJ, Bensing JM, Andela MG. Patient preferences for genders of health professionals. *Soc Sci Med*. 1997;44:1531–1540.

26. Delgado A, Lopez-Fernandez LA, Luna JD. Influence of the doctor's gender in the satisfaction of users. *Med Care*. 1993;31:795–800.

27. Mavis B, Vasilenko P, Schnuth R, et al. Female patients' preferences related to interpersonal communications, clinical competence, and gender when selecting a physician. *Acad Med*. 2005;80(12):1159–1165.

28. Mast MS, Hall JA, Roter DL. Disentangling physician sex and physician communication style: their effects on patient satisfaction in a virtual medical visit. *Patient Educ Couns*. 2007;68(1):16–22.

29. Andrews C. Modesty and health care for women: Understanding cultural sensitivities. *Comm Oncology*. 2006;3(7):443–446.

30. Fadiman A. *The Spirit Catches You and You Fall Down*. New York: The Noon Day Press; 1997.

31. Portes A, Rumbaut R. *Immigrant America: a portrait*. 2nd ed. Berkeley: University of California Press; 1997.

32. United Nations High Commissioner Refugee Agency. gtrf Retrieved at http://www.unhcr.org/en-us; 2016.

33. Fulford KWM. Values-based practice: a new partner to evidence-based practice and a first for psychiatry? *Mens Sana Monographs*. 2008;6(1):10–21.

34. Ramer L, Richardson JL, Cohen MZ, et al. Multimeasure pain assessment in an ethnically diverse group of patients with cancer. *J Transcult Nurs*. 1999;10(2):94–101.

35. Waitzkin H. *The Politics of Medical Encounters: How Patients and Doctors Deal With Social Problems*. New Haven, CT: Yale University Press; 1991.

36. Fineman N. The social construction of non-compliance: implications for cross-cultural geriatric practice. *J Cross Cult Gerontol*. 1991;6:219–228.

37. Kauffman KS. The insider/outsider dilemma: field experience of a white researcher "getting in" a poor black community. *Nurs Res*. 1994;43(3):179–183.

38. Bushy A. Rural determinants in family health: Considerations for community nurses. In: Bushy A, ed. *Rural nursing*. Vol. 23. Newbury Park, NY: Sage; 1991.

39. University of Montana. The National Rural Bioethics Project, Ethics in rural health care settings: Decisions and obligations – "It's a matter of priorities." Retrieved at: http://www.umt.edu/bioethics/healthca re/resources/educational/casestudies/ruralfocus/decisions.aspx.

40. Nelson JA, Gingerich BS. Rural health: access to care and services. *Home Health Care Manage Pract*. 2010;22(3):339–343.

41. Care of the dying. *A Catholic Perspective*. St. Louis: The Catholic Health Association of the United States; 1993.

42. Haddad LG, Hoeman SP. Home healthcare and the Arab-American client. *Home Healthc Nurse*. 2000;18(3):189–197.

43. Campinha-Bacote J. Patient-centered care in the midst of a cultural conflict: the role of cultural competence. *Online J Issues Nursing*. 2011;16(2):1.

44. Kleinman A. *Patients and Healers in the Context of Culture*. CA: University of California Press.

45. Endo JA. *Addressing Race in Practice*. Institute for Health Care Improvement; 2016. Retrieved from http://www.ihi.org/communities/blogs/_layouts/15/ihi/community/blog/itemview.aspx?List=7d112 6ec-8f63-4a3b-9926-c44ea3036813&ID=308.

46. Bensimon EM, Dowd AC, Witham K. Five principles of enacting equity by design. Association of American Colleges and Universities. 2016;19(1):1–8.

47. Tervalon M, Murray-Garcia J. Cultural humility versus cultural competence: a critical distinction in defining physician training outcomes in multicultural education. *J Health Care Poor Underserved*. 1998;9(2):117–125.

48. Bechtel GA, Davidhizar RE. Integrating cultural diversity in patient education. *Semin Nurse Manag*. 1999;7(4):193–197.

CHAPTER 6

Respect in the Institutional Settings of Health Care

Prelude

If you are in the ER waiting room at around like 9 AM or 10 AM, you will see an influx of patients with the buses that sort of hit the front door and so the buses will unload and an exodus of patients will come and register and that's sort of their project for the day to make it to Highland and out. Almost anyone in our system comes through the ED.

THE WAITING ROOM[1]

Health care does not exist in a vacuum. Health care exists within institutions, perhaps in a system of institutions, and within society at large. Like a set of Russian nesting dolls (matryoshka dolls), with each larger doll holding a smaller and smaller one until we reach the tiniest doll, a doll that could represent the patient surrounded by family and intimate friends, then surrounded by acquaintances, neighbors, and perhaps health professionals, in hospitals or clinics, in a neighborhood or city, each level encompassing more people and challenges to the delivery of health care. This chapter focuses on some key insights regarding the complexity of the health care system where you will exercise your professional skills. You will almost inevitably work in an institutional environment, which exists to provide health care services. Your ability to understand and respect the basic structure, operations, and aims of health care institutions is essential to patient outcomes, as well as your professional success and satisfaction in your work. Understanding the environment in which you work will contribute to how you are viewed by patients, colleagues, and the wider community.

It follows that readers of this book will be influenced by their work environment, as well as influence that environment by participating in its everyday activities. A good starting place for

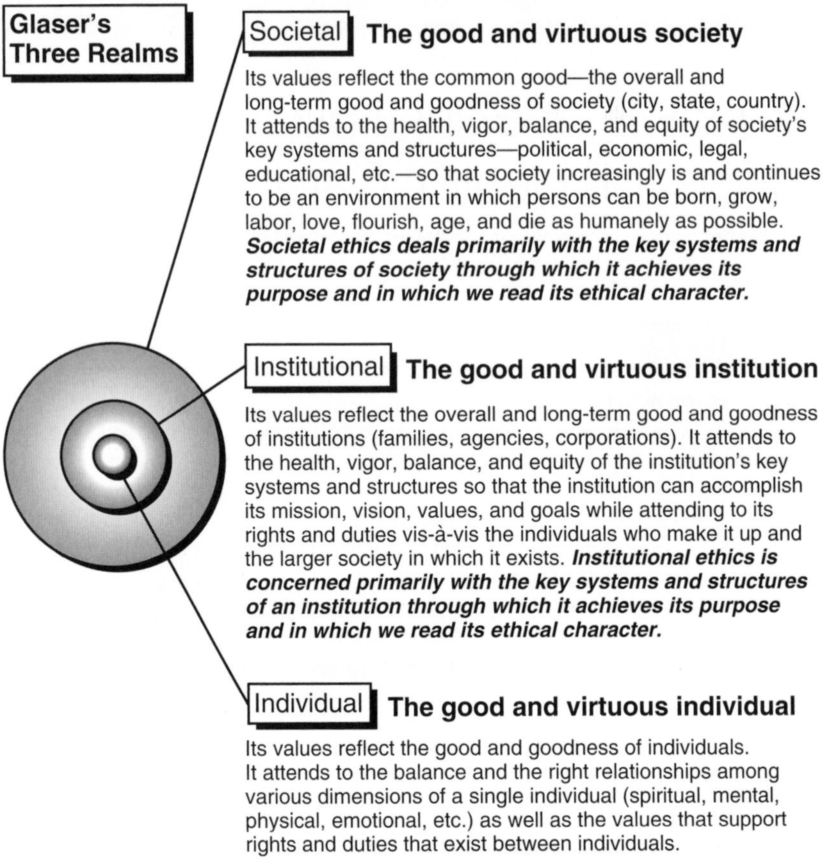

Glaser's Three Realms

Societal | The good and virtuous society

Its values reflect the common good—the overall and long-term good and goodness of society (city, state, country). It attends to the health, vigor, balance, and equity of society's key systems and structures—political, economic, legal, educational, etc.—so that society increasingly is and continues to be an environment in which persons can be born, grow, labor, love, flourish, age, and die as humanely as possible. *Societal ethics deals primarily with the key systems and structures of society through which it achieves its purpose and in which we read its ethical character.*

Institutional | The good and virtuous institution

Its values reflect the overall and long-term good and goodness of institutions (families, agencies, corporations). It attends to the health, vigor, balance, and equity of the institution's key systems and structures so that the institution can accomplish its mission, vision, values, and goals while attending to its rights and duties vis-à-vis the individuals who make it up and the larger society in which it exists. *Institutional ethics is concerned primarily with the key systems and structures of an institution through which it achieves its purpose and in which we read its ethical character.*

Individual | The good and virtuous individual

Its values reflect the good and goodness of individuals. It attends to the balance and the right relationships among various dimensions of a single individual (spiritual, mental, physical, emotional, etc.) as well as the values that support rights and duties that exist between individuals.

Fig. 6.1 Glaser's three realms.

respectful interaction, then, is to become familiar with basic characteristics of such institutions and then address key characteristics of institutional relationships within them. It will also benefit you at this point to become aware of some key policies and practices designed to command respect from all who engage with the institution, whether employees or those seeking goods and services, so we introduce them in a general way in the final sections of this chapter.

Characteristics of Institutions

Glaser describes three realms of social activity—individual, institutional, and societal—each having an impact on the health professional's effectiveness and sense of well-being. Institutions sit at the interface between the individual and the larger society (Fig. 6.1).[2] All institutions comprise individuals and groups. An institution as a "whole" interacts with other institutions and societal entities such as government agencies, the legal system, etc. When we think of a health care institution, often an image of a building such as a hospital or a clinic comes to mind, but these are not the only types of institutions that exist in health care. Professional associations such as the American Occupational Therapy Association or the American Medical Association are institutions as well and influence professionals within the association and interact outside the association with the public at large. Other institutions in health care that have major influence on health professionals and patients are educational institutions that prepare health professionals for their roles in health care, insurance providers, and pharmaceutical and device manufacturers, to name a few.

Ideally, institutional policies and practices reflect deep respect for values that guide individual health professionals personally and professionally but also encourage them to be responsive to the basic societal expectation that patients should be the top priority. In turn, health professionals will not only engage in respectful interpersonal relationships with patients and families but also be loyal and respectful of management and administrative policies of a variety of institutions.

Additionally, institutions have obligations to society, not just to the well-being of the institution. As Glaser argues,

> [Hospitals] need to become a more vigorous part of the community of concern shaping our health care system and less an agent of special interest pressure. They need to invest time in understanding health issues from the perspective of community good, not merely from the viewpoint of the organizational benefit. They need to take time to develop some consensus about what an adequate health system for our society would look like: what percentage of the GNP we can reasonably spend on health care—relative to other needs of the common good.[2]

Of course, hospitals are not the only health care institutions in which health professionals work. In fact, increasingly more health care is delivered in some type of ambulatory or community-based setting that is often less hierarchical than traditional hospital settings and geographically separated.

DIVERSITY OF FACILITIES

The institutional realm of health care is a complex web of ideas and values expressed in numerous types of health care facilities. Health professionals work in hospitals, ambulatory care clinics, home care, long-term care facilities, rehabilitation settings, research centers, diagnostic laboratories, schools, hospices, industrial settings, and military first response units; among sports teams; and on cruise ships, to name a few. What is fitting for one type of facility may look quite different from another.

Moreover, the organization of health care is not completely a *rational system*. Rational systems are oriented expressly to the pursuit of one specific goal and have a highly formalized social structure designed to meet that goal.[3] An example is an airport, where the single goal is to move people and goods from place to place. The institutions of health care can be more illustrative of an *open system* in which shifting and sometimes competing interest groups negotiate for their goals to be met. There are numerous entry and exit points in the health care system, which makes it an "open" system in that sense as well. Patients come to the health care environment from their homes to a clinic and then perhaps to a hospital or same-day surgery center. Elderly patients, for example, someone with a broken hip, can travel the range of institutions in health care, arriving in an ambulance through the emergency department (ED), which is a common entry point to traditional health care, as noted in the quotation at the outset of this chapter, to the operating room, general medical floor, discharge to rehabilitation in a skilled nursing facility, and then perhaps home to live independently with visiting therapists and nurses.

When you enter a program of professional preparation, the basic type of institutional setting where you will work may be determined in part by the focus of your profession. For example, a focus on maintenance and health promotion may mean you will practice in a school, occupational health setting, or free-standing clinic that provides wellness education. If you are drawn to acute care, rehabilitation, chronic health, or end-of-life care needs, it is likely you will find work in a hospital, rehabilitation center, nursing home, hospice, or home care.

REFLECTIONS

- In what type of health care setting can you see yourself working? Why? What are the attractions—for example, the patient population, type of care delivery such as fast-paced or extended time with patients, urban or rural setting?
- Think of the health care settings you have experienced as a patient or student. Which ones made you want to spend time there? Why?

Institutional environments have changed and will continue to do so during your professional career. Attention to where you find the best fit for your practice will require attentiveness to changing styles and designs of institutional environments. The very structure of hospitals and clinics reflects these changes, with consultation rooms designed to accommodate members of the interprofessional team, the patient, and the patient's extended support system, for example.

The types of services that specific institutions within health care systems provide are often highly regulated. For example, let us take a closer look at one hospital, Highland Hospital, which is the subject of the documentary film *The Waiting Room*. Highland Hospital is part of the Alameda Health System, which is "an integrated public health care system with over 800 beds and 1000 physicians across nine major facilities throughout Alameda County."[4] There are two hospitals, a psychiatric pavilion, and a large number of ambulatory clinics within this particular health system. Highland Hospital has a Level II Trauma Center and the ED referred to in the opening quote to the chapter. To achieve the Level II designation, the hospital must meet certain state-developed standards that are then verified by the American College of Surgeons. These standards often include comprehensive trauma care and 24-hour availability of specific medical specialties and support personnel, as well as other supportive services. Highland Hospital's ED is the most trafficked in the country, partly because of its location in Oakland and the high levels of violent crime there and because of the socioeconomic status of many of the ED's patients who come to Highland to get primary care. This is a mere snapshot of one hospital in one health system out of the 386 general acute care hospitals in the state of California alone.[5]

Characteristics of Institutional Relationships

The ability to show and receive respect in the work environment requires an understanding of several characteristics of relationships that take place in health care institutions compared with other types of relationships. To highlight this point, we examine an important characteristic of health care institutions that distinguish them from some others you participate in—namely, their public rather than private nature.

PUBLIC-SECTOR AND PRIVATE-SECTOR RELATIONSHIPS

Public-sector relationships are interactions reserved for engagements within institutions of public life, whereas private-sector relationships are reserved for the world of family, friends, and other intimates.[3] Individuals generally separate their lives into these two worlds of relationship. Public-sector relationships are designed to serve a useful purpose and then dissolve, whereas private-sector ones are more likely to continue. Student and professor or patient and health professional relationships belong to the world of public-sector relationships. Social boundaries that are maintained in a public-sector relationship permit rapid introduction and rapid separation, promoting cooperation around a common goal. All public-sector relationships are characterized by abrupt changes from extreme remoteness to extreme nearness with the expectation that the relationship will be temporary. Students who become close during their years of formal preparation go their separate ways on graduation. Professionals in attendance at a conference of their professional organization come from different worksites to learn, share their own research or expertise, enjoy socializing, and then depart back to their own practice settings.

REFLECTIONS

- Think about public-sector relationships you have engaged in during your life. How did they benefit you? Jot them down for further reflection as this chapter unfolds.
- Are your relationships with fellow students or professionals more akin to private-sector or public-sector relationships? Why?

Opportunities for involvement in each other's lives and well-being and the boundaries of respect that must be honored with patients, families, and peers are addressed throughout this book, especially in Section 1.

The physical structure of an institution helps enable an effective private-sector or public-sector relationship. Hospitals, clinics, or schools, for instance, unmistakably are public buildings. What are some of the clues for this conclusion? Sometimes the environment where health care is administered mingles private-sector and public-sector environments. For instance, there are private spaces in health care for examinations or procedures and public waiting areas. On a different scale, a home visit to a patient requires that you go to his or her residence, be welcomed in as a guest would be, make your way across the living room among discarded pages of the morning paper, trip over the sleeping dog, and move a bathrobe from a comfortable overstuffed chair to sit down. You have entered a profoundly private-sector environment. However, your presence and professional conduct represent the type of public-sector relationship that takes place within health care institutions, and this usually suffices to set the tone for a public-sector interaction.

Patients and families lose some freedoms when entering a health institution such as where they should wait, what they must wear, or how long they can visit. Even within one's own home, the presence of health professionals limits freedom in some ways. The underlying question about any limitation on a patient's freedom should be the reasonableness of the limitation. In other words, are the restrictions there to protect the well-being of patients or are the rules in an institution there to make the staff's work easier?

REFLECTIONS

Suppose you are scheduled for a series of diagnostic tests for a possible serious health problem. You will have several appointments over more than one day. Each test includes directions for what you need to do to prepare for that specific test, such as refrain from eating or drinking at least 8 hours before the test, shower with a specific antibacterial soap the morning of the test, etc. Of the following questions, which ones do you think would be of concern to you?

- What should I wear?
- Do I need someone to accompany me and take me home after the test?
- Will there be pain and how will this be managed?
- Can my partner accompany me in the prep area before the test?
- When will I get the results of the tests? Who will share the results? How will the information be conveyed—in person, on the phone, through an electronic patient-accessible medical record?

These concerns will vary based on the type of condition and the value system of the individual. However, the important point is that the patient will have concerns about what restrictions the institution will impose.

Your own autonomy as a health professional in an institution where you work as a professional will also be shaped by the structure and how authority is divided. They may include policies for securing employment, regulations regarding employee conduct, expectations regarding the number of people in your care, and other institutional peculiarities. These will either enable or inhibit your ability to satisfy your professional and personal goals. Obviously, a crucial component of your professional choices is to find an institution that is consistent with your personality and value system. As you consider an institutional environment, paying attention to Glaser's three realms should help you identify areas where personal, institutional, and societal values overlap and where they may create potential conflicts.

Health professionals are also key sources of institutional change who can help create ways that respect can be expressed in humane and person-centered environments. As people talk about ways in which their autonomy and other values can better be honored within the confines of partial institutions, you can think of ways to help bring about those changes.

Working with the Administration

All employees in institutions have the opportunity and obligation to work well with their team members and administrators. The administration's role is to safeguard the interests of the institution and its components. In health care institutions, the administration comprises a wide range of groups and individuals, including institutional trustees, boards of directors, and the central administration (including a chief executive officer [CEO] and chief financial officer [CFO], human resources director, and departmental and unit supervisors responsible for operations or services). The range and duties of the administration should reflect the needs of the institution as determined by its mission, goals, and functions. Health care institutions will include at least the following administrative areas:

1. quality care mechanisms to ensure that patient and family rights are respected
2. officers for enforcing legal compliance with federal and other policies and regulations
3. accountability mechanisms ensuring qualifications of professional employees
4. risk management personnel regarding concerns of liability and malpractice
5. means of ensuring that employees get due payment for their services

Taken together, like other well-working institutions, there will be personnel and mechanisms devoted to care delivery oversight, quality assurance, financial solvency, legal compliance and assurances that legal rights are honored, public relations, and efficiency.

These administrative supports should always be designed to allow constructive participation of professionals to ensure their mutually shared goal of good health care. For example, general goals or aims of health care institutions have been widely adopted and focus on optimizing four dimensions of performance, sometimes referred to as the "quadruple aim," as follows: (1) improving the health of populations, (2) enhancing the patient experience of care, (3) reducing the per capita cost of health care, and (4) improving work and life balance.[6] At the same time, differences in the scope of accountabilities determined by their respective roles lead to understandable conflict at times. To illustrate how differently administration and health professionals might look at the same set of challenges, we invite you to consider the following case, first from the point of view of the professional and patient relationship and then from the administrator's point of view.

Case Study

Mary Jacobs is the coordinator of the large pediatric division of Metro Rehabilitation Center. She is single and the mother of two children. She has mortgage payments and car payments to make, but thanks to her job, she feels quite secure financially.

Mary has worked at the Center for 15 years. The first 12 years she worked as a staff professional in the adolescent unit, with increasing supervisory and student clinical teaching responsibilities. Three years ago, she was tapped by the administration for her present position, which includes departmental administrative responsibilities, as well as continuing to treat patients. Although her position has many benefits, she realizes her primary concern still lies with the patients and their families.

At the same time, she likes the idea of being able to further shape a service with an excellent reputation. She believes that the 3 years overall have been both personally and professionally rewarding.

Mary reports directly to the Vice President for Patient Services (Carole Nash), though most of her day-to-day activities revolve around the team, support personnel, and patients. She meets with Carole once a month. She is painfully aware that the pediatric unit has been under increasing financial duress, because of two competing pediatric rehabilitation units in the area. She is not entirely surprised when Carole tells her that as a result of financial pressures at Metro, Mary must lay off two professional staff and four support staff by the end of the fiscal quarter (within the next 6 weeks). But as she walks back to her unit she begins to resent having to upset such a well-working team and deal with the negative impact on morale. Central to her concern is that the upset will have a detrimental effect on patient care quality. She must admit that she also resents her unit being asked to make cuts when she is aware that overall the census is down at Metro Rehab.

The next morning Mary calls the Vice President's office to ask if she can discuss this situation with Carole further. Carole's administrative assistant replies that he will check but wants to warn Mary that Carole herself did not make the decision independently. He believes "the final decision already has been made." A bit later Carole drops in to see Mary. She says that she appreciates how difficult this is for Mary and her staff but adds, "With the present situation in the pediatric unit, there should be no question in your mind, either, about what had to be done. As you know, I, too, come from a clinical background, so I'm sure you feel torn. I wish we had the resources to launch an aggressive campaign to counter our competition, but we don't. So, I finally agreed with Metro's board of directors that yours is one area we should downsize. Ethically speaking I am torn, but it's the kind of hard decision administrators sometimes must make. I am sorry."

As is often the case in health care settings, clinical and administrative roles are not entirely separate, so at some level both Mary Jacobs and Carole Nash can see the other's point of view. Viewed from Mary's perspective as a health professional who identifies with her caregiving role more than her administrative one, reflect on the following:

	Strongly Agree	Agree	Not Sure	Disagree	Strongly Disagree
1. Mary has a right to expect that her concerns be listened to by the higher administration.					
2. If Mary can show that patient care quality in her unit will be decreased by the downsizing, Carole should go back to the board to advocate for finding another place to cut personnel.					
3. Mary's concern that a decrease in team morale might have a detrimental effect on patient care is a legitimate concern.					
4. If Mary does not succeed in making her case, she should resign.					
5. If Mary does not take the recommended action, she is likely to lose her job.					

- What values, duties, and other considerations are appropriate for Mary Jacobs to consider in making judgments about the situation?
- When should she share her problem with others, and whom should they be? Why?
- What alternatives are open to her other than resigning if she is unsuccessful in reversing Carole's decision?

Viewed from Carole Nash's perspective as an administrator, reflect on the following from the point of view of institutional loyalties:

	Strongly Agree	Agree	Not Sure	Disagree	Strongly Disagree
1. Carole's major responsibility is to be sure Metro Rehabilitation Center stays financially stable, even though some difficult decisions must be made.					
2. The board's plan to cut personnel to help sustain the financial health of Metro Rehabilitation Center outweighs Mary's concern about the negative effect on her team's morale.					
3. Carole should meet with the members of Mary's unit before giving Mary the task of terminating personnel.					
4. Administrators in high positions such as Carole's would make more objective, rational decisions if they did not have a health professions background.					

- What basic administrative values, duties, and other considerations are appropriate for Carole to consider in her position as she responds to this administrative problem?
- Should Carole have shared the information with Mary that the decision came from the Metro Board of Directors instead of representing it as being her decision? Why or why not?
- What, if any, alternatives are open to Carole to help ensure that the positive aspects of the outcome will be optimized and the damage minimal?

This case is just one type of situation in which health professionals and administrators may have to negotiate decisions that are not 100% acceptable to either party. The better the communication channels and the more transparent the policies and processes for mediating difficult decisions, the more likely it is that the highest possible level of mutual acceptance will be reached.

Respecting the Interface of Institutions and Society

In addition to the constraints and opportunities you, your colleagues, and patients will experience from the design of the institution and its administrative practices and policies, your daily professional relationships in that institution also will be affected by laws and regulations that govern health care settings. The following pages illustrate some of the most widespread and important categories. They are examples only and not intended to be up-to-date in all cases because the details may change at any time. As a professional you are responsible for keeping current with all laws and regulations regarding your profession.

LAWS AND REGULATIONS REQUIRING PROFESSIONAL COMPETENCE

In an effort to protect society from incompetent practitioners, all health care institutions that want to remain accredited by national and regional accrediting boards must take steps to ensure that their professional staff is well qualified to do the work they say they can do. In the United States, laws of every state include professional licensing, certification, and registration mechanisms, whereby a person must pass a national certifying or board examination and meet other qualifying criteria to practice in that state. In other countries, provincial or national laws may be the rule. Some institutions go beyond the minimum requirements established by their government bodies by adding continuing education requirements for their own professional employees. Also, national certifying bodies (e.g., specialty boards in medicine, nursing, physical therapy, and other health professions) have requirements pertaining to specialized and continued competence. Today many health professionals are personally responsible for negligence and other types of conduct that lead to malpractice claims, so institutions increasingly are requiring individuals to maintain personal malpractice insurance. These requirements should not have a negative impact on your work and may even have a positive effect because they have been developed over the years to help ensure that the basic tenets of professional respect are maintained for all who require your services.

LAWS AND REGULATIONS TO PREVENT DISCRIMINATION

Several nondiscrimination laws developed in the second half of the 20th century continue to have direct bearing on health care institutions in the United States, and similar ones have been crafted in other countries as well. Consider a few key examples:

- *Title VII of the Civil Rights Act* (1964) prohibits employers from refusing to hire an employee on the basis of race, color, sex, religion, or national origin.
- *The Equal Opportunity Act* buttressed and expanded Title VII in 1972.
- *The Equal Pay Act of 1963* required that men and women receive equal pay for performing similar work.
- *The Age Discrimination and Employment Act* (1967) prohibits discrimination against persons 40 to 70 years old.
- *The Rehabilitation Act (Section 504) of 1973* required all employers to have an affirmative action plan that includes hiring impaired persons. Superseding this act was the Americans with Disabilities Act of 1990, which states that institutions with more than 25 employees cannot use a physical examination to deny employment.

Understandably, policies continue to be introduced all the time, and older ones evolve.

OTHER LAWS AND REGULATIONS

In addition to laws ensuring your professional competence to practice and prohibiting discrimination, others have a direct bearing on your relationship with patients. As Chapter 3 emphasized, prohibitions against some types of conduct such as touching a patient in ways not consistent with what your practice requires for diagnostic and treatment purposes, sexual intercourse with or sexual harassment of patients are often written into licensing laws, as well as being reiterated in institutional policies and the ethical codes of professional organizations.

With the advent of the AIDS epidemic, numerous laws and policies were implemented nationally and within institutions to try to decrease the accidental transmittal of infections through body substances to health professionals, among patients, or to others. The most notable of these in the United States was the *universal precautions,* a federal mandate introduced in 1985 and later adjusted to be known as *standard precautions* by 1996. They require all health professionals to protect themselves and others by wearing certain types of protective clothing in treating any patient, including gowns and gloves. Goggles or other personal protective equipment may have to be added while treating patients with infectious diseases and by adhering to strict methods for handling and disposing of body fluids, bandages, and needles. The requirements for the amounts and types of protective devices vary by the mode of transmission of the organism and likelihood of body fluids being transferred from patient to health professional or vice versa.[7]

Depending on your area of service as a health professional, you may be regulated by other additional laws and regulations. In the United States, if you work in a clinical or laboratory area where blood and other body fluids are handled, you will be subject to an institution's safety standards set out by the Occupational Safety and Health Administration (OSHA). If you work with patients or clients who have sexually transmitted or other infectious diseases, you will be required to report this information to your state's department of health or similar governing body. In the United States, if your patient population falls within reimbursement guidelines established by Medicare and Medicaid regulations, what you may offer in reimbursable services will be governed by those regulations. Similar concerns of reimbursable services are an issue in almost all settings today.

Additionally, there have been dramatic changes in the number of individuals covered by health insurance since the passage of the Patient Protection and Affordable Care Act (often referred to as the Affordable Care Act [ACA] or simply "Obamacare") in 2014. Before the passage of the ACA, large numbers of people—around 49.9 million in the United States in 2010—went without health insurance.[8] By 2014, 33 million went without insurance for the entire year.[8] The increase in coverage occurred both with private insurance (mandated by the ACA) and Medicaid (for which coverage increased in states choosing to expand coverage). Thus more Americans had access to health care services than ever before. The election of President Donald Trump in January 2017 resulted in proposed changes to the ACA, as promised repeatedly in his campaign, ranging from eliminating the act and starting anew to other less dramatic revisions to parts of the regulations associated with the ACA. Only time will tell if and what changes to ACA will occur, but any changes are certain to have an impact on health care institutions and the health professionals who work there.

Laws and regulations regarding the documentation of patient status, patient progress, and other patient information will affect the everyday practice of your profession. The medical record (whether electronic or hard copy) is a legal document, as are many other types of reports and statements you prepare for billing, quality assurance reviews, and other activities requiring data about patients and clients (Fig. 6.2). Sometimes professionals treat documentation as a means of protecting their own interests legally. However, self-interest should not be a priority when documenting a clinical encounter. Rather, think of your documentation as an accurate accounting of interactions between you and the patient. Preparation of your documentation, like all other aspects of your interaction within the institution, should be undertaken first with respect for the patient's dignity and rights and then with respect for the type of professional you want the world to know you are.

Although this sampling of regulations and policies is not intended to be exhaustive, and focuses on situation in the United States, it illustrates that your relationship with society and the institution within which you practice is part and parcel of what you are able to do.

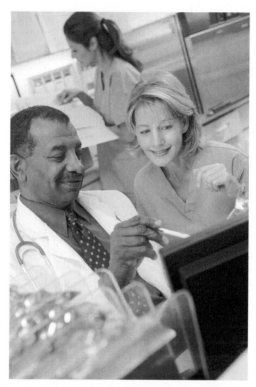

Fig. 6.2 Professional colleagues discuss information in the electronic medical record. (© monkeybusinessimages/iStock/Thinkstock.com.)

LAWS, REGULATIONS, AND CHANGE

We conclude this section with a short reminder that laws and regulations are always in a state of flux. They deserve to be followed if you judge them to enhance your capacity to be respected and show respect in all your professional interactions. If they present major difficulties for you practically or ethically, you should reflect seriously on how you can help bring about their change. Like every generation of health professionals before you, you have an opportunity throughout your career to help shape a better environment for the health professions by working to change unworkable, unfair, or otherwise inadequate laws, regulations, and other policies. As we introduced in Chapter 1, the professional's freedom to initiate and carry out a person-centered course for each patient is the ultimate expression of respect, and all institutional activities must reflect that goal.

The process of changing unacceptable laws, regulations, and policy requires willingness, persistence, and courage. Some steps toward that end include:

- Document problems diligently, both individually and as a unified interprofessional care team.
- Gain an understanding of the informal opinion leaders and formal authorities in the type of situation you want to change.
- Identify interprofessional colleagues and lay organizations with whom you can link arms to develop effective strategies for addressing your issue.

- Be flexible and prepare to negotiate anew as new information comes your way.
- Stay with the project until change is accomplished or you understand why it cannot be.

Patients' Rights Documents

In health care institutions patients, too, have rights and incur responsibilities. Some that are protected by law have been mentioned. However, other rights not addressed by legal guidelines have come to be accepted as important.

Rights often named include the right to:

- considerate and respectful care
- accurate and complete information
- participation (directly or through a legally appointed spokesperson) in health care decisions
- privacy and confidentiality (within constraints of the law). There are rights to information about the institution itself (e.g., who owns it and what its overall services are) and the right to have continuity of care.

All US readers of this book should be aware of the *Health Insurance Portability and Accountability Act (HIPAA)* regulations, which originally went into effect in 2003. The regulations, called the *New Federal Medical-Privacy Rule,* were designed to help protect patient privacy. They have had a profound effect on health professionals and health care institutions regarding the type of confidential information that can be transmitted into medical records and other information systems. The rule also contains requirements regarding information about research subjects. The following types of details are among the most important that may not be photocopied or faxed without specific authorization to do so by the patient: psychotherapy records, counseling about domestic violence, sexual assault counseling, HIV test results, records regarding sexually transmitted diseases, and social work records.[9] Moreover, as a health professional you are not allowed to provide current medical status and information about a patient to third parties, even family members, without the patient's explicit consent.

The Health Information Technology for Economic and Clinical Health Act (HITECH) of 2009 expanded and strengthened these privacy laws and went into full effect in 2013. This law stipulated new obligations on covered entities, business associates, and subcontractors. The act also designated funding to expand national electronic patient records with measures to ensure privacy and security.[10]

REFLECTIONS

- What rights and responsibilities of patients do you think should be included in nationally binding documents in your country of employment?
- What do you see as strengths and challenges with the HIPAA regulations?

GRIEVANCE MECHANISMS

In recent years, several professional organizations and institutions have created grievance mechanisms to assist patients who believe their rights or other reasonable expectations are not being honored. Some institutions employ patient representatives, or ombudsmen, whose job is to listen to patients' problems and try to help solve them. Institutional ethics committees bring together health professionals and patients and their families as they try to determine what to do next in complex life-and-death decisions or to help resolve conflicts among various members of the group. The following case illustrates the types of differences that can arise around seemingly straightforward policy decisions within an institution and the negative impact of such decisions on patients.

Case Study

You work in a long-term care facility that recently experienced an outbreak of scabies (a highly communicable skin disease caused by an arachnid, *Sarcoptes scabiei*, the itch mite). When the usual public health measures fail to prevent new and recurring cases, the decision is made by a committee of senior health professionals in the facility to treat all patients and staff with permethrin. One patient, Cora Grosklaus, who is 82 years old, alert, and oriented, has refused the treatment. She understood the treatment process to kill the mites—that is, the permethrin cream would be applied from the neck down, left on overnight, and then washed off. This application would have to be repeated in 7 days. This treatment is considered to be the safest and most effective treatment for scabies. Regardless of the explanations the staff has provided about the importance of the treatment for her well-being and that of others, Mrs. Grosklaus will have none of it, stating, "I will not submit to such humiliating treatment."[11]

If you were a member of the team caring for Mrs. Grosklaus, how might you have gone about explaining to her the importance of the application?

Where might a breakdown in communication have occurred, and what could have been done to possibly prevent this unhappy state?

The measure being undertaken is believed by the health providers to benefit Mrs. Grosklaus, as well as be an important public health measure. What should be done if, like the team described earlier, you got nowhere in convincing her?

Sometimes health care institutions feel trapped by patients (or, in this case, long-term care facility residents) who refuse treatments that health professionals think are necessary for the patients' well-being. Sometimes individuals do just the opposite of Mrs. Grosklaus and insist on treatments that health professionals believe will not benefit them or will harm them. At other times, patients insist on going home before the health professionals think they are ready. In the latter case, they are said to have left "AMA"—against medical advice. They may be asked to sign a document confirming they have been informed of the physician's judgment but are choosing to act contrary to his or her advice.

The good news is that great strides have been made toward recognizing and respecting patients' preferences as an integral aspect of patient-centered decision-making in health care institutions. At the same time, problems do remain. A part of the process of preparing to be a professional is to learn how to recognize, analyze, and help patients move toward an acceptable decision when differences create distress for the parties involved.

Grievance mechanisms for employees also are available. Disputes about policies or practices, salary increases, work hours, and termination of employment are frequent reasons employees seek recourse through institutional processes designed for airing their disapproval and coming to resolution.

An important area of employee protection has been implemented in recent years for personnel whose grievance involves their perception of wrongdoing by others in their institution. *Whistle blowers* disclose to a person or public body, outside the normal channels and management structure, information concerning unsafe, unethical, or illegal practices.[12] In the past the necessity of "blowing the whistle" on an incompetent, unethical, or impaired colleague was often suppressed by the realistic fear of reprisal by the institution. Fortunately, today many institutions have developed processes and policies to protect the interests of everyone involved until the matter is investigated and resolved.[13] This is consistent with Glaser's statement in the graphic of the three realms that the good and virtuous institution "attends to the health, vigor, balance, and equity of the institution's key systems."[2] To uphold this goal, adequate mechanisms must be in place to help ensure that an employee who documents the misconduct or debilitating condition of another employee is protected, as well as the person or unit against which the grievance is made.

Summary

Respect within health care institutional environments requires the cooperation and responsible participation of individuals, institutional leaders, and society. Professionals' efforts at providing high-quality care in a well-working setting will be fruitless without support from institutional leaders. At the same time, respect is so fundamental that you have an opportunity and duty to exercise it at all levels: as an individual professional, as an employee of the institution, and as a citizen. Today numerous legal regulations and guidelines help shape health care institutions in ways that protect and honor the interests of everyone involved. When institutional policies, practices, or processes threaten to diminish or destroy a respectful environment, a professional's obligation extends to help constructively change the situation.

See Section 2 Questions for Thought and Discussion on page 263 to apply what you've learned in this section to a variety of case scenarios.

References

1. In The Waiting Room, "Exodus." A project of Open'Hood, 2012. Retrieved at:www.whatruwaitingfor.com/2010/03/exodus.
2. Glaser J. *Three Realms of Ethics*. Kansas City, MO: Sheed and Ward; 1994:30.
3. Scott WR. *Organizations: Rational, Natural and Open Systems*. Englewood Cliffs, NJ: Prentice Hall; 1981.
4. Alameda Health System. http://www.alamedahealthsystem.org/about-us/our-history.
5. California Health Care Foundation. California health care almanac quick reference guide, California Hospitals – 2103. Accessed on February 14, 2017 from http://www.chcf.org.
6. Bodenheimer T, Sinsky C. From triple to quadruple aim: care of the patient requires care of the provider. *Ann Fam Med*. 2014;12(6):573–576.
7. U.S. Department of Health and Human Services. Public Health Service, Centers for Disease Control and Prevention. *MMWR Morb Mortal Wkly Rep*. 1987;36(suppl 25):55–65.
8. ASPE Issue Brief: Overview of the Uninsured in the United States: A Summary of the 2011 Current Population Survey, September 2011. Available at http://aspe.hhs.gov/health/reports/2011/cpshealthins2011/ib.shtml. Accessed August 14, 2013.
9. Federal Register: 67:53182–53273, 2002.
10. Salz T. HIPAA: training critical to protect patient practice. *Medical Econ*. 2013;25(Sept):43–47.
11. Smith M, Strauss S, Baldwin HJ. *Pharmacy Ethics*. Binghamton, NY: Pharmaceutical Products Press; 1991:534. Case adapted from p. 534.
12. Mannion R, Davies HT. Cultures of silence and cultures of voice: the role of whistleblowing in healthcare organisations. *Int J Health Policy Manag*. 2015;4(3):503–505.
13. Miceli MP, Pollix-Near J, Dworkin TM. *Whistleblowing in Organizations*. New York: Routledge; 2008.

Respect for the Patient's Situation

Section 3 examines closely the person who seeks professional services—the patient—and does so in two different but connected ways. Just as history does not exist in nature but is created in the telling, so, too, autobiography and the patient's case history emerge out of interactions, which means that they are at the same time both less and more than the "facts" of the case.[1] Chapter 7 focuses on how we understand our patients by examining the ways the patients' stories are created. Illness and injury are milestones in patients' lives. The clinical record is one place where the experience of the patient is set into words by individuals other than the patient, words that are shared with the whole health care team. The format, syntax, perspective, and language we use to tell the patient's story deserve your attention as much as the content. It becomes apparent that it is not enough to merely describe the chronology of events that bring patients to us.

You will want to understand why things happened the way they did, what meaning the patient gives to the experience, and what the patient expects from you. To come closer to understanding the meaning your patients give to their life experiences, you will depend on your ability to communicate that is explored in Section 4.

Chapter 8 examines the patient in regard to how his or her intimate and close personal relationships are affected, specifically the role of traditional and contemporary families as collaborators in the patient's care. In this chapter, you will gain a better understanding of how families define themselves, how they function, and how to best interact with them across care delivery systems.

We also explore how a family's health and functioning are affected by the uncertainties of illness or injury of one of its members. Alterations in roles and responsibilities are common in close relationships, and health professionals must partner with patients and families to optimize health outcomes within the context of each family culture. Health professionals are in a unique position to help patients, families, and friends express their stressors, fears, needs, and concerns related to care, finances, and social burdens of health care.

Ask yourself the following questions as you read about the patient's story and the various relationships that make up a patient's life:

- How do my attitudes and conduct convey respect toward a patient?
- What do I need to know about patients to effectively work with them and the significant people in their lives to set reasonable patient- and family-centered goals consistent with their deepest values?
- How can I best honor and support the patient in the context of his or her intimate and close personal relationships?

Reference

1. Greenhalgh T, Hurwitz B. Why study narrative?. In: Greenhalgh T, Hurwirtz B, eds. *Narrative based medicine: dialogue and discourse in clinical practice.* London: BMJ Books; 1998.

Respecting the Patient's Story

Prelude

When you have mouth sores you think very carefully before even trying to take a bite of food; even something as innocuous as a yogurt smoothie is like swallowing a handful of nettles. This also happened to be the time when my hair truly fell out. Because I couldn't eat my weight had dropped alarmingly. I happen to be one of those people who look a wreck when I have a mere head cold; I look horrible out of all proportion to my symptoms. This time when I looked in the mirror I was truly alarmed. This was not a case that the Look Good–Feel Better people could solve.

J. HOOPER[1]

For many decades, most health professionals believed that if they carefully observed a patient and listened to the patient's responses to the numerous questions they posed, they could arrive at an accurate clinical diagnosis and treatment plan. However, this approach to understanding the patient's experience or story to offer effective interventions is not sufficient for several reasons. First, asking an established list of questions to arrive at a diagnosis of any type shapes the story along health care lines, not the lived experience of the patient.

Second, the patient's role is passive in this traditional model of interviewing and ignores the fact that a "new" story of what is wrong, what needs to be fixed, or what needs attention is being unilaterally created by the health professional. This chapter offers a different way of viewing what happens during interactions between health professionals and patients, as well as an understanding of the roles both play in creating the patient's story.

Human beings experience illness, injury, pain, suffering, and loss within a narrative, or story, which shapes and gives meaning to what they are feeling moment to moment.[2] One may say that our whole lives are enacted narratives. Another way to understand this is to think about life as an unfolding story. *Narration* is the forward movement of the description of actions and events that makes it possible to later look back on what happened. And it is through that backward action that we can engage in self-reflection and self-understanding.[3] Illness and injury are milestones in a person's life story. "The practice of medicine is lived in stories: 'I was well until . . .' 'It all started when I was doing . . .' are common openings of the medical encounter."[4] Think about an illness or injury "story" from your own life. How does your story begin? Is your story a tragedy or a comedy? Who has a starring role? Who has a supporting role? All of these elements of an illness or injury story tell us a lot about who you are as a person, how you see the world, and what is important to you. The same is also true of the patients you encounter in professional practice.

Much of this book has emphasized that health professionals are called into a particular relationship with patients because of the importance of an illness experience or serious injury. The setting of that relationship is the patient's story. This chapter will help you grasp the importance of paying attention to the unique and personal story of a particular patient's life beyond the more general suggestions we have offered so far. Because the final focus of all of our efforts in health care is the patient, the insights that arise from viewing the patient's account of what is meaningful about an illness or injury experience are essential to delivering high-quality, compassionate care. Furthermore, narrative analysis or narrative theory can offer ways for health professionals to understand the stories that patients tell from a variety of perspectives. We highlight how different voices offer different stories of the patient's predicament. We briefly explore some of the basics of narrative theory and apply it to health care communications, such as textbooks, scientific journal articles, and the medical record. We go beyond professional, scholarly literature to the humanities to include some examples of literature such as poetry and short stories to give you an opportunity to read and think in different terms about patients' and health professionals' experiences.

Who's Telling the Story?

When a patient enters the health care system, regardless of the place of entry, an exchange of stories begins. It might be hard for you to consider the patient's "history" portion of a traditional history and physical examination to be a kind of story, but it is. So are the entries in a medical record and the scientific explanation of a particular pathological condition in a textbook. Even within the health record, for example, many individuals who are members of the health care team contribute their voices and perspectives to the single entity of the patient's health record.

Montgomery has convincingly argued that all knowledge is narrative in structure.[5] Although her work focuses on the physician and patient encounter as a story, her insights apply to all health professional and patient encounters. In these encounters, the patient tells the story of an illness or injury, which she notes is an interpretive act in that the patient chooses certain words and not others and reports some incidents and not others. The health professional then interprets the story and translates it into a list of possible diagnoses. Frank[6] suggests that the physician's story is guided by the notion of "getting it right." "Diagnostic stories are about getting patients to the appropriate treatment as quickly as possible."[6] From the patient's perspective, however, getting it right from the professional's perspective may or may not be what is important. For example, a patient who has a chronic illness such as multiple sclerosis might have a story that is guided by figuring out how to cope with the unpredictable nature of the disease, or a dying patient might want to address challenges to his or her faith. Getting to a correct diagnosis does not seem like the appropriate response to either of these patients' stories. The act of interpretation begins by really listening to what the patient is trying to say. The health professional must listen with a narrative ear.

Narrative theory helps us understand what patients are experiencing and to appreciate or adopt others' perspectives.[7-9] Narratives pull elements such as events, characters, and setting(s) together in a meaningful way. If we think about a novel as one type of narrative, the preceding explanation makes sense in that we expect that every novel will include events, characters, and setting(s) arranged in some manner. The novel will also include a plot, point of view, and motivation so we can understand why the characters act the way they do. It is only when we apply these components of narrative theory to written communication within the health care setting that things get confusing because the genres are so different. One way to help clarify the application of narrative theory to clinical practice is to begin with the narrator, or the person who tells the story. You will see that when the narrator shifts, so does the content of the story and the arrangement or prioritization of the various elements of the story.

FROM THE PATIENT'S PERSPECTIVE

One way to highlight the different ways that the same story can be viewed is to look at it from various perspectives. For example, how is a cerebral vascular accident (CVA) seen from the perspective of the patient, written about in the medical record, and described in a medical textbook? Before we look at these different "stories" about a CVA, consider the most basic differences in language here regarding what we call the neurovascular injury in question, a *cerebral vascular accident*, or, in common language, a *stroke*. Think of all the metaphoric meanings of the word "stroke" that are stripped away by the use of the clinically sterile term *cerebral vascular accident*. Even this technical term uses a word that leaves room for interpretation because an accident connotes a variety of meanings. An accident is unintended, not foreseen. Think about how we would view this diagnosis if the term were cerebral vascular *event* rather than *accident*. What is the difference between an event and an accident? Next consider how health professionals distance themselves even further from the patient's experience by replacing "cerebral vascular accident" with the acronym "CVA." We will now return to the patient's perspective with a personal written account from a man who had a stroke. He recounts his experience in the past tense. This is common because most patient stories are recollections.[10] The following is an excerpt from a much longer account of the stroke that changed this person's life:

> On May 23rd, 2004, I was reading a Hopalong Cassidy novel by Clarence Mulford, the best western author ever, late at night when an artery on the right side of my brain burst and began bleeding into my skull. I suddenly experienced the mother of all headaches. Headaches for me were rare. I'd had fewer than five in my entire life. As I read, the words on the page broke apart into individual letters that started crawling off the page like ants off a paper plate. It was a hallucination, and it wouldn't be my last. I walked to the bathroom to get some aspirin, the only pain reliever on hand. I felt "removed," very "spacey." I looked in the mirror as I passed by and was shocked by what I saw. My mouth drooped on the left side. Suddenly my bowels knotted up and my stomach did a flip. My face looked like melted wax. I suspected I was having a stroke because of the droop. I remember seeing Kirk Douglas after his stroke. Following a short bout of diarrhea, I vomited. This worried me because I'd seen many animals let go from both ends when they were fatally injured. My left leg wouldn't work, and my left arm felt like it was made of wood. Walking was impossible. I fell more than a dozen times while returning the thirty plus feet to my bed. Each time I got up, only to fall again. I refused to just lay there. My thinking was confused and clouded, but I vaguely knew I was in trouble.[11]

The description is written in the first-person voice. *Voice* is the personality of the writer coming through the words on the page. Voice can give the reader an indication of the uniqueness of the person who is speaking in the text. When a writer uses the first-person voice, it feels as if the writer is talking directly to the reader. The story begins with what could appear to be an unnecessary detail in that the patient tells us what he was reading and his opinion of the author's work. Although we do not need to know which western novel he was reading or even if he was reading at all, this information gives us some insight into how the patient marked the moment the stroke began and a bit about his values and interests.

REFLECTIONS

- What did you notice first about the patient's story? What does the patient's choice of words (e.g., "artery," "hallucination," "vomited") tell you about him?
- What sorts of emotional reactions, if any, did you have to the patient's story?
- Consider another story, this time a verbal account from a Ted Talk, from Jill Bolt Taylor, a neuroanatomist who also suffered a stroke (http://www.ted.com/speakers/jill_bolte_taylor).
- How are these two stories similar or different?

This is probably not the first time the patient told the story of his stroke, although it could be the first time that he wrote about his experience. In the telling and retelling of landmark experiences such as the trauma associated with a stroke, "the narrative provides meaning, context, and perspective for the patient's predicament. It defines how, why, and in what way he or she is ill. It offers, in short, a possibility of understanding which cannot be arrived at by any other means."[12] When a patient begins to tell you the story of his or her illness, you might be able to discern whether this is a familiar, often told story or if the patient is still trying to figure out what happened and make sense of the experience. Clearly, only in retrospect could the patient know that "an artery on the right side of my brain burst." He includes this information in his written account to help make sense out of what happened, but he could have easily left that clinical explanation out of his story and just provided the facts of what progressed that night.

HEALTH RECORD

Beginning with the patient's direct experience of the trauma that he has undergone, let us move forward in time to a different setting and interpretation of the story of his CVA and what is happening to him. The patient reports that he was eventually discovered by his brother and taken to an emergency department at a local hospital. In a hospital, one of the vehicles for communication between health professionals who care for a specific patient is the health record. The health record might be handwritten but is today more commonly an electronic health record (EHR). How might the patient's story continue in the EHR? Here are three typical entries, the first from the nurses' notes, the second from the medical progress notes, and the third from physical therapy. Assume that they were written 3 days after the patient was admitted to the hospital.

Daily Nursing Note–7/18/20__ Impaired physical mobility; impaired verbal communication R/T aphasia; unilateral neglect; fear and anxiety

9:00 A.M.

AM Assessment Notes: Pt. irritable and tearful. Repeatedly asked for "book" but no books found in bedside stand. Pt. then pointed to note with brother's name and phone number. Pt. calmed down when reassured brother would visit soon. Pt. neglects L arm when moving in bed. Pt. required moderate assistance with breakfast. Poor appetite.

Plan: Continue to support pt.; consult with speech, occupational, and physical therapy as needed; use every encounter to support communication; obtain picture board; remind pt. to attend to L arm and leg affected by sensory alteration.

Physician's Progress Note–7/18/20__ Dx: R hemisphere hemorrhagic infarct.; Pt. stable; echo, CXR, repeat MRI; contact speech/OT/PT for rehabilitation assessment.

Physical Therapy Notes–7/18/20__:

S: Pt. teary. No c/o pain.

O: Pt. alert, oriented to place and person. Cooperative, but impulsive. ROM is within normal limits. Flaccid paresis in left upper limb. Left lower limb strength is 2-/5 in hip extension, hip adduction, and knee extension. Minimal spasticity noted in left lower limb extensors. Pt. demonstrates denial of left upper and lower limb. Could not assess sensation due to emotional lability. Pt. requires maximal assist for bed mobility and transfers supine to sit at EOB. Sitting balance is poor. Standing not attempted.

A: Left hemiparesis. Dependent in mobility secondary to left-sided weakness and perceptual deficits affecting all activities of daily living. Good rehabilitation candidate with goal to achieve ability to perform bed mobility and transfers with minimal assist and ability to locomote via walking with assist.

P: Recommend for inpatient stroke rehabilitation when medically stable.

REFLECTIONS

What do you notice first about these versions of the patient's story?
- Do you understand all the terms and language?
- Do these more objective, clinical renderings of the patient's illness give you different insights into what you can do to help the patient?
- How do these clinical narratives compare to the patient's accounts in content and tone?

Clearly, there is a difference in how the patient and health professionals describe what is going on. In Chapter 10, we discuss the use of jargon in health care and how it serves a useful purpose of facilitating communication between health professionals but also works to distance patients from providers. The jargon in these sample entries from a fictitious medical record almost becomes impenetrable to a novice in the official language of health care. Did you understand the terms and abbreviations? What is "flaccid paresis"? Did you know that "R/T" means "related to," that "echo" is shorthand for "echocardiogram," and that "CXR" is an acronym for "chest x-ray"?

Although the patient describes his experience of having a stroke in the first-person voice, the EHR refers to him in the third person. He is now "Pt.," which is shorthand for "Patient." In the assessment notes from the physical therapist, the patient is almost completely invisible in the account. We will discuss point of view in more detail later in this chapter. It is sufficient here to note the type of voice used in writing and the implications of using a particular voice. Third-person voice distances us from what is going on in the narrative. The EHR may even move further away from these textual accounts to drop boxes that merely require a check or click to categorize the diagnosis or problem and the plan of care from a range of standardized choices. The fact that a patient is upset and "teary" would likely have no place in a health care record that is largely based on billable categories of care. One final comment about all health records, whether written or electronic—they are essentially monologues, with each member of the health care team entering information, and offer little opportunity for collaborative interaction.

Consider one more version of the patient's story, this one even further removed from the personal experience of a CVA. In a current medical diagnosis textbook, the clinical signs and symptoms of an intracerebral hemorrhage (ICH) are described as follows:

Although not particularly associated with exertion, ICHs almost always occur while the patient is awake and sometimes when stressed. The hemorrhage generally presents as the abrupt onset of focal neurologic deficit. Seizures are uncommon. The focal deficit typically worsens steadily over 30 to 90 minutes and is associated with a diminishing level of consciousness and signs of increased ICP such as headache and vomiting. The putamen is the most common site for hypertensive hemorrhage, and the adjacent internal capsule is usually damaged. Contralateral hemiparesis is therefore the sentinel sign. When mild, the face sags on one side over 5 to 30 minutes, speech becomes slurred, the arm and leg gradually weaken, and the eyes deviate away from the side of the hemiparesis. The paralysis may worsen until the affected limbs become flaccid or extend rigidly. When hemorrhages are large, drowsiness gives way to stupor as signs of upper brainstem compression appear. Coma ensues, accompanied by deep, irregular, or intermittent respiration, a dilated and fixed ipsilateral pupil, and decerebrate rigidity. In milder cases, edema in adjacent brain tissue may cause progressive deterioration over 12 to 72 hours.[13]

What does this final version of the experience of a CVA tell you? How does this technical version mesh with the two different patient accounts? The authors of the medical text are not concerned with a specific patient who has an ICH, a more specific diagnostic term than CVA. The description is objective, one written for health professionals—hence the use of highly abstract terms—and one that can be applied to all patients who suffer this type of stroke. The symptoms are described as a matter of clinical, scientific fact, not of personal experience. You might be thinking, "Perhaps this is not all bad. A general description helps a health professional learn what to expect when a patient has had a cerebral hemorrhage." The danger lies in accepting the textbook description as "fact" or the truth as opposed to just one more interpretation of what a CVA is and means to individual patients. To assist you in scrutinizing the narratives you encounter in clinical practice, turn now to some basic concepts from narrative theory.

Awareness of Literary Form in Your Communication

When you see a poem on a page, even if you do not know anything about poetry, you recognize it as a poem because of its form and structure (i.e., the way it looks on the page). Because it is a poem, you also know that the words the poet chose are important. In poetry, every word matters. It is unlikely that you look at the writing in your textbooks, even this one, in the same way. Yet any type of written communication (whether on paper or digital) has a form and structure, subtle or obvious. By paying attention to these aspects of the various types of written communication you encounter in clinical practice, you can develop an appreciation for how language is used and its impact on your thinking and behavior. Two assumptions from narrative theory applicable to narratives encountered in health care are that (1) language is not transparent and (2) language does not reflect the whole reality of what is going on.

LANGUAGE IS NOT TRANSPARENT

The language of narrative does not function like a clear glass that lets messages pass between sender and receiver. In other words, it is not transparent.[14] No language is neutral or "colorless." This is true of any narrative, whether it is a story, a case study, or an article in a scholarly, professional journal. Scientific writing (this includes the writing in a patient's health record) does not call attention to itself the way language does in a poem, play, or novel. As you saw in the sample entries in the medical record of the patient who had the CVA, there were no metaphors, similes, or figures of speech. The nurse did not write, "I walked into the room and found the patient sobbing his heart out." The physical therapist didn't note, "The patient is as helpless as a newborn kitten." Yet if the nurse and therapist used this type of language, we would understand what they meant regarding the patient's grief and vulnerability. Professional writing in health care is devoid of these kinds of richer descriptions, but it is based on and created in a particular context for a particular purpose. The closest we get to an emotion in the nurses' notes is in the phrase "Pt. found tearful" or the physical therapist's observation "Pt. teary," but there is no mention of grief, loss, or frustration, just the fact that tears are present. However, the decision of the nurse and the physical therapist to mention the tears in their notes indicates that the emotional state of the patient is as important to them as his physical condition.

In Chapter 10 you will discover that one skill you must learn in your professional preparation is to write in a technical, objective manner to communicate with other professionals. Robert Coles describes an interaction with one of his teachers when he was in medical school. Although it involves physicians in training, it is applicable to all health professions. "He remarked that first-year medical students often obtain textured and subtle autobiographical accounts from patients and offer them to others with enthusiasm and pleasure, whereas fourth-year medical students or house officers are apt to present cryptic, dryly condensed, and, yes, all too 'structured'

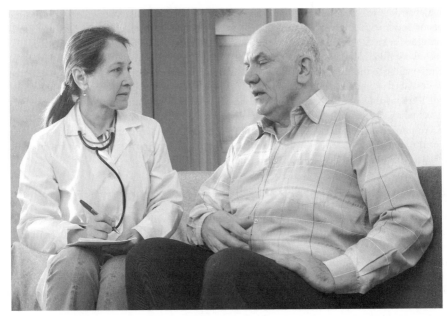

Fig. 7.1 A health professional listening while a patient shares his story. (© JackF/iStock/Thinkstock.com.)

presentations, full of abbreviations, not to mention medical or psychiatric jargon. No question: The farther one climbs the ladder of medical education, the less time one has for relaxed, storytelling reflection."[15] How and what one writes or conveys verbally about the patient's story of illness or injury is a choice and should be a conscious one. Although you need to learn enough jargon to know what colleagues are saying, you do not have to be limited by it. Rita Charon, a general internist trained in literary theory, does not begin patient interactions with a battery of questions. Instead, she begins her interactions this way (Fig. 7.1):

> *I find that I have changed my routines on meeting with new patients. I simply say, "I'm going to be your doctor. I need to know a lot about your body and your health and your life. Please tell me what you think I should know about your situation." And patients do exactly that—in extensive monologues, during which I sit on my hands so as not to write or reflexively call up their medical record on the computer. I sit and pay attention to what they say and how they say it: the forms, the metaphors, the gaps and silences. Where will be the beginning? How will symptoms intercalate with life events?[16]*

REFLECTIONS

- Why do you think Charon states she has to "sit on her hands" while the patient is telling his or her story?
- What is the hardest part of listening to a patient's story for you? Why?

LANGUAGE CREATES REALITY

Rather than reflecting reality, language creates reality.[14] For example, without thinking much about it, most health professionals would say that a patient's history in a medical record states the case as it is. In other words, the history is simply recorded observation. Yet the language used creates the reality of the case insofar as it frames the kinds of questions we ask about it, how we seek answers, and how we interpret what we find. It also sets limits on what we observe or even consider. Refer to the structure of the physical therapist's notes. Did you know what the letters S, O, A, and P that preceded the physical therapist's entries meant? The SOAP charting method is one way to record information in clinical records. The words being abbreviated by SOAP are *subjective* (usually a direct quotation from the patient), *objective* (the health professional's observations or description of the situation), *assessment* (the health professional's interpretation of the situation), and *plan* (actions to be taken to solve the problem presented).[17] The opening step in SOAP charting, subjective, involves interpretation on the part of the health professional because a choice is made about which quote to include among the many things a patient might say. The quote is an important choice because it is a springboard for the rest of the entry. Furthermore, the whole structure of SOAP charting requires one to think of patients as individuals with problems that need professional resolution, which shapes our thinking about the patient and what we attend to in our interactions.

Language also can be used to exclude others. A clinical ethicist noted this manipulation of language on medical rounds:

> *As I began to watch this process more carefully, it became apparent that the physicians spoke a language which was quite understandable when they thought the ethical issues were fairly clear and where there would probably be some consensus but resorted to high code when they felt uncomfortable with the decision(s) before them or when there was dissent in the group.[18]*

So, when things were easy and comfortable within the group, everyone spoke the same language. When things got tough, the physicians switched to a technical language that allowed them to distance themselves from the discussion and enabled them to dominate it as well.

The use of extremely technical language, or "high code," creates an atmosphere that prevents people who do not understand the key to the code from participating in the conversation. In addition, scientific language and technical information are more often highly valued than what the patient has to say, as poet and physician Jack Coulehan notes:

> *Witness the time devoted on rounds to discussing serum magnesium levels as compared to the time spent discussing the patient's experiences. When the patient's narrative (variously called "subjective," "qualitative," or "soft" data) conflicts with laboratory or radiographic findings (considered "objective," "quantitative," "hard" data), the narrative is usually given the lesser weight; it might well be ignored or minimized and the patient attacked for being a "poor historian."[19]*

Although the language may vary from profession to profession, generally speaking, the health professional's language tends to prevail over that of the patient.

Contributions of Literature to Respectful Interaction

Health care practice is a rich metaphor for so many archetypal human dramas, featuring such riveting themes as life and death, loss and hope, and love and hate. All of these human experiences and emotions play out in different scripts, some meaningful and others trivial, each experience providing its own opportunity for wonder at the infinite capacity for human invention. There is an increasing emphasis on the use of literature, a specific type of narrative, in health professions education. A recent study by Doherty, Chan, and Knab[20] evaluated students' attitudes about a literary account of an illness experience and if they applied lessons from a common fictional reading to the delivery of patient-centered care. Several themes emerged from this narrative learning experience. Those with significance to the health professional and patient interaction include seeing family members as stakeholders, applying lessons to clinical practice to better see the patient as a person, and taking alternative perspectives to step into the shoes of the patient.[20] The premise is that studying literature about illness, death, or caregiving will help you, the student, relate more personally to patients, hear patients' stories more clearly, and make decisions that reflect a humane appreciation of patients' situations.[21] Reading novels, stories, plays, and poetry is a means of participating imaginatively in other lives; it encourages you to construct your own stories in relation to the ones you are reading. Consequently, you will come to know yourself better, too.

LITERARY TOOLS

Narrative literature, and by this we mean language used in an intensified, artistic manner, can be used to offer a fresh way for you to understand the encounter between health professional and patient. You can use some simple literary tools such as point of view, characterization, plot, and motivation to examine narrative literature and, as you have seen, the usual types of narrative writing in health care communication, such as the patient's medical record, consultants' reports, and even interprofessional clinical rounds in the hospital.

Point of View

Point of view is a good place to begin when reading any type of literature because it gives you an immediate sense of who is speaking to you through the poem or story. As you think about point of view, here is a simple question to get you started: Who is the narrator of the piece? Put more simply, who is telling the story? In a health record, the point of view is always third person. Health professionals talk about the patient in the third person, even avoiding pronouns whenever possible; that is, the patient is referred to as "Pt." and not as "him" or "her." In the excerpt from *Harrison's Principles of Internal Medicine,* 18th edition, that described a CVA earlier in this chapter, the point of view is that of an omniscient, authoritative narrator but one who is almost invisible. The personal voice is deeply hidden in scientific and professional writing, yet it is there and exudes authority.

Characterization

Also in stories that engage us, characters bring their whole intricate selves to the story. For instance, if the character in a story or a drama is a physical therapist, you will also learn that he is a son, maybe a husband and father, a friend, and a softball coach. You may also learn that he smokes and has tried to quit many times, cheats at cards, and loves pizza. As the narrative unfolds, you appreciate how multiple, often conflicting, interests and identities figure in the twists and turns of his motivations and decisions. You follow along, getting the feel of his prejudices, fears, passions, and pains. Then, if you are lucky, the magic of transference will take you on a journey into the story and eventually into the byways of your own life, but from some new and different angle. The lived quality of narrative is what makes it plausible. "I could be him," feels the reader. "I've been there, too." On the other hand, some characterizations can cause discomfort, which can teach us about our "unspoken, unacknowledged, and often unknown fears, biases and prejudices."[22] As you studied in the discussion of transference in Chapter 2, learning about what makes you uncomfortable is equally valuable as the characters or principles that you identify with when reading a novel, short story, or play. All of this knowledge has implications for your interactions with patients who may be similar to you or very different from you.

Plot and Motivation

Narratives of clinical interest tend toward plot in their structure rather than the more basic narrative of a simple story. In his oft-cited work, *Aspects of the Novel,* E.M. Forster explains the difference between a simple story and a plot: "in a story we say 'and then—and then' . . . in a plot we say 'why'?"[23] Why do the people in a clinical narrative make certain choices and act in specific ways? You can examine the motives of the individuals in clinical narratives in the same way you can those of characters in a short story or novel. Once again, you may have to try harder to find motivation in clinical narratives because so much work goes into hiding the feelings or emotional reactions of health professionals. Even emotional outbursts by patients are written to appear objective and "clinical." Consider the "plan" portion of the nurse's note presented earlier in the chapter: "Continue to support pt.; consult with speech, occupational, and physical therapy as needed; use every encounter to support communication; obtain picture board; remind pt. to attend to L arm and leg affected by sensory alteration."

REFLECTIONS

- What can you discern regarding feelings in the plan portion of the nurse's notes?
- Is there any indication of the feelings or emotional reactions of the nurse?

POETRY

Literature written from the patient's perspective is particularly helpful to health professionals to gain insights into the illness or disability experience. Poetry is one form of literature that deliberately calls attention to the specific words in the poem, as well as how the words are placed on the page. There are many definitions of poetry, but the following description of poetry perhaps captures it best: "Poetry gives pleasure first, then truth, and its language is charged, intensified, concentrated."[24] The following poem explores the poet's experiences as a patient with a colostomy. We suggest that you read the poem at least twice before reading the questions to help you appreciate it. After you have read through the poem, you should be able to recognize who is speaking, what his situation is, and to whom he is speaking. These are just a few questions to help you begin to understand the poem and find meaning to take away to help you in clinical practice.

A RARE AND STILL SCANDALOUS SUBJECT
From Susan Sontag's *Illness as Metaphor*

The title of my confession
is "Colostomy." The word,
cured and salted,
sizzles on my tongue.

This is shame:
standing naked at the sink,
unsnapping the adhesive flange
from my abdomen.

I couldn't have imagined
the stoma, the opening,
red glistening intestine.
Peristalsis moves it like a caterpillar, hatched
from a visceral cocoon.

My life depends on the stoma,
which insists on gratitude,
gurgling, "Listen to me,"
but I place my hand over it,
even now when I am alone.
—R. Solly[25]

REFLECTIONS

- Before reading on, take each stanza in turn. What mood is the author trying to convey?
- Refer to the poem's title, "A Rare and Still Scandalous Subject." The title is taken from a book by Susan Sontag. What is the "subject" in the title the poet is talking about?
- What is it like for the narrator of the poem to live with a colostomy?
- Why is the poem a "confession"?

SHORT STORIES

A short story should be complete, which means it should have a beginning, a middle, and an ending. Stories should also have proportion (i.e., the parts of the story should be in proportion to one another). Generally, more time is devoted to the beginning than the ending. Finally, a story should be compact. Every incident in a story must point to a solution, favorable or unfavorable, to the problem introduced at the beginning of the story.[26] The same literary tools that apply to poetry also apply to fiction. It is important to understand that the narrator in both poetry and fiction is not necessarily the author. Authors can create narrators who are more or less involved in the story and more or less reliable. Consider the following short story about a nurse and long-time patient in an intensive care unit.

Morning Visitors

Mr. Johnson doesn't look so good today. I noticed it as soon as I walked into the room this morning. As I go through his chart, all the numbers are the same. His vital signs and his laboratory results are all rock stable. He's been here a long time, not looking very good, but today he looks a little greener or bluer or whiter, or something. Perhaps the smell in the room has changed, or the ventilator sounds a little more high-pitched. I can't put my finger on what it is, but something is different . . . . His immobile features give me no clues for what's giving me this sense of deterioration.

Even in a coma he seems to be maintaining a dignified expression. I imagine him saying, "Don't worry, dear, I'm fine," but I feel uneasy as I go about his familiar morning care and medications. He looks like such a nice man, and he would no doubt be mortified by the spectacle of his stuffing coming out, as he leaks onto the bed like a sawdust doll.

Mrs. Johnson, the wife, is very gracious and soft-spoken. Her clothes are elegant and her hair is always beauty-parlor perfect. Her face is wrinkled but still beautiful, and her eyes are clear blue. She comes in every day and asks the same questions. Things don't change much. She stands quietly by his bed, always refusing to sit down, and squeezes his hand.

I recognize the even sound of her heels before she enters the room. I've fixed him up to look nice for her visit, but he still looks below par. She enters, scans the room, and then looks as though she smells smoke. We discuss his lungs, his vital signs, the plan of the day, the usual things. There is no concrete change to offer her, as we look at each other's worried faces.

"I don't know why, but he doesn't look as good today," I finally say.

"No, he doesn't. He looks sadder today," she says positively.

She goes to take her place by the bed, and I take my cue to leave the room for awhile. She always leaves at the same time, before the next round of medications and treatments. She wouldn't dream of being a bother.

I imagine the two of them going out for dinner, probably to a nice place where they know the owners and order the same dishes each time. They eat slowly, drink slowly, talk quietly, enjoy each other's company . . . . He squeezes her hand under the table.

The consciousness in Mr. Johnson's brain is like an eel languidly *S*-ing through smooth dark weeds. A few rays of light from the water's surface make little spotlights on the sea bottom, but mostly the eel *S*-es along in dull monotonous ecstasy.

A cluster of neurons in the frontal lobe simultaneously galvanize themselves for the struggle to be Mr. Johnson. "I am not an eel!" they cry. Mr. Johnson floats to the surface. One lidless eye just manages to break the surface tension of the water and take in the upper world. A spaghetti of plastic tubing threaded through a bank of blinking pumps is above his head, and the tubing snakes toward his head and chest. His chest is being mechanically inflated with bigger whooshes of air than feel comfortable.

Mr. Johnson gasps like a fish beached on a merry-go-round. The ventilator shrieks in outrage at having its cycle thrown out of phase. His vital signs climb upward on the monitor until the alarms are all going off.

Mr. Johnson's bedside is usually a harmonious humming of happy machines, but right now all the alarms are going off. I scurry over to see what's going on and I'm happy to see that his vital signs have gone up instead of down. I walk closer to his bed and see one eye is barely open and darting around like a sardine. His body tenses up and one arm stirs, just a little. The hand on the awakened arm starts groping around.

I take and squeeze his hand, partly to keep it from grabbing any of the equipment, and speak directly into his good ear.

"Mr. Johnson, you're in the intensive care unit." His eye darts toward me and stays but looks unfocused.

"You've been here about a month. Your heart is healing. You're doing okay. Your wife comes every day to be with you. She just left."

These are the most encouraging things I can say without lying.

"Mr. Johnson, can you squeeze my hand?"

He squeezes my hand spasmodically, and then he suddenly looks gray and exhausted. His hand and arm go limp, his eye closes, and his vital signs sink back down to their usual numbers.

Mr. Eel Johnson sinks back to the sea bottom. He thrashes around a moment and then goes back to S-ing through the smooth dark weeds.[27]

REFLECTIONS

- From this short story, what do you know about the narrator of the story?
- Did he or she treat Mr. Johnson with respect? Why or why not?
- What emotions and reactions is the author trying to evoke in you, and how is this accomplished?
- The author uses strong imagery in the story, the ocean floor and sea creatures, to contrast with the clinical images of intensive care. What insights do these images provoke?
- The machines in the intensive care unit react with emotion. Why would the author use such a device? What does it tell you about the use of technology in cases like Mr. Johnson's?

The story form of narrative expands beyond the basic facts of most health care interactions into the experience of the event, creating an opportunity for reflection on your reaction to challenging patients, especially those like Mr. Johnson who cannot verbally communicate.

ILLNESS STORIES/PATHOGRAPHIES

A third type of literary narrative is the *pathography*, a form of autobiography or biography that describes personal experiences of illness, treatment, and sometimes death. "What it is like to have prostate cancer," or "How I live with multiple sclerosis," or "What it means to have AIDS" are examples of the typical subjects of pathography that help us understand the experience of illness and endow it with meaning.[28] Some pathographies have developed on the Internet on discussion forums or blogs. The "Leukemia" narrative is one example of an electronic narrative in a discussion group format that evolved from an introductory post in 1991 from Phil Catalfo, the father of a 7-year-old son, Gabe, who was diagnosed with leukemia. The discussion group on the WELL (Whole Earth 'Lectronic Link) health conference site allowed for an ongoing discussion between Phil Catalfo, who interpreted his son's illness experience and his own experience as a father of a terminally ill child, and numerous respondents who added to the story as it continued through the course of Gabe's illness and eventual death. The whole discussion is archived on the WELL site.[29] The Internet allows for, and perhaps encourages, this type of interactive and public form of a pathography.

Refer to the quote by Judith Hooper that opened this chapter. Hers is not the usual description of a patient's experience with chemotherapy after breast cancer surgery. Hooper's pathography from which this quote is taken would probably be characterized as an "angry pathography," even though it is laced with sarcastic humor. In angry pathographies, the author expresses frustrations and disappointments with the health care system in general and with particular programs or health professionals. Pathographies can be satirical or more commonly, of the the testimonial type, in which the author offers uplifting advice and guidance to others who are faced with the same disorder or problem that they, seemingly, have conquered. A particularly interesting form of pathography are those written by health professionals who become patients. The insights gained by health professionals who are patients are often dramatic as in this account by a radiologist who was diagnosed with stage IV lymphoma. Here is her account about a relatively minor issue from a health professional's perspective and how she sees it now that she is the patient.

> *Innocently, I had always thought that once a port is in, getting injected through the port would feel the same as injecting IV tubing after the IV is in place—i.e., painless. Unfortunately, the port is under a tiny layer of skin which has lots of nerve endings. The term "access the port" is a euphemism for "I'm going to take a dagger and stab you in the heart." No local anesthesia of any kind—no injection, no cream, no freezing spray, nothing. It made me appreciate how much pain patients go through with the procedures we inflict on them.[30]*

Pathographies offer you yet another type of narrative to help you understand your patients and their struggles.

Where Stories Intersect

After exploring all the various ways a story can be told, you might wonder: "What is the true story?" The health professional must listen carefully to the patient's story but also understand that the patient does not know the "whole truth" either. There are clearly differences between the patient's experience and the health care professional's explanation of the experience. So how do we get coherence, if not the true story? The first step to a coherent, richer account could be to recognize the dialogical nature of narrative as Frank affirms:

> *We tell stories that sound like our own, but we do not make up or tell our stories by ourselves; they are always co-constructions. Stories we call our own draw variously on cultural narratives and on other people's stories; these stories are then reshaped through multiple retellings. The responses to these retellings further mold the story until its shape is a history of the relationships in which it has been told.[6]*

The kind of exchange described by Frank among a patient, health professionals, and family members produces a fuller interpretation of the patient's story than any one person could produce, including the richest account a patient could offer.[31-33] Certainly viewing the interview process as "building" a history rather than "taking" a history from a patient is a step in the right direction. Building suggests collaboration and the positive outcome of mutual work rather than taking something from the patient and making it your own.[34]

Summary

Literary explorations of the subjective and interpersonal responses of patients, family members, and health professionals to the tensions encountered in health care settings can engage you in your own personal questions and reflections about your response to similar situations in professional practice. Narrative, in all its forms, offers a way of seeing the deeper, subtle nuances involved in your interactions with patients, families, and peers, thereby improving the chances that the opportunities for showing them due respect are not missed or behaviors misguided.

Your role in your patients' stories will vary from assisting them to recover to witnessing their deaths. Whatever roles you take, recall that you also bring your own unfolding story to the relationship. You will build a story with each patient you encounter that becomes another part of the unfolding narrative of both of your lives.

References

1. Hooper J. Beauty tips for the dead. In: Foster P, ed. *Minding the Body: Women Writers on Body and Soul.* New York: Anchor Books; 1994.
2. Donald A. The words we live in. In: Greenhalgh T, Hurwitz B, eds. *Narrative Based Medicine: Dialogue and Discourse in Clinical Practice.* London: BMJ Books; 1998.
3. Churchill LR, Churchill SW. Storytelling in the medical arenas: the art of self-determination. *Lit Med.* 1982;1:73–79.
4. Hatem D, Rider EA. Sharing stories: narrative medicine in an evidence-based world. *Patient Educ Couns.* 2004;54:251–253.
5. Hunter KM. *Doctors' Stories: the Narrative Structure of Medical Knowledge.* Princeton, NJ: Princeton University Press; 1991.
6. Frank AW. From suspicion to dialogue: relations of storytelling in clinical encounters. *Med Humanit Rev.* 2000;14(1):24–34.
7. Bruner J. *Acts of Meaning.* Cambridge, MA: Harvard University Press; 1990.
8. Sharf BF, Vanderford ML. Illness narratives and the social construction of health. In: Thompson T, Dorsey A, Miller K, Parrott R, eds. *Handbook of Health Communication.* Mahwah, NJ: Lawrence Erlbaum; 2003:9–34.
9. Charon R. *Narrative Medicine: Honoring Stories of Illness.* New York: Oxford University Press; 2006.
10. Robinson JA, Hawpe L. Narrative thinking as a heuristic process. In: Sarbin TR, ed. *Narrative Psychology: The Storied Nature of Human Conduct.* New York: Praeger; 1986.
11. Little ME. *Stranger in the Mirror.* Bloomington, IN: Author House; 2006.
12. Greenhalgh T, Hurwitz B. Why study narrative? In: Greenhalgh T, Hurwitz B, eds. *Narrative Based Medicine: Dialogue and Discourse in Clinical Practice.* London: BMJ Books; 1998.
13. Smith WS, English JD, Johnston SC: Chapter 370. Cerebrovascular diseases. In: Longo DL, Fauci AS, Kasper DL, Hauser SL, Jameson JL, Loscalzo J, eds. *Harrison's principles of internal medicine.* 8th ed. Retrieved February 20, 2017, from http://www.accessmedicine.com/content.aspx?aID=9145753.
14. Donley C. Whose story is it anyway? The roles of narratives in health care. *Trends Health Care Law Ethics.* 1995;10(4):27–31.
15. Coles R. *The Call of Stories: Teaching and the Moral Imagination.* Boston: Houghton Mifflin; 1989.
16. Charon R. Narrative medicine: attention, representation, affiliation. *Narrative.* 2005;13:261–270.
17. Weed LL. Medical records that guide and teach. *N Engl J Med.* 1998;278:593–600.
18. Rogers J. Being skeptical about medical humanities. *J Med Humanit.* 1995;16(4):265–277.
19. Coulehan J. Pearls, pith, and provocation: teaching the patient's story. *Qual Health Res.* 1992;2(3):358–366.
20. Doherty RF, Chan P, Knab M. Getting on the same page: an interprofessional common reading program as foundation for patient-centered care. *J Interprof Care.* 2018;20:1–8.
21. Davis C. Poetry about patients: hearing the nurse's voice. *J Med Humanit.* 1997;18(2):111–125.
22. Wear D, Aultman JM. The limits of narrative: medical student resistance to confronting inequality and oppression in literature and beyond. *Med Educ.* 2005;39:1056–1065.
23. Forster EM. *Aspects of the Novel.* New York: Harcourt, Brace; 1927.
24. Drury J. *Creating Poetry.* Cincinnati: Writers' Digest Books; 1991.

25. Solly R. A rare and still scandalous subject. (Unpublished. Reprinted with permission of the author.)
26. Mueller L, Reynolds JD. *Creative Writing: Forms and Techniques*. Lincolnwood, IL: National Textbook; 1992.
27. Shay E. Morning visitors in Cortney Davis and Judy Schaefer. In: *Between the Heartbeats: Poetry and Prose by Nurses*. Iowa City: University of Iowa Press; 1995:169–171.
28. Hawkins AH. *Reconstructing Illness: Studies in Pathography*. West Lafayette, IN: Purdue University Press; 1993.
29. Catalfo P: Leukemia, introductory posting (16 January 1991), topic originally numbered 453, health conference, the WELL (Whole Earth 'Lectronic Link). Retrieved December 19, 2011, from http://www.well.com.
30. Liberman L. *I Signed as the Doctor: Memoir of a Cancer Doctor Surviving Cancer*. 2009. Booklocker.com.
31. Poirier S, Rosenblum L, Ayres L, et al. Charting the chart—an exercise in interpretation(s). *Lit Med*. 1992;11(1):1–22.
32. Brody H. "My story is broken, can you help me fix it?" Medical ethics and the joint construction of narrative. *Literature Med*. 1994;13(Spring):85–87.
33. Manoogian MM, Harter LM, Denham SA. The storied nature of health legacies in the familial experience of type 2 diabetes. *J Fam Communic*. 2010;10:40–56.
34. Haidet P, Paterniti DA. "Building" a history rather than "taking" one: a perspective on information sharing during the medical interview. *Arch Intern Med*. 2003;163:1134–1140.

Respect for the Patient's Family and Significant Relationships

Prelude

A special pattern of communication developed between Robin and Mark (her father) during his hospitalization. Each morning Mark phoned home to tell her about the animal picture on the sugar packet that he had saved from his breakfast tray. One morning Robin explained to Mark that she had a cold, and then, with 3-year-old directness, asked, "What do you have, Daddy?"

After a pause he replied, "I have cancer."

She handed the phone to me and said, "I think Daddy's crying." Though he had never hesitated to discuss his illness with others who asked, he was deeply shaken by the weight of Robin's question and the implications of his answer.

S.A. ALBERTSON[1]

In this excerpt from a book portraying a young family coping with the fatal illness of a father and husband, we suddenly see a moment when the patient breaks down unexpectedly, touched deeply by the implications of his beloved young daughter's innocent question. The personal life of a patient exists in a web of activities and intimate or close personal relationships that help provide status, meaning, support, and a sense of belonging to this person. Respect for this fact is immensely important if you are to reach the goal of maintaining the patient's dignity and achieving a truly caring response during your professional interactions with him or her.

This chapter focuses attention on patient relationships and family. In today's society, the patient identifies who "family" is and determines how they will participate in his or her care and decision-making. In times of illness or injury, a patient's relationships with family, close friends, business associates, neighbors, and others who are important to the patient are greatly affected. Special attention in this chapter is devoted to family members or other persons who become caregivers for the patient because their relationship is often dramatically challenged by the new situation. We offer suggestions about how and when you can become a source of support and encouragement to a patient and those close to them as they go through stressful and often difficult times.

Family: An Evolving Concept

In the past, mainstream health care in the United States focused exclusively on the patient as the sole recipient of care. It was not commonplace to attend to families as the focus of care. Today we know how important it is to care for patients, especially youth and elders, in the context of their families. The family is implicitly and explicitly recognized as a critical context surrounding and influencing its members and, in turn, being influenced by its members. Care can best be accomplished if it is considered a collaborative venture between the family and the interprofessional care team. Patient and family-centered care is "an approach to the planning, delivery, and evaluation of health care that is grounded in mutually beneficial partnerships among health care providers, patients, and families."[2] This approach leads to better health outcomes, improved patient and family care experiences, increased clinician satisfaction, and wiser allocation of resources.[3,4] The components of patient and family-centered care in Box 8.1 provide a context for recognizing the family's central role. If you are to work with families as collaborators in maintaining the health of family members who are ill, injured, or impaired, you must understand how families define themselves, how they function, and how best to interact with them.

Family Defined

The term *family* has been defined in a variety of ways. How would you define family? It is safe to say that your notion of what constitutes a family is influenced by your values, culture, upbringing, and professional perspective. The most common type of familial bond is through spousal and

---

BOX 8-1 ■ Core Concepts of Patient- and Family-Centered Care

- *Dignity and Respect.* Health care practitioners listen to and honor patient and family perspectives and choices. Patient and family knowledge, values, beliefs, and cultural backgrounds are incorporated into the planning and care delivery.
- *Information Sharing.* Health care practitioners communicate and share complete and unbiased information with patients and families in ways that are affirming and useful. Patients and families receive timely, complete, and accurate information in order to effectively participate in care and decision-making.
- *Participation.* Patients and families are encouraged and supported in participation in care and decision-making at the level they choose.
- *Collaboration.* Patients and families are also included on an institution-wide basis. Health care leaders collaborate with patients and families in policy and program development, implementation, and evaluation; in health care facility design; and in professional education, as well as in the delivery of care

Reprinted with permission from the Institute for Patient- and Family-Centered Care: http://www.ipfcc.org.

blood relationships. Families may include several generations of blood kin, a mix of stepparents and children, or a combination of friends who share in household responsibilities and childrearing. One area of growth in family units is same-gendered parents, and one change has been the shift from nuclear to extended families.

As society evolves through scientific and social advances, it must redefine what is meant by "family." New Mexico's Memorial Task Force on Children and Families and the Coalition for Children offer the following definition:

We all come from families. Families are big, small, extended, nuclear, multigenerational, with one parent, two parents and grandparents. We live under one roof or many. A family can be as temporary as a few weeks, as permanent as forever. We become part of a family by birth, adoption, marriage, or from a desire for mutual support. As family members, we nurture, protect, and influence one another. Families are dynamic and are cultures unto themselves, with different values and unique ways of realizing dreams. Together, our families become the source of our rich cultural heritage and spiritual diversity. Each family has strengths and qualities that flow from individual members and from the family as a unit. Our families create neighborhoods, communities, states, and nations.[5]

REFLECTIONS

- Who are the members of your family?
- Name two ways your family contributes to your health and two ways your family distracts from your health.
- If you were acutely ill, which member of your family would you call first and why? How does this family member support you in your day-to-day life?

A definition of family should be inclusive and allow the members to define themselves as a family unit, acknowledging the variety of cultural styles, values, and alternative structures that are part of contemporary family life. In fact, families define a unique culture—that is, a unique behavioral complex that is socially created, readily transmitted to family members, and potentially maintained through generations.[6]

Family Structure and Function

Family structure and function have important influences on health. Family structure involves the characteristics that make a family unique. This includes family composition and household roles. According to the latest U.S. Census, the average household size was 2.58. Of the households, 33% included people under 18 years, and 25% included people 65 years and over. Multigenerational family households (three generations of relatives or more living together) are on the rise, as are unmarried partner households.[7]

To work with families, you also must understand how families function. An individual's physical and emotional health and cognitive/social functioning is strongly influenced by how well the family functions.[8,9] There are numerous family theories describing how families operate and how they respond to events both internal and external. Most health professionals use a combination of family theories in their work with families, but all have in common the fact that the focus of health care shifts from the individual member who is ill, injured, or disabled to the family as a unit of care. In this chapter, we focus on a particular method of viewing the family—the family health system approach.[10] According to this approach, care is directed toward five processes: (1) interactive, (2) developmental, (3) coping, (4) integrity, and (5) health. The Case Study of Ian will help show how the family health system model applies to a particular child and his family.

Case Study

Ian is a low-birth-weight infant with short bowel syndrome (SBS). SBS is characterized by maldigestion, malabsorption, dehydration, electrolyte abnormalities, and both macronutrient and micronutrient deficiencies. Owing to new multidisciplinary approaches and advances in medical and surgical treatments, the SBS survival rate has improved from an average of 70%, to as high as 90% in recent studies.[11] Ian will require long-term parenteral nutrition (PN); that is, he will not be able to take food orally and will be dependent on intravenous solution to provide the bulk of his nutritional needs. Ian is the first child of Dylan and Adrianna Chapel, both in their early 30s. After a stay in the neonatal intensive care unit, Ian was sent home with his parents, who have provided care since that time with the help of a home care agency and a nutritional support company. The Chapels do not have other family members nearby. Most of Ian's care falls to them.

Ian is now an active 2-year-old. Mrs. Chapel is the primary caregiver during the day and most evenings. She works weekends as a nursing assistant at a local assisted living center to supplement their family income. Mr. Chapel works as a paralegal in a law firm and attends law school at night. The Chapels' insurance coverage is through a group plan at the law firm where Mr. Chapel works.

Assume you are assigned to work with the Chapel family during an on-site educational experience with the home care agency providing primary care. The goal of your interaction with Ian and his family is to help promote family adaptation to his chronic condition (SBS) and empower the Chapels to develop and maintain healthy lifestyles. By reviewing the five processes listed earlier, you can get a picture of the family's functioning and possible areas for intervention.

INTERACTIVE PROCESS

The *interactive* process of the family is composed of communication, family relationship, and social supports.[10] In your assessment of the interactive process of the Chapel family, you will explore the types of communication patterns they use; the effect of Ian's illness on the communication of the family both internally and externally; the types of relationships within the family; and the quality, timing, amount, and nature of social support they receive. Open communication should be encouraged. One aspect of care could be to assist the Chapels in mobilizing the informational and emotional support they need to cope with Ian's illness. Because the Chapels do not have family support in the immediate community, they may have to rely on informal support systems, such as friends and co-workers, and formal support systems, such as respite care agencies, to assist them in the care of their child. Perhaps there are other children who have SBS or who must rely on parenteral nutrition in the community. The caregivers of such children may have or could form a support group to help troubleshoot common problems and offer advice.

DEVELOPMENTAL PROCESS

Assessment of the developmental process includes the family developmental stage and individual developmental stages. The Chapels, as a family, are in the second stage of family development as described by Duvall in his classic work.[12] Stage II of the family life cycle involves integrating an infant into the family unit, accommodating to new parenting roles, and maintaining the marital bond. Ian is moving from infancy to becoming a toddler, and soon he will be increasingly interested in his environment and want to explore it. Ian will become increasingly mobile and develop language during this stage. (You will be introduced to basic development needs of toddlers later in Chapter 11). All of this is influenced by the presence of his chronic condition.

It is appropriate for you as a member of the interprofessional care team to assess how well developmental tasks are being achieved. You will educate the Chapels in the developmental milestones Ian should achieve and the tasks involved. For example, Ian needs freedom of mobility to explore objects in his environment and learn to walk, so his nutritional solution could be placed in a backpack to allow him to move more freely. Children with SBS also may require frequent visits to the bathroom throughout the day when the time comes for toilet training. To decrease the Chapels' frustrations, you could plan for this next developmental milestone and work with them to plan a structured routine that is consistently implemented and results in success for all involved, especially the child. There is some evidence that about 10% to 15% of children with SBS will experience neurological or developmental delays.[13] Thus you will also want to watch for possible developmental delays to plan for early therapeutic interventions.

COPING PROCESS

Coping has been identified as problem-solving, adaptation to stress and crisis, and management of resources.[10] Coping helps us lower our anxiety so that we can meet the demands of the day. Each person has a different coping style when dealing with uncertainty. Coping styles can be both problem focused and emotion focused. In general, coping styles depend on what a person is like as a person and his or her role in the family.[14] The uncertainty of illness presents a variety of stressors for families. In your work with the Chapels, you should assess their ability to handle stress and the impact that Ian's illness has on everyday activities while reinforcing a coping style fitting for them.

REFLECTIONS

Which of these questions would most help you show respect for the Chapels' predicament?
- How do the Chapels conceptualize and manage Ian's diagnosis as a family? What meaning does it have?
- Has Ian's illness caused a change in the family's life plans? For example, did Mrs. Chapel plan on returning to full-time work outside the home after the birth of her son?
- If the family planned on Mrs. Chapel returning to work, can the family adapt to the loss of income, or are support services available to allow Ian to be cared for during the day so that Mrs. Chapel can work?
- Were the Chapels intending to have several children? Have Ian's care needs changed their family planning?
- What else do you want to know to care for the Chapel family?

Overall, you would want to assess how the family deals with crises in general. You can support the Chapels' coping processes by:
1. offering advice on the progression of the illness,
2. discussing the normal feelings of frustration and guilt that accompany the care of a chronically ill or disabled family member, and
3. offering resources to help the family cope more effectively, such as respite care and other support groups.

The Chapels will also have to cope with financial stressors. Even with the best health insurance, there are lifetime limits on coverage; in addition, there are many out-of-pocket expenses related to the care of a child with this diagnosis. Although most children experience small bowel adaptation over time and can be weaned from parenteral nutrition, some children suffer liver dysfunction, and many require extensive intestinal rehabilitation, including intestinal lengthening procedures and transplantation.[11,15] Thus the Chapels may be facing years of out-of-pocket expenses and expensive hospital stays, procedures, and medications. This kind of financial pressure can be stressful for any family.

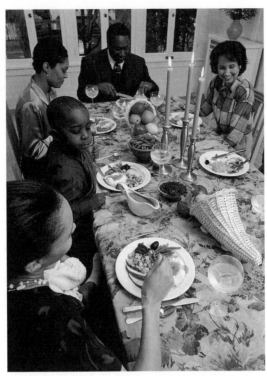

Fig. 8.1 The process of family life involves family values, rituals, history, and identity. (© *Ryan McVay/Photo-disc/Thinkstock.com.*)

INTEGRITY PROCESS

The integrity process of family life involves family values, rituals, history, and identity.[10] These aspects of the family process greatly affect its behavior. Family rituals, one facet of the *integrity* process, provide a useful framework for assessing threats to a family's integrity. Family rituals include celebrations and traditions such as activities surrounding birthdays, religious holidays, or bedtime routines for children (Fig. 8.1). Suggestions for evaluating family rituals include assessment of the following:[16]

- *Does the family underuse rituals?* Families who do not celebrate or mark family changes such as birthdays, deaths, anniversaries, and so forth may be left without some of the benefits that accompany rituals, such as bringing the family together or marking changes in life and family roles.
- *Does the family follow rigid patterns of rituals?* In families who are inflexible, things are always done the same way, at the same time, and with the same people. Families who are rigid may have difficulty responding to changes that disrupt routines and rituals occasioned by illness and injury.
- *Are family rituals skewed?* A family with skewed rituals tends to emphasize only one aspect of family life (e.g., religion) and ignore others. For example, a family might spend all its time celebrating with the father's side of the family on religious holidays and ignore the different rituals cherished by the patterns practiced on the mother's side.
- *Has the ritual process been interrupted?* For example, a child born with a physical or cognitive impairment or congenital condition may threaten family identity and permanently disrupt family rituals. In the case of the Chapels, they have elected to stay home for traditional

family holidays because almost all holidays involve a focus on food. For the foreseeable future, Ian cannot tolerate most food orally, so the Chapels should consider what this interruption in ritual means to their life together and may have to develop other rituals at holiday time that do not focus so prominently on food.

- *Are the rituals hollow?* Rituals performed just for the sake of performing them have lost their life and may be stressful for the family rather than a source of joy and strength.

In addition to changes in ritual that occur over time in families, many role changes also occur, particularly when chronic illness or impairment is involved. For example, Mrs. Chapel has become the primary caregiver. She may or may not have expected to take on this role. Essential interventions include helping the Chapels redefine major family roles and maintain their new responsibilities.

HEALTH PROCESS

The final process of family experience is related to health. This process includes health status, health beliefs and practices, and lifestyle practices.[10] Assessing a family's definition of health and how they define the health of the individual members is a key step in this process.

> **REFLECTIONS**
>
> - Besides the responsibilities involved in caring for a child who requires parenteral feedings, what do the Chapels do to maintain their own health?
> - How do the Chapels deal with health problems? To whom do they turn?

Interventions in the health process include education, encouragement, and counseling regarding the short- and long-term aspects of Ian's care. The situation of Ian and his parents illustrates the family health system as one useful approach to the care of patients and families. The family health system applies to all families, whatever the composition and stage of familial development. You are encouraged to explore other models of working with a family and their effectiveness in achieving optimal family health. Regardless of the model you choose, it is clear that family relationships are an important consideration in understanding the conduct of any patient and for developing an effective mode for respectful interaction with that patient.

Facing the Fragility of Relationships

At this point in your training, you are acutely aware that living with illness or disability is not just an individual journey but one that has a profound impact on a patient's friends and family. Families are deeply influenced by the health and wellness of each member of the familial unit, so any significant change in a person has the power to alter his or her status and roles in various relationships. Like a mobile, when one person in a relationship changes, every component necessarily moves, and everyone must pull together to find a viable new balance point. As patients become aware of changes, they often express concerns of abandonment or fears that they will be unable to contribute to their key relationships in meaningful ways. Whatever else characterizes close relationships during times of illness or injury, one sure thing is that there will be stress. *Stress* usually conjures up only negative feelings, and dictionary definitions support this meaning. But psychologists and others have probed the dynamics of what happens when the stakes are high or the chips are down: Stress is, at its core, a psychological motivator. Stress can have results that are destructive or that enhance individuals and relationships. Rambur and colleagues[17] divide stressful experiences and conditions into negative outcomes of *distress* and positive ones of *eustress*. In this section, we ask you to consider some areas of potential distress with some suggestions for helping all involved to realize eustress opportunities as well.

Among the potential sources of distress during the fragility brought about by change are the patient's concern that others will lose interest in helping to sustain his or her dearest relationships. In some cases, the loss of interest is experienced more fully as actual disdain toward the patient. Loved ones and friends who are thrust into the role of caregiving often grapple with similar concerns.

Concern That Others Will Lose Interest

We all hope that our families, friends, and associates will take our problems to heart—fortunately they usually do. However, sometimes patients are unpleasantly surprised by the degree of indifference they feel many people show to the struggle they went—or are going—through. You know from your own experience that this feeling is not limited to persons who become patients. More generally speaking, it can be dismaying to realize that, no matter what momentous event you have been through or are still experiencing, most people in your life do not want to know much about it!

Others' apparent lack of interest may be due to many reasons. For instance, when there is good news to share, some might be jealous of your good fortune or feel that their security is threatened by your success; when the news is bad, some may be threatened by that, too, thinking, "There but for the grace of God go I." For that matter, some really do not care much in the first place, even though it was easy and enjoyable to show interest when things were moving along in the usual familiar groove.

REFLECTIONS

Almost everyone has experienced the apparent lack of interest in one's good or bad fortune.
- Can you think of an incident in your own life when you were surprised by this?
- How did it make you feel? Describe, if you can, some of the emotions and responses it brought up in you.

In extreme circumstances, most people do turn more inward and become self-absorbed, and patients are no exception. Therefore sometimes a distressed patient becomes extremely boring or demanding, driving others away. Friends and loved ones may assume that the patient no longer really cares about them and lose interest in maintaining the relationship for that reason. As one exhausted wife exclaimed, "I have turned into a service organization! I love Dick but I can't keep this up. He was never demanding like this, and I find myself coming to see him less and less because of it! He panics every time I begin to leave!"

Over the years the authors have learned never to be surprised when a patient or family member suffers a profound emotional blow because of a breakdown of an important relationship. However daunting it may seem, it is always worthwhile to try to offer comfort and hope in such situations. For instance, if you see it coming, you can try to help prepare patients for a disappointment they might encounter if their expectations regarding important relationships seem unrealistic. Just by talking directly to the patient about an obvious absence of someone who previously was present on a regular basis may give the person an opening to discuss his fears or the reality of what is happening. Of course, to pry deeply into the particulars of a patient's intimate or close personal relationships (or the apparent increasing dissolution of one) also can be an unwelcome intrusion into the patient's privacy if the timing is not right. The point is that gentle probing may lead to an opportunity for the patient to talk through and think more expansively about the situation. In fact, sometimes allowing a patient to talk about family, friends, or other social contacts will help him or her start remembering things about the relationships that are treasured and help the patient's focus to turn to strengthening those relationships during this unusual time.

Family members, partners, or friends who become caregivers often go through their own worries about whether others are losing interest in the patient or are becoming indifferent to the negative stresses on the relationship the patient and caregiver(s) are experiencing. Their concerns are founded on their observation that longtime friends and associates are backing off. This seems to be especially true in situations in which the one being cared for has undergone a serious and long-standing change in appearance or abilities.

The social functions and activities that partners, families, and friends enjoy with others often dwindle, isolating the patient and caregivers from familiar sources of enjoyment and their feeling of belonging within their larger communities. The loss of a job can further distance them from longtime associates and patterns. For many it is easier to stay away than to face the hard realities with the affected persons. Internal divisions within families also may erupt, often over differing hopes and expectations about who will take responsibility for various aspects of caregiving. The patient may begin to feel as if he or she has caused all the distress and withdraw further from contributing to the vitality of key relationships.

Shunning by Others

Unfortunately, a special burden falls on relationships when the patient has a condition that carries a social stigma of some sort. Loss of a social life may be accompanied by a loss of status. In most such cases, what appears to be a loss of interest may be an even deeper disdain and rejection. People who have a diagnosis of AIDS are prime examples of such a group who (by virtue of their illness) may lose their social life or job security. Although great strides have been made in the United States and elsewhere to educate about AIDS, and laws and policies have been put in place to prevent discrimination against the person and family, this disease still has the power to marginalize patients and their loved ones from their communities and important relationships.

AIDS is by no means the only condition associated with societal attitudes that may be informing why others appear to be losing interest in a patient and those in close relationship with him or her, or worse, shunning him or her. This attitude is also prevalent in substance use disorders. In fact, social stigma toward individuals with substance use disorders exceeds stigma toward those with mental illnesses or physical disabilities across cultural contexts.[18] Unfortunately, it is also common for health professionals to have negative attitudes toward individuals with substance use disorders, contributing to suboptimal health care.[19] Sometimes people close to the patient are also expected to feel ashamed for accusations that they had a role in allowing, causing, or worsening a patient's predicament. An example was relayed to us by a colleague who was teaching a 2-week summer course in another city when her adult son overdosed. She recalls the following conversation on hearing the news that her son was in the intensive care unit:

Hospitalist: Your son has overdosed and is in the intensive care unit.

Woman: Oh no! What happened?

Hospitalist: [Explains some medical details.] Was he well when you left?

Woman: He seemed fine! We know he struggled with abstinence in the past, but thought it was under control since he has been under the care of the addictions team. [More questions about his condition.]

Hospitalist: His primary care doctor has told me that he has had trouble staying on his treatment program in the past. Has he been attending his check-ins and support group?

Woman (still shaken): I think so! I've been gone for 2 weeks but . . . .

Hospitalist: Oh, yes. Young adults often fall off the wagon when their parents are gone.

The woman said that, whether the doctor was intentionally trying to shame her for not being there when her son overdosed, just by that conversation she was afraid she would be shunned by his professional caregivers when she returned.

What can you do in your role to help decrease the deleterious effects of others' loss of interest or shunning of the patient or loved one? Some straightforward suggestions include:

- Listen to your own comments with a reflective third ear to think about how they might be coming across to the patient or caregivers. Do they sound off-putting? Blaming?
- Facilitate contact with patient and/or family support groups of similarly affected persons.
- Be prospective as a resource, suggesting additional supports available at your worksite such as religious counselors, psychologists, or social workers who are skilled in dealing with the negative stresses caused by the situation.
- Speak up to counter destructive shame-inducing attitudes and behaviors in the larger society.

You may think of other ways to decrease the distress related to both patients and their loved ones who are concerned about real or imagined loss of interest by others or who are feeling shunned and therefore increasingly isolated.

Weathering the Winds of Change

Patients also justifiably worry about other relationship-related effects of serious illness or impairment from injury. Unfortunately, the change a person undergoes during illness or injury may in some cases cause him or her to become almost a stranger to loved ones.[20] In extreme cases, the established patterns of old relationships become unrecognizable in the present situation. For example, a spouse who sustains a traumatic brain injury may act like a child; a longtime business partner with bipolar disorder may become suspicious or abusive toward family, trusted associates, or clients; or a young man known for his bravado may become fearful of hanging out with the guys after a heart attack, convinced they will see him as a has-been.[21]

REFLECTIONS

Think about a relationship you hold dear—and would count on the most—if you were to become a patient with a serious illness or injury.
- What do you think would be your greatest worry in terms of the changes you knew your condition could impose on your loved one?
- List one or two people you could call on to help you and the other person make it through the hard times of such a change.

Now put yourself in the position of a family caregiver for your loved one.
- What type of condition that your loved one might incur would be the greatest challenge to your relationship as it now stands? Why (i.e., what values and behaviors have seemed to sustain the "core" of the relationship during other stressors)?

These types of exercises can help you imagine the challenges and concerns patients and their closest resources are facing and sympathetically acknowledge that most people must navigate stresses in their intimate relationships when one person in it is changed by illness or injury. This recognition is extremely important because all too often the health of family or other caregivers has been ignored to the detriment of everyone involved, especially when the new situation requires an intense, long-term (or even lifelong) commitment. You may ask how important it is for you in your professional caregiver role to gain an understanding of the family or close friend caregiver's situation. The answer is extremely important. The US Department of Health and Human Services estimates that family and friend (called *informal*) caregiver services will be one of the biggest changes this society will see as the baby boomer generation (those born between 1946 and 1964) ages. Informal caregivers provide assistance with a variety of health-related tasks, including assisting family and friends with self-care and other activities of daily living, cooking and home management tasks, transportation, medication management, medical encounters, and financial activities such as bill paying. In 2011 alone, 18 million informal caregivers provided 1.3 billion hours of care monthly to the more than 9 million older adults receiving informal assistance.[22]

The majority of informal caregivers provide care for a relative or loved one. Most family caregivers rise to the occasion with remarkable courage, good spiritedness, and, if all else fails, resignation. Still, study after study reveal that the everyday reality of life for most family caregivers begins with the belief that they have an unbounded obligation by their wedding vows and commitments as parent, spouse/partner, son, or daughter, or "only living relative."[23] Despite this, physical, emotional, and financial demands of caregiving can be high.

Positive outcomes of caregiving include the confidence that one's loved one is well cared for and feeling closer to the recipient.[24] Negative outcomes include consequences to mental and physical health, including:[23,25]

- A frequent occurrence of negative stress-related or distress-related disorders
- Serious physical injury from lifting or lack of good judgment because of exhaustion
- Social isolation
- Increased rates of depression and anxiety
- Increased risk factor for death (especially among older caregivers)

Family members or other informal caregivers who drop out because they literally cannot take it any more often face acute guilt for abandoning their loved one and often find their action another source of shunning by their already dwindling sources of community support. A burgeoning new industry of caregiver supports and technologies, as well as other professional services, is popping up everywhere to provide respite and help support caregivers in these uncompensated roles.

Enduring the Uncertainties

The issues facing close relationships we have been discussing contain elements of uncertainty. This theme is so fundamental that we now turn to uncertainty to consider it directly. At some time in every recovery or adjustment process, a patient's uncertainties loom before him or her (Fig. 8.2). Whenever that happens, the reverberations race through intimate and close personal relationships. As a young child put it to one of the authors, "My sickness is like a ghost that hangs around our house. I'm doing OK, then it can creep up on me and 'Pow!' because I can't see it coming. When that happens everybody in my family has to change their plans." His condition was characterized by roller coaster–like exacerbations and remissions, keeping everyone in suspense about what would be possible for all of them from day to day.

One persistent theme is uncertainty about the unsettling effect of it on the patient's close personal relationships. This manifests itself in many ways that health professionals must be prepared to interpret and try to respond to respectfully. Behavior changes or comments by the patient will often give you clues.

Patients who have dark doubts about what lies ahead may be asking a deeper question, although not always directly: "Will you stay with me through this situation, whatever the outcome?" You can respond by assuring the person that you and your colleagues will do everything you can for her or him within your role. Such a question should also be an opportunity for you to gently explore whether this qualm is coming from uncertainty about whether persons important to the patient will be there at some critical juncture or whether they all will be able to make it through their ordeal without your skilled assistance. What can you do then and there to make a sincere effort to decrease their distress? You can:

- Make time to provide them with as much certainty about their condition and its future course as your own information and role allow.

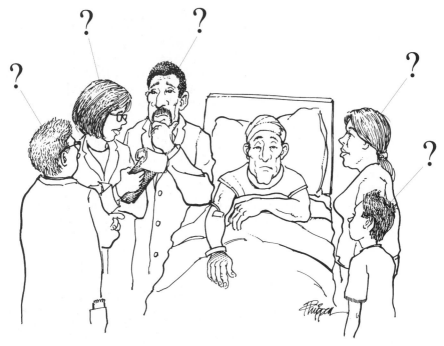

Fig. 8.2 Varying degrees of uncertainty is a problem patients face during recovery or adjustment, and negative stress reverberates into his or her significant relationships, as well as presenting challenges to professional caregivers.

- Collaborate with members of the interprofessional care team, and refer to others who are more qualified to respond to questions.
- Exercise restraint by not giving questionable information, instilling false hope around areas of your own uncertainty. The truth will do. The desire to comfort patients by providing false certainty will lead to their feeling of distrust or betrayal in the long run.
- Assure the patient that although the patient's condition may not improve, you will always care for him or her. When goals of care shift from cure to comfort, patients and families need to know that you will be by their side. Uncertainty can arise around longstanding habits of who makes decisions between a couple or among family members. The Case Study below presents an apt example.

Case Study

Oscar works in a chemical processing plant, his occupation since he was a teenager. He did not get the chance to finish high school because his dad died in a plant accident and he had to become the breadwinner for his mom and three siblings. He says that one of his biggest accomplishments, which "woulda made my dad proud!" was to get his GED in the evening school offered through the plant. His youngest brother, Walter, lives with him and has since their mom died about 20 years ago. Walter was let go from school after the sixth grade on the basis that he was "slow," though Oscar always doubted this "diagnosis." Oscar thought a better explanation is that when Walter lost his baby teeth, his adult teeth never came in. When he tried to talk, the other kids laughed and made fun of him, calling him "grandpa" because so many of the old people in this impoverished town were without teeth or dentures. Walter was in his middle teens by the time anyone mentioned the possibility of dentures to Oscar. A social worker at the local community clinic helped to get the dentures for Walter, but to this day, his childhood experiences have left scars on his personality and self-esteem. Whenever he makes even a small mistake, he suffers, calling himself a "dumbbell." Fortunately, since receiving dentures his pronunciation, nutrition, and appearance have improved.

Oscar was able to get Walter work at the plant, and Walter has done well there. Over the years, his co-workers have grown used to his self-effacing personality, have come to appreciate his hard work and big heart, and know that there is more to him than may meet the eye initially. Oscar watches out for him, too, menacingly confronting anyone who treats Walter disrespectfully.

Over the past several months, Walter has been wheezing. Oscar notes that he is going to bed earlier and earlier, always with some "lame excuse." Some of the guys ask Oscar if Walter is OK because he seems short of breath and is sweating so much. Oscar finally convinces Walter to go to the company clinic. The nurse practitioner who sees Walter and Oscar allows Oscar to stay with Walter while he undergoes tests. However, when the tests come back, the physician asks Oscar to leave the room and shares the bad news with Walter that he has emphysema. He explains that it is in its early stages, and the physicians think that he may benefit from entering a clinical trial of a medication that they hope will help relieve the progressive deleterious symptoms of the condition. Walter is paralyzed by this news, saying that Oscar should make that decision and insists that the doctor tell Oscar everything he has just said. The doctor gently tells Walter that he feels it may be best if Walter makes his own decision.

But Walter grows stony cold and looks distrustful. Once included, Oscar listens authoritatively, saying he will take responsibility for making the decisions about what will happen next and declines the offer of a social worker who would be willing to talk with the brothers. He refuses the literature about the study. They both just laugh when the young physician asks if they would like to talk with a chaplain about this. But later, while Walter is filling out some paperwork, Oscar confides to the nurse practitioner who had seen them together on their initial visit that he knows the physician disagrees with his making the decisions, and he is frightened he might make the wrong one.

Again, when they discuss it among themselves the health care providers are uncertain about what to do, understandably reluctant to turn over the decision-making authority to Oscar for a decision that is so important to Walter's life and well-being. To them, ethically and legally Walter is a competent, middle-aged adult and should be making his own decisions even though both he and his brother seem to assume that Oscar will do so.

REFLECTIONS

- If you were one of the health professionals in this situation, can you think of ways you might bring more certainty into these brothers' understanding of why the professionals are hesitant to accept the decision-making arrangement?
- What, if any, additional information about their relationship would you need to help decrease your team's uncertainty about how to proceed?

The dynamic between Walter and Oscar sometimes can be observed in some cultures and among some older patients. For those in marital relationships, their conviction that the husband "is the boss" and makes the decisions is all that some couples can fathom. For a husband suddenly to be left out of the information loop and lose his decision-making authority role may be extremely disorienting to both parties, adding a new level of uncertainty to an already difficult period in their life together. The actual dynamic of a relationship is not always easy to unravel. For instance, some caregivers of elderly parents may appear to have overridden the patient's self-confidence sufficiently for them to become beholden to the other.

What can health professionals do to decrease the negative stress of their own uncertainties as much as possible when concerns arise over who will speak for the patient?

- Family meetings approved by the patient can become an avenue of fact finding and clarification for all involved.
- Ethics committees or ethics consultants are a mechanism to help navigate situations that the professional caregivers find unethical or illegal and therefore cannot accept.
- Documenting such patient requests in the patient's electronic medical record signals to other members of the health care team why you are relying on someone other than the competent patient in decisions about his or her health care regimen.
- The help of professionals qualified to detect unhealthful relational dynamics should be sought for the benefit of all involved.
- Remind the interprofessional care team that the goal of any such discussion and discernment is not ultimately to decrease your own distress but to do so only when the patient's distress has been fully addressed.

Having reviewed some important uncertainties patients and their loved ones face, as well as the ripple effect of uncertainties you face in such situations, we turn in the next section to economic challenges and how these challenges affect the patient's intimate and important personal relationships.

Close Relationships and Health Care Costs

In today's health care arena, at least in the United States, health care expenditures are largely affected by current law and existing regulatory environments. In recent years, the Patient Protection and Affordable Care Act's expansions of eligibility for Medicaid and the creation of state Marketplaces (in which people can purchase health care coverage) represented some of the largest expansions of health insurance in the United States since the establishment of Medicare and Medicaid in 1965.[26] Despite this, many patients struggle to afford health care, and many of their significant relationships are dramatically affected by costs associated with health care–related expenses.

Some purport that except for the wealthiest today, persons in relationships touched by serious illness or injury are forever more vulnerable to severe financial duress.[27] This may come about by the cost of the initial health care episode, the necessary changes in employment made by the person or family caregiver, or the decreased likelihood of being able to find health insurance coverage for future conditions and ongoing maintenance. An adult's values may include that of being a good provider for those dependent on him or her, but the loss of opportunity to earn money for a time (or permanently) may be compounded by the high cost of medical and other health care bills. Patients who decide to make a highly desirable change in life direction or lifestyle with a loved one may feel prohibited from doing so by the reality of the desperate financial distress the illness or injury has caused.

Their distress may express itself in depression or cause patients to make health care choices you do not understand. It is well known that many instances of so-called nonadherence on the part of patients are occasioned by the cost of medications, treatments, devices, or services. High deductibles and copays often present financial challenges. Patients need to weigh those goods against that same money being spent for food, housing, or other necessities for themselves and their children or others dependent on those resources.

As a health professional, you are in a good position to be an advocate on behalf of patients and their family or other caregivers. Fortunately, many health care educational programs include courses designed to help you understand the financial mechanisms supporting or constraining what you can offer in the way of services and assurances. This can give you some certainty about how, and if, to talk realistically about what is available. Beyond that, what does advocacy entail in such a situation?

1. Inform patients and their caregivers of available institutional resources (e.g., social workers and case managers) who can help them maneuver through the confusing web of bureaucratic procedures they must traverse to receive essential services.
2. Be attuned to community services that patients, families, and others in caregiver relationships with the patient may be able to access.
3. Educate yourself regarding the basic language and concepts of health care financing and how it operates in your area of expertise so you can contribute to discussions and strategies about it in areas relevant to your role. Attend educational conferences or inservice sessions addressing these areas of your professional practice.
4. Document instances in which you are forced by inadequate or unjust policies to say "no" to interventions or services you know will strengthen the relationships most critical to the patient's quality of life. For example, in the United States, Medicaid, Medicare, or private insurance reimbursement practices often control the number of days the patient is eligible for treatment, placing both professional and family caregivers in an untenable position.
5. Judiciously gather empirical data regarding treatment effectiveness and patient outcomes to assist policy-makers in creating cost-effective approaches to care.
6. Work directly with your colleagues and professional organizations to influence legislation or other policy in your institution, state, or province and nationally.
7. Implement innovations in your workplace to address the strengths and weaknesses of cost-containment policies.

In short, although many of the family's financial burdens will remain outside of your sphere of responsibility or influence, these steps can be taken for you to advocate for them and for all coming down the road in similar situations.

Revaluing Significant Relationships

Bookstores brim with titles such as *Ten (or a Hundred) Places to Visit Before You Die*. On the scale of opportunities for deep human flourishing, an even more compelling book should be *Ten People to Spend More Time with Whether or Not You Are Dying*. Having reviewed some questions and problems patients and their loved ones face, this final section of the chapter ends on a positive note, turning to the enrichment that can be realized in relationships touched by adversity. Although families and health professionals often focus on the negative effects of stress related to illness or injury, there are, gratefully, some positive aspects that can sometimes motivate, leading to "eustress."[17] "*Eu*" is a Greek prefix meaning "good" or "positive" or "beauty."

A stressor can shock one into putting priorities in order and focus on what is important. In his poignant book, *When Breath Becomes Air*, neurosurgeon and author Paul Kalanithi illustrates this point, stating "The tricky part of illness is that, as you go through it, your values are constantly changing. You try to figure out what matters to you, and then you keep figuring it out."[28]

Many people faced with illness or injury discover that it prods them to reflect on the value of significant relationships, past and present. In the epilogue to the above-mentioned book, Paul's wife, Lucy, reflects on their relationship and the marital trouble they experienced before Paul's diagnosis. Knowing that most of her family and friends were unaware of that trouble before the publication of the book she reflects on their relationship, writing "We each joked to our close friends that the secret to saving a relationship is for one person to become terminally ill. Conversely, we knew that the trick to managing a terminal illness is to be deeply in love—to be vulnerable, kind, generous, and grateful."[29]

REFLECTIONS

Although it is difficult to place yourself in a future situation, try to reflect on the following:
- If you learned that you had a serious medical condition that would likely lead to your death in, say, the next year or so, do you think there are relationships you would like to mend or enrich?
- Can you name a relative or close friend whom you would probably spend more time with?
- Are there things you would like to say to someone dear to you?
- Are there relationships you would now feel free to shed?
- Are there old friends, relatives, or others you would want to call or go to visit?

This reflection may give you a glimpse of the urgency with which you might invoke the help of others if you thought they were a resource for fulfilling one or more of your relationship-related goals. As a health professional, you will sometimes be brought into the patient's thoughts or plans as the person reflects about things done and left undone regarding his or her relationships.

Longstanding breaches with a friend or loved ones are the biggest challenge for most patients. We have noted that sometimes a patient is surprised to feel a stirring to make amends. Of course, sometimes a past trauma weighs so heavily on a patient or family member that he or she never fully recovers from it and their relationship remains mired in anger or grief. At other times, the illness or injury highlights a deeper burden of estrangement the person has been carrying. Fortunately, there is hope that today our increasing understanding of depression and of profound delayed responses to serious earlier trauma (post-traumatic stress syndrome) will provide an escape for many more people who in the past have been locked into these burdens.

The good news, too, is that most people do recover or adjust sufficiently to take stock of what is important in their lives. A young couple may decide their differences are not that important after all and try to make a new life together. A man who felt he was too busy for golfing may decide to take the opportunity to resume regular golf games with his long-time buddies and the camaraderie that they enjoy. An older woman may decide to move out of a secure but harsh job environment to find a new position where she believes she will find more support and her impairment will be more accepted. Religious beliefs and images can help provide meaning to the patient's experience and aid in healing or adjustment of intimate and close personal relationships, too.

Sometimes patients will ask your advice or even intervention, and at times you may feel you are faced with a dilemma about what to say or how much to get involved. A good general rule is to be mindful of the nature of respectful health care provider and patient relationships. You have been gaining some ideas about that as you have read and reflected on the chapters in this book. Some helpful guidelines for maintaining appropriate professional boundaries are discussed in more depth in Chapter 3. However, any written guidelines also assume you recognize that whatever you can reasonably do will mean a lot to that patient. The result is that often you will have the satisfaction of watching patients or former patients use their conditions, however unwelcome they were initially, as opportunities to think things over and start afresh, in the process rejuvenating or bringing new perspectives to their close relationships.

Summary

The personal life of the patient involves a web of activities, roles, and relationships that help provide status, meaning, support, and a sense of belonging to this person. Today, the term *family* is defined in a variety of ways. Guided by the principles of patient- and family-centered care, health professionals must understand how families function and how to best interact within the context of each family culture. The family health systems approach offers one such method to optimize health outcomes for the delivery of efficient, effective, and compassionate care.

The most immediate intimate relationship for most people is their family; therefore, showing respect for the patient and assessing the stressors facing the patient mean thinking about how his or her predicament affects the family and vice versa. Shifting the focus of health care from the individual member who is ill, injured, or disabled to the family as a unit of care is key to compassionate care. Despite this shift, the fragility of relationships is often increased by the fears and realities facing patients, their loved ones, and other supporters. Sometimes they see interest and support falling away; they may suffer from the changes that are taking place and from the uncertainties that lie ahead. Financial burdens are almost always an added stress. In all instances, the patient's responses are influenced by those closest to him or her. In turn, those near the patient become enmeshed in the concerns, new responsibilities, and changes. Those who become family or other "informal" caregivers represent a growing group of persons who can be at risk for injuries, burnout, and other debilitating conditions and require the health professional's respect and considered attention to help them all nurture their most treasured relationships. The good news is that illness or injury also may become an opportunity for relationships to draw on their past strengths and find renewed vitality and vision. One of the most critical and ultimately satisfying contributions you can make in your professional capacity is to engage in behaviors that express genuine care for everyone in the patient's circle of key relationships.

See Section 3 Questions for Thought and Discussion on page 263 to apply what you've learned in this section to a variety of case scenarios.

References

1. Albertson SA. *Endings and Beginnings: A Young Family's Experience with Death and Renewal.* New York: Random House; 1980.
2. Institute for Patient- and Family-Centered Care. What Is Patient and Family-Centered Care. http://www.ipfcc.org/about/pfcc.html. Accessed July 5, 2017.
3. Johnson BH, Abraham MR. *Partnering with Patients, Residents, and Families: A Resource for Leaders of Hospitals, Ambulatory Care Settings, and Long-Term Care Communities.* Bethesda, MD: Institute for Patient- and Family-Centered Care; 2010.
4. Committee on Hospital Care and Institute for Patient and Family Centered Care. Patient and family-centered care and the pediatrician's role. *Pediatrics.* 2012;129(2):394–404.
5. Developed and adopted by the Young Children's Continuum of the New Mexico State Legislature, June 20, 1990; contributed by Polly Arango, Family Voices founder.
6. Sparling JW. The cultural definition of family. *Phys Occup Ther Pediatr.* 1991;11(4):17–28.
7. Lofquist D, Lugaila T, O'Connell M. *Households and Families: 2010 Census Briefs.* U.S. Department of Commerce Economics and Statistics Administration. U.S. Census Bureau; 2012.
8. Schor E. Family pediatrics: report of the task force on family. American Academy of Pediatrics. *Pediatrics.* 2003;111:S1541–S1571.
9. Lu C, Yuan L, Lin W, et al. Depression and resilience mediates the effect of family function on quality of life of the elderly. *Arch Gerontol Geriatr.* 2017;71:34–42.
10. Anderson KH. The family health system approach to family systems nursing. *J Fam Nurs.* 2000;6(2):103–119.
11. Duggan C, Stamm D. *Management of Short Bowel Syndrome in Children.* Hoppin, AG, ed. UpToDate. Waltham, MA. UpToDate Inc. http://www.uptodate.com. Accessed August 13, 2018.
12. Duvall EM. *Family Development.* 5th ed. Philadelphia: Lippincott; 1977.
13. Beers SR, Yaworski JA, Stilley C, et al. Cognitive deficits in school-age children with severe short bowel syndrome. *J Pediatr Surg.* 2000;35(6):860–865.
14. Doherty RF, Kwo J, Montgomery P, et al. *Maintaining Compassionate Care: A Companion Guide for Families Experiencing the Uncertainty of a Serious and Prolonged Illness.* Boston: MGH Institute of Health Professions; 2008.
15. Khan FA, Squires RH, Litman HJ, et al. Pediatric intestinal failure consortium. predictors of enteral autonomy in children with intestinal failure: a multicenter cohort study. *J Pediatr.* 2015;167(1):29–34.
16. Imber-Black E, Roberts J, Whiting R. *Rituals in Families and Family Therapy.* New York: Norton; 1988.

17. Rambur B, Vallett C, Cohen JA. The moral cascade: distress, eustress and the virtuous organization. *J Organiz Moral Psychol.* 2010;1(1):41–54.
18. Kennedy-Hendricks A, Barry CL, Gollust SE, et al. Social stigma toward persons with prescription opioid use disorder: associations with public support for private and public health–oriented policies. *Psychiatr Serv.* 2017;68:462–469.
19. van Boekela LC, Brouwersa EPM, van Weeghela J, et al. Stigma among health professionals towards patients with substance use disorders and its consequences for healthcare delivery: systematic review. *Drug Alcohol Depend.* 2013;131:23–35.
20. Zuckerman C. 'Til death do us part: family caregiving at the end of life. In: Levine C, ed. *Always on Call: When Illness Turns Family Into Caregivers.* New York: United Hospital Fund of New York; 2000.
21. Akin C. *The Long Road Called Goodbye: Tracing the Course of Alzheimer's.* Omaha, NE: Creighton University Press; 2000.
22. Freedman VA, Spillman BC. Disability and care needs of older americans: an analysis of the 2011 national health and aging trends study. Report to the HHS/ASPE, office of disability, aging and long-term care policy. 2013. Available at: http://aspe.hhs.gov/daltcp/reports/2014/NHATS-DCN.cfm.
23. Purtilo R. Social marginalization of persons with disability. In: Purtilo R, ed. *Have HAMJ Ten: Ethical Foundations of Palliative Care for Alzheimer Disease.* Baltimore: Johns Hopkins University Press; 2004.
24. Spillman BC, Wolf J, Freedman VA, et al. *Informal Caregiving for Older Americans: An Analysis of the 2011 National Study of Caregiving.* U.S. Department of Health and Human Services Assistant Secretary for Planning and Evaluation Office of Disability, Aging and Long-Term Care Policy; 2014. Available at: https://aspe.hhs.gov/system/files/pdf/77146/NHATS-IC.pdf.
25. Family Caregiver Alliance. *Caregiver Statistics: Health, Technology, and Caregiving Resources;* 2016. https://www.caregiver.org/caregiver-statistics-health-technology-and-caregiving-resources. Accessed July 3, 2017.
26. Decker SL, Lipton BJ. Most newly insured people in 2014 were long-term uninsured. *Health Aff.* 2017;36(1):16–20.
27. Sered SS, Fernandopulle R. *Uninsured in America: Life and Death in the Land of Opportunity.* Berkeley: University of California Press; 2005.
28. Kalanithi P. *When Breath Becomes Air.* New York: Random House; 2016:160–161.
29. Kalanithi P. *When Breath Becomes Air.* New York: Random House; 2016:216.

Respect Through Communication

The most immediate "tool" you have available for respectful interaction is your own communication, whether that tool is used verbally or nonverbally and with colleagues or patients. Effective communication among health professionals is an integral component of interprofessional collaboration and team-based health care. Interprofessional communication is important because of the increasing complexity of patient status and the risk for errors in hospitals and other health care settings. Good communication can create a safer environment, improve patient outcomes, decrease redundancies in care, and reduce patient and societal costs. Chapter 9 provides an overview of the Interprofessional Education Collaborative's Core Competencies for Interprofessional Collaborative Practice[1] that represents in its membership 15 associations of schools of health professions. Elements of collaborative skills in addition to communication such as mutual respect and trust, shared planning, and decision-making by interprofessional teams are discussed. Barriers to effective interprofessional communication and methods to improve collaborative practice are explored.

What you say, how and when you say it, and how you communicate nonverbally through gestures and other types of physical messages will set the tone for everything else that happens in the health professional and patient relationship. Chapter 10 focuses on components of respectful interaction in verbal and nonverbal aspects of communication. As you read and reflect on all the types of messages you give and receive, think back to Sections 1 and 2, especially to the parts of those chapters addressing values and culture. It is almost certain that you will work with colleagues and patients from countries and backgrounds different from your own. There also will be differences in levels of health literacy and basic literacy, as well as facility with the various technological tools for communication and engagement such as the Internet, smart phone applications, patient portals, and social media tools. These differences in language, literacy, and understanding are evident as we attend to patients and listen to or read what they choose to include in their stories and what is left unsaid. Consider how the challenge of communicating both verbally and nonverbally, face-to-face or from a distance, is enhanced and influenced by these factors.

Reference

1. Interprofessional Education Collaborative. *Core Competencies for Interprofessional Collaborative Practice: 2016 Update.* Washington, D.C.: Interprofessional Education Collaborative; 2016.

CHAPTER 9

Respectful Interprofessional Communication and Collaboration

Prelude

When nurses did talk with physicians in these spaces, it was to provide or obtain information. At the physicians' stations, nurses provided data or requested orders. In one exchange at the physician station, a nurse approached a physician and informed him, "You know that guy in 47 is diabetic?" and the physician's response was, "Yes. Well, no I didn't. And he's my patient." In a different exchange, a nurse approached the physician's station to ask, "What am I doing with 42?"

DEAN, GILL, AND BARBOUR[1]

In previous chapters, you were introduced to some basic components of respectful interaction with patients, families, and others. Often the discussion focused on you as an individual professional. Still, you could observe from our examples—and likely from your own experience—that much interaction between professionals and patients today does not occur between a sole health care provider and a patient. In contrast, your interventions often are one of several provided by a group of you working together on the patient's behalf. In this situation, we have referred to you as a member of an interprofessional care team. In the following pages, we examine in more depth the concepts, dynamics, and processes of care provided by multiple professionals working together to care for a patient and your role as an effective member of such teams bonded by common goals and purpose.

Begin by examining the physician and nurse communication in the quote at the opening of this chapter. The setting in this opening summary of dialogue between physicians and nurses is in a busy emergency department. Communication is brief and to the point. These health professionals have reduced the patients to room numbers. There are also boundaries indicated by designated spaces—for the physicians, the physician's station; for the nurses, the nurse's station. That gives you an idea of the context of the interaction. The participants each go about their individual role-specific activities. Where these parallel activities converge, questions are asked and answered but there is little additional discussion. We assume they all are motivated by the common goal of delivering quality care and ensuring the safety of their patients and that working together is necessary to achieve such ultimate goals. They may conclude that this is exactly what they are doing. In this type of perfunctory exchange, the interactions could be considered multidisciplinary because more than one discipline is involved. However, we will give you several reasons why such an exchange is not a truly interprofessional approach and therefore falls short of achieving the broad goals of providing high-quality care and ensuring safety.

Focus on Interprofessional Collaboration

Attention to the importance of working together effectively took root because of the increasingly complex needs of patients along with an emphasis on reducing errors in health care and a fragmented health system. These problems led the call for *interprofessional collaboration*. The Institute of Medicine (IOM; renamed the National Academy of Medicine) in 2001 recommended that health professionals who worked together in interprofessional care teams be better equipped to address the challenging needs of contemporary patients.[2] The next year, the IOM specifically called for greater focus on interprofessional education in their report *Who Will Keep the Public Healthy? Educating Public Health Professionals for the 21st Century* and repeated this appeal in a 2010 report.[3,4] Likewise, The Joint Commission, an independent, not-for-profit organization that accredits and certifies health care organizations and programs in the United States, noted the damaging effects that poor workplace communication can have on patient care and the need to improve interprofessional communication because of the increasing number of errors in health care.[5,6]

The term *interprofessional collaborative practice* brought these ideas into further usage. The World Health Organization defined it accordingly: "When multiple health workers from different professional backgrounds work together with patients, families, carers, and communities to deliver the highest quality of care."[7] Initially this formal, intentional "working together" was thought to be necessary mostly for specific, complex patient care situations, and indeed there are some practice environments in which interprofessional care teams have been the norm since their inception. Examples are rehabilitation, hospice, geriatric care, and mental/behavioral health settings.[8] Perhaps because of the multifaceted and often chronic nature of the health problems experienced by patients cared for in these specialties, as well as the focus of care on common goals, interprofessional care teams were more prepared to share their expertise and perspectives to work toward achieving the patient's maximum level of independence and recovery from an injury. Interprofessional collaboration is now widely recognized as the basis for all effective care delivery.

Why are interprofessional collaboration and communication so critical to the delivery of high-quality, patient-centered care? As has been mentioned several times, patients today generally have multiple health problems and therefore require the expertise and care of more than one health professional to address their needs. Research has affirmed that collaborative interprofessional practice improves efficiency, reduces errors, promotes patient satisfaction, and enhances job satisfaction among health professionals (Fig. 9.1).[9,10] Poor interprofessional collaboration has the opposite impact on patient care in a variety of ways, including errors, increased hospital costs, unnecessary readmissions, pain, and suffering.[5,11]

Core Competencies for Interprofessional Collaboration

About the same time as the call for interprofessional collaboration was being promoted from a variety of constituencies in health policy and accreditation, the Interprofessional Education

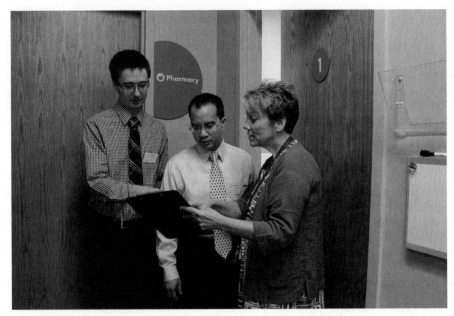

Fig. 9.1   Members of interprofessional care team on rounds. (*Courtesy of Maren Haddad.*)

Collaborative (IPEC) formed and developed core competencies for interprofessional collaborative practice specifically for the prelicensure/precredentialed future health professional.[12] Recall the professional competencies for all health professionals presented in Chapter 2. Note the differences and similarities between the individual professional competencies and the following interprofessional core competencies.

IPEC defines *interprofessional competencies* in health care as "integrated enactment of knowledge, skills, values, and attitudes that define working together across the professions with other health care workers, and with patients, along with families and communities, as appropriate to improve health outcomes in specific care contexts."[12] The four initial competency domains included interprofessional communication, values/ethics, roles and responsibilities, and teams and teamwork. IPEC updated the 2011 competencies in 2016 to integrate population health competencies and respond to the changes in the health care system, including the focus on the Triple Aim, and the implementation of the Patient Protection and Affordable Care Act in 2010.[13] The original four domains now fall under the single domain of interprofessional collaboration (Fig. 9.2).

The IPEC competencies are now incorporated into almost all health professions' accreditation standards. What began with the participation of six national associations of schools of health professions that created the core competencies expanded to 15 members in 2016. The following are a few examples of what these standards look like from physical therapy and pharmacy. The following standard is from physical therapy and will become effective in 2018: "The didactic and clinical curriculum includes interprofessional education; learning activities are directed toward the development of interprofessional competencies including, but not limited to, values/ethics, communication, professional roles and responsibilities, and teamwork."[14] Similarly, interprofessional education is required by the Accreditation Council for Pharmacy Education (ACPE) in the following standard, "The curriculum prepares all students to provide entry-level, patient-centered care in a variety of practice settings as a contributing member of an interprofessional team. In the aggregate, team exposure includes prescribers as well as other healthcare professionals."[15]

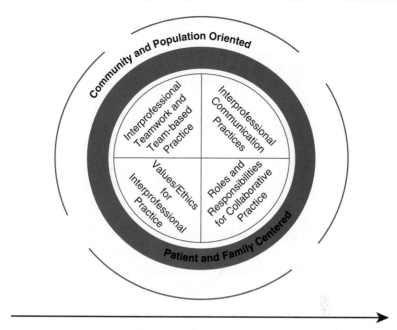

The Learning Continuum pre-licensure through practice trajectory

Fig. 9.2 Interprofessional collaboration competency domains. (*Copyright © 2016 IPEC Interprofessional Education Collaborative.*)

Most health profession programs include a required standard on interprofessional education like these. Integrating interprofessional competencies into accreditation standards ensures that today's health professions student is effectively prepared to function as a member of the interprofessional care team.

INTRAPROFESSIONAL COLLABORATION

Not only do health professionals consistently interact with colleagues from other disciplines, but also they interact with members within the same broadly defined discipline but at different levels. Problems with coordination and communication can occur even among those who share a similar understanding of their professional obligations and shared ownership of patient care interventions. For example, an Occupational Therapist Registered (OTR), Certified Occupational Therapy Assistant (COTA), and Occupational Therapy Aide are all part of the profession of occupational therapy, but each may not necessarily effectively draw on each other's specific contributions to increase efficiency to provide direct service to patients. An early study regarding how to improve intraprofessional collaboration within occupational therapy noted, "If team members' needs are not satisfied, dysfunctional intraprofessional teams result."[16] The needs that they identified were mutual respect, mastery or effective performance, and personal growth and professional socialization. Similar findings were the outcome of a study of licensed practical nurses (LPNs) and registered nurses (RNs). An LPN expressed the following feelings of being devalued by her RN colleague on the team: "She has more years at school than me but I think that when we talk rationally together we can come to an agreement calmly for the sake of our patient and not to see where me or she is right."[17] The LPN seems to be asking for mutual respect and the opportunity to contribute to the care of the patient. Because many professional disciplines include members at the assistant or technical level, there is a need to strengthen these intraprofessional relationships in the same manner as interprofessional collaboration. However, even though they might share a common knowledge base, intraprofessional factions exist within every profession and challenge communication through contrary views and cultures. Generally, methods to improve interprofessional interactions apply equally well to intraprofessional interactions.

Elements of Collaborative Skills

Key elements of successful collaborative interaction are built on an understanding of one's own professional identity and perhaps select character traits. The following are prerequisites or essential attributes that one should possess and develop before embarking on interprofessional collaboration.

INDIVIDUAL ATTRIBUTES TO COLLABORATION
Self-Awareness

The first personal attribute for successful collaboration is the ability to reflect on personal knowledge, skills, and abilities and is built on an understanding of your personal identity based on your own value set, as introduced in Chapter 1. Self-awareness also requires examination of biases, motivations, and emotions that have an impact on your personal and professional growth. "Each individual brings to the team a unique personality and position, which reciprocally affects team function."[18] Also, individuals bring ongoing expectations and hopes, mostly subconscious, to the work environment.

An important component of self-awareness for any health professional is professional identity, which is more than completing a specified course of study and passing a licensure examination. To be a full member of a profession means one must behave like a member of that profession. What does it mean to behave like a member of a profession?

First, at its most basic level, members of a profession share a language; that is, they know the way to talk in a kind of shorthand with members of that profession. As we note in Chapter 10 health professionals share a general culture of health care with its common language that is often foreign to patients. In addition, each profession has its own language that is sometimes reduced to acronyms that only full-fledged members of that profession understand. For example, the term *MTM* is common parlance in pharmacy practice, but only a member of the profession or someone who took the time to translate this acronym would know that it means "medication therapy management." MTM is at the heart of pharmacy practice and refers to a broad range of health care services provided by pharmacists.

Second, one behaves like a member of a health profession when one asks the types of questions those within that profession ask. For example, we would expect a social worker to ask questions about income, living conditions, or sources of family and community support but might be surprised if an oncologist did so. Certain questions are particularly relevant to each health profession's scope of practice.

Third, to behave like a member of a profession one should understand and explain things the way a member of the profession does.[19] We return to these components of professional identity that profoundly affect successful collaboration when we discuss differences in communication styles among professions.

Competence

The second individual attribute necessary for collaborative work is being secure in your abilities in your own discipline, an attribute that acts as a benchmark of respect for the patient introduced in Chapter 2.[20] Sometimes discussions of professional competence that emphasize individual experience and confidence overlook the fact that it also includes the ability to successfully work with others. Being competent in your field allows you to explore and appreciate the contributions of other disciplines. In fact, curiosity and a willingness to learn about the unknown or unfamiliar are assets in interprofessional collaboration.

Trust

Just as trust between professionals and patients is essential for respectful interaction, individuals also must be able to trust other members of the team. "The ability to trust originates from self-knowledge and competence."[21] Trust is often described as a prerequisite to teamwork of any type and begins with the idea that we approach other members of the team as if they are competent and have good intentions. It is easier to establish trust when the members of the team share similar backgrounds and cultures. However, in health care, the members of the team are from different professional backgrounds and new starting points for trust need to be established, such as a clear understanding of the norms and expectations for the professions on the team and a history of successful interpersonal exchanges among team members.[22] Therefore you must have the inclination to trust other members of the team and appreciate that trust continues to develop over time.

Commitment to Team Goals and Values

The fourth individual attribute is commitment to a unified set of team goals and values that provides direction and motivation for individual members.[21] Later we discuss the importance of a shared goal or aim as part of successful collaboration. Here we are talking about the personal sense of responsibility you feel as a member of a team. When you are committed to a commonly agreed on cause or project, you feel responsible to the other members of the team and are thus often willing to work harder to reach a goal if that is necessary. Sometimes commitment is expressed by the metaphor of "having each other's backs," in that we will support each other even when the going gets tough.

Flexibility

Flexibility is defined as "the ability to maintain an open attitude, accommodate different personal values, and be receptive to the ideas of others."[21] Flexibility requires you to keep an open mind and a willingness to see things in different terms. Often the complexity of a patient's predicament requires a novel approach that is much more likely achieved by all members of the team contributing their various perspectives.

Acceptance

Finally, one must be accepting of differences among the members of the team. It is easier and more comforting to be among the familiar; however, our differences make us better. In health care, today, a health professional cannot avoid working in an interprofessional environment, so our choice really comes down to whether we want to work together well or badly. At times, territorial issues of different professions, as well as different world views, conspire to make this a difficult task.[23] All members of the interprofessional care team must move beyond tolerance to acceptance and understanding. When grounded in the principles of dignity and respect, members of the team can clarify specific values that are central to one's own profession with other members of the team. It is likely that just as there is blurring across professional boundaries, there also will be blurring or, perhaps better put, sharing of core values that can help with cross-disciplinary understanding.[24]

REFLECTION

Consider the individual attributes for participating in successful collaboration with other members of the health care team—that is, self-awareness, competence, ability to trust, commitment, flexibility, and tolerance.
- Which of these attributes to do you possess, and which do you need to develop more fully?
- You are participating in morning rounds on an inpatient unit with an interprofessional care team. At one point, you realize that you strongly disagree with the recommendation of another member of the team. Which individual attributes would be particularly helpful in resolving the differences of professional opinion and maintain good interprofessional collaboration?
- How else might you communicate your disagreement to your teammate?

TEAM SKILLS FOR COLLABORATION

In addition to individual attributes, skills more specific to team collaboration also are essential for optimum patient-centered outcomes. A team is defined as "a small group of interdependent people who collectively have the expertise, knowledge and skills needed for a task or ongoing work."[25] This definition of a team is particularly important for health professionals who may be used to working in a hierarchical structure because the definition emphasizes interdependency. The term *interdependency* highlights that the team does not exist to help meet the needs or aims of those at the top of the organizational hierarchy but rather to fulfill mutually agreed on common goals for the welfare of the patient, family, or community. A team needs expertise in the following skills if it hopes to succeed in attaining such goals.

Mutual Respect

The IPEC core competencies specifically refer to mutual respect as a requirement for working with individuals of other professions.[13] As noted previously, such respect is built on the personal trust among members of the team that develops into mutual respect over time. For mutual respect to exist, there must be a culture of "status-equal" basis. All members of the team need to see each other as peers with the capacity to step into the leadership role at any time that specific expertise or skills are needed. Additionally, all members of the team must believe in the value of what the other members of the team bring to the table.

Communication Skills

All the basic verbal and nonverbal communication skills discussed in Chapter 10 come into play in interprofessional communication, with the added challenge of differing language and communication styles among health professions. For example, nurses lean toward being very descriptive and detailed in their communication whereas physicians are generally brief in the information they provide about the patient's situation or treatment.[26] Thus physicians might think when nurses are speaking, "I wish they would get to the point," which can be frustrating to nurses who value a fuller understanding of a patient's story that, from their perspective, is essential to planning patient care. A qualitative study of communication between physicians and other health professionals on an inpatient unit explored current patterns of communication by observing interprofessional and intraprofessional exchanges.[11] Physicians in the study exhibited a consistently terse communication style in which they offered brief reports on their patients' medical status, requested information, or informed the team of patient-related orders. Most of the deliberative communication in which a patient's case was discussed beyond basic medical issues was between members of nonmedical professions such as nursing, occupational therapy, social work, etc. When physicians did have more in-depth discussions about a patient, it was most often with another physician, not a health professional from another discipline.

Negative communication is a problem that often reflects a lack of respect or a resistance to changing the traditional hierarchy in health care. Negative communication includes disparaging comments such as intimidating or condescending language, deliberate delays in responding to requests, reluctance to work as a team, and impatience with questions.[27] At a minimum, efforts should be directed at eradicating such negative communication, which clearly affects the quality of the exchange of information across professions. Communication should be clear and precise, calm and supportive, respectful, and responsive. Members of the team can contribute to positive communication by sharing pertinent information, listening attentively, respecting others' opinions, using common language, and providing feedback as well as accepting feedback.[28]

Shared planning and decision-making are essential to good teamwork. However, health professionals often get stuck in their disciplinary silos and focus on specific tasks or decisions that are important to the values of their profession and ignore or discount the larger picture. These types of isolated decisions about specific treatments or tests do little to achieve overarching goals for the patient, which should serve as a central focus of the team. Shared planning requires compromise. Members of the team must anticipate that there will be differences in perspectives that can lead to conflict but do not have to do so. Reasoning from alternative approaches or angles about a given situation should be encouraged initially and then ideally be part of a team's culture. The establishment of mutually understood and agreed upon goals, even though such goals may change at some future time, is necessary for members of a team (including the patient and family) to think that they are achieving something.

Interprofessional Communication and Collaboration: Challenges and Opportunities

Clearly with so many variables that affect a more collective approach to professional and patient interactions there are barriers and opportunities to refine what an individual health professional can accomplish in providing respectful, patient-centered care.

BARRIERS TO EFFECTIVE INTERPROFESSIONAL APPROACHES
Time Constraints

One of the first barriers to interprofessional communication and collaboration that overworked, busy health professionals mention is that they do not have the time to meet with other members of the interprofessional care team, let alone really learn about the unique or special contributions of other professions. Additionally, there is often no physical space for different members of the team to meet where they can privately air differences and think they are not being overheard or interrupted. It is common to see health professionals conduct "hallway consultations" or "corridor consults," terms applied to unplanned encounters between two or more different members of the team who stop and obtain quick, informal feedback or urgently request information to guide their decision-making. Protected time, dedicated space (literally space to meet), and support for formal discussions for shared planning and decision-making are essential for true collaboration. Although hallway consultations will not disappear, they should not be the only means for members of the team to communicate.

Lack of Shared Structures for Communication

Another barrier to interprofessional communication is a lack of an agreed upon conceptual structure for such dialogue among colleagues. As noted previously, different health professions have their distinct ways of communicating based on underlying values, understanding of their professional obligations and skills, and habits they acquire by observing the actions and conduct of other members of their specialty. A promising example is that considerable research and effort have been focused on the improvement of the *handoff* of a patient when the patient's condition warrants a change involving health

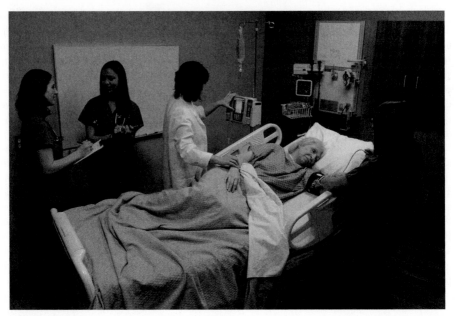

Fig. 9.3 Interprofessional communication is critical during handoffs between health professionals. (*Courtesy of Maren Haddad.*)

disciplines because of a change in the patient's status or when one shift in an institution is ending and a new one beginning. A handoff is "the transfer of patient information and responsibility between health care providers" and is a critical point of vulnerability to communication error (Fig. 9.3).[29] As you can see, if done well, it is an excellent opportunity to ask questions and participate in shared decision-making so the patient's high quality of care remains seamless. To provide structure and improve the transfer of information at the handoff, a variety of common mental models have been proposed and studied, such as *SBAR*, which stands for Situation, Background, Assessment, and Recommendation; *SBIRT*, which stands for Screening, Brief Intervention, and Referral to Treatment and is often used in emergency departments; and *I-PASS*, which is a mnemonic for Illness Severity, Patient Summary, Action List, Situation Awareness, and Contingency Planning and Synthesis by Receiver.[29-31]

All such mental models are an attempt to create a standard language that is not "native" for any one of the professions involved, so there is lower risk for miscommunication and a stronger focus on the patient's situation. Although proven very useful for minimizing communication errors at handoff and clearly useful for assessment and communication of patient status, some have noted that these models are not very helpful for the breadth of information that composes a holistic picture of the patient such as social or psychological factors that have great potential to influence patient care.[32]

Uncertainty

Uncertainty about one's own contributions and those of others can be a barrier to interprofessional communication too. Even with competency and confidence, you also need to know the roles and responsibilities of other members of the team. Often members of an interprofessional care team operate on unconscious stereotypes about other professions and misunderstandings about boundaries and scopes of practice. There also can be overlap between professions and role blurring. Additionally, some teams change every week or month. Turnover in team members can be a real challenge to all involved. It contributes to uncertainty and can lead to lack of continuity in the delivery of safe, efficient, effective, and compassionate care.

The traditional assumption that the physician is always the designated leader of the interprofessional care team is another barrier that persists in health care. Collaborative practice works best when leadership is assigned because of specialized knowledge or technical skills that are relevant to the specific decision at hand. Clearly, there is no one person on a team today who possesses all the specialized knowledge and technical skills needed in a complex case, so informed leadership should shift as the situation dictates. Even given this reality of the need to share the leadership role to best serve overall goals for the patient, there are members of the team who are reluctant to give up their authority or are fearful of accepting the responsibility of a leadership role. For an interprofessional care team to work effectively, members of the team must be able to speak up, not just ask for permission or give orders. It is only through the elimination of established but unnecessarily inflexible power structures and assumed roles that members of the team can see the whole picture, not just focus on what they need to get done within their individual scope of practice.

Gender and Social Class

Differences in *gender* and *social class* among health professionals also are a long standing barrier to effective communication and collaboration. These differences and the stereotypes that accompany them inform role expectations that have historical and social roots. Health professionals are influenced by these abiding images of their professional roles such as the analytic, knowledgeable, objective decision-maker, which is connected to traditional masculine traits versus the caring, compassionate, hands-on traits of femininity. As was discussed in Chapter 5, such gender stereotypes as well as those connected to race, culture, etc., limit the varied and complex contributions that all health professions offer to the team. For true collaboration, all members of the team must be considered equal partners who possess an array of knowledge, skills, perspectives, and abilities.

Geography

Finally, *geography* is a barrier to interprofessional communication. Proximity yields familiarity. When members of a team are in one place, there is more of a chance for the development of trust and socialization. Geographic barriers can be overcome by distance technology, but more effort is required to establish relationships built on shared experiences both within and outside of the work environment.

OPPORTUNITIES FOR IMPROVING INTERPROFESSIONAL APPROACHES

Some, but certainly not all, key elements for effective collaborative practice are listed in Box 9.1. As you read the case involving Dr. Halamek and the Collins family, note where these elements are present or lacking.

BOX 9.1 ■ Key Elements of Effective Collaborative Practice

- Cooperation
- Assertiveness
- Responsibility
- Communication
- Autonomy
- Coordination

From Norsen L, Opladen J, Quinn J: Practice model: collaborative practice, *Crit Care Nurs Clin North Am.* 7(1):43–52, 1995.

Case Study

David Halamek, MD, is a new pediatrician in a large children's ambulatory clinic that includes the full range of health professionals among the clinic's staff. Because he just became a member of the clinic practice, Dr. Halamek is seeing patients who were new to him or new to the clinic. One of these families is the Collins family, who were making their first visit to Dr. Halamek. There was not much in the background information Dr. Halamek received before he saw the Collins family. He knew there were two children, ages 2 and 4, and that this was a visit for a routine physical for the 4-year-old. He also saw in their materials a recent evaluation from one of the occupational therapists at the clinic regarding the 2-year-old, Mia. The note from the occupational therapist said: "Mia has left hemiparesis resulting from an intracranial hemorrhage secondary to prematurity. She has full PROM and AROM in her left upper extremity, but there is mild to moderate increased tone. She has a well-controlled reach with the left arm, but her hand tends to close before reaching the object she is trying to grasp. She likely needs orthotic intervention to improve manipulation of objects."[33] Dr. Halamek also noted that there were no records of immunizations for either child. At the outset of the visit, Dr. Halamek asked Mrs. Collins if she could remember the vaccinations her son had previously received. She told Dr. Halamek that her son had never received any vaccinations and that she did not plan on ever vaccinating her children because she had heard from several reliable sources that they were the cause of autism. Dr. Halamek informed Mrs. Collins that her views about the connection between autism and vaccinations were based on faulty information. He had encountered parents like Mrs. Collins before, so he had a copy of the now infamous journal article that featured a retraction of previously published false data on the alleged connection between vaccines and autism. He gave the copy of the article to Mrs. Collins. But Mrs. Collins did not want to discuss it. After moments of frustration and further attempts to convince Mrs. Collins about the importance of immunization for her children and others, Dr. Halamek told Mrs. Collins that he would not be able to treat her children if she was unwilling to agree to the approved immunization schedule. Mrs. Collins picked up Mia, grabbed Todd's hand, and left the room. One of the other pediatricians and a nurse practitioner were standing in the hallway as Mrs. Collins huffed out of the office. When Dr. Halamek stepped out of the examination room, they inquired what happened. He explained that Mrs. Collins refused to immunize her children. He then said, "I had no choice but to tell her that I couldn't care for her children under those conditions." His colleagues looked surprised at Dr. Halamek's story. The nurse stated, "There are other options, the first of which is to work with the other members of the team in complicated situations like this. We have been working for months with Mrs. Collins to get Mia the services she needs. I am going to worry sick about that little one." The pediatrician added, "We are all part of a team here, so no one has to or should make decisions alone. We need all the help we can get to resolve stressful situations like this." Dr. Halamek was not entirely convinced that this was a "team" decision because he felt a personal and professional responsibility to his patients and to other patients in the waiting areas who might be at risk from children who have not been vaccinated.

REFLECTIONS

- What barriers to effective interpersonal collaboration were at play in the case?
- Which members of the interprofessional care team should have been involved in setting goals, specifically about how to approach the subject of immunizations, for the Collins family? Why?

Consider what might have occurred in this case if Dr. Halamek had worked with other members of the team to make a collaborative decision on how best to work with the Collins family. Let us rewind the case, back to the beginning when Dr. Halamek looked at his new patients for the day and noticed that there were no records of the Collins children's immunizations. How might the following skills of effective teams make a difference in communicating with Mrs. Collins about vaccinations? Note that the focus here is not which approach to working with vaccine-hesitant parents is the best in this case but on the contributions of effective interprofessional teamwork in providing quality patient-centered care.

Cooperation

Cooperation is defined as "acknowledging and respecting other opinions and viewpoints while maintaining a willingness to examine and change personal beliefs and perspectives."[34] Starting from a place of collaborative practice means that the members of an interprofessional care team rely on the expertise and talents of each member and their contributions to the plan of care. The team participants must be able to cooperate with each other, which means that they must acknowledge and respect other opinions and viewpoints perhaps different from their own. Dr. Halamek acted independently as a solo health professional and relied on his own experience and knowledge on the topic of vaccine refusal. For him it was a matter of lack of accurate information on the part of Mrs. Collins, and he acted to correct the problem. He did not consider that others in the clinic likely have encountered vaccine-hesitant parents and may have different ideas about the reasons for Mrs. Collins's refusal and effective interventions. In fact, effectively communicating with parents about vaccination is a common and sometimes challenging issue in pediatric care. By seeking the input of colleagues such as other pediatricians, the pharmacist, the nurse practitioner, or even the clinic's legal counsel in some cases, Dr. Halamek could have discovered valuable information about how the clinic views the use of vaccines and how they routinely approach vaccine-hesitant parents. However, cooperation is more than the process of getting advice from others who have something to contribute to a decision. Cooperation means that you view the issue from the perspective of the team, mindful of what others can and should contribute that you cannot.

Assertiveness

Assertiveness also is required for effective collaboration. Individuals on the interprofessional care team do not only have to speak with confidence but also make sure that their voice is heard. Dr. Halamek's colleagues demonstrated assertiveness when they told him, "There are other options, the first of which is to work with the other members of the team in complicated situations like that," and "We are all part of a team here, so no one has to or should make decisions alone. We need all the help we can get to resolve stressful situations like this." Their comments are focused and clear. They affirm values of teamwork and interdependence that undergird a philosophy of practice of which Dr. Halamek is now a part.[34] They do not tell Dr. Halamek that he was wrong in the way he handled the situation, rather they use broad statements offering him an opportunity to gain from their support, not the kind that place Dr. Halamek in a defensive position. They are not being aggressive, which could be demeaning to Dr. Halamek, who may already be frustrated and embarrassed after Mrs. Collins's exit.

Responsibility

Each individual member of the interprofessional care team has responsibilities for certain tasks and duties related to patient care. There are also shared or mutual responsibilities that the team must fulfill. This means that individual members of the team must accept and share responsibilities and actively participate in group decision-making and support the decision approved by consensus.[34] This element of collaborative practice means that once a decision is made, all members of the team must be supportive even if it does not fully reflect that person's views or perspective. Getting to consensus depends on autonomy and good communication among team members, so individuals believe their input has been fairly considered in the decision-making process. It is especially important that all members of the team are supportive when a decision requires reconsideration based on new information. In the case of Dr. Halamek, there was no group decision-making involved. It is possible that there was past group decision-making and consensus on the part of the clinic personnel to follow a protocol for working with vaccine-hesitant parents depending on where the parents fell on the continuum from cautious acceptance to outright refusal.[35] This is a good example of the importance of educating new members of a team into the existing culture—that is, explaining what protocol the team follows in specific cases.

Communication

Communication, which is the "effective sharing of important information and exchanging of ideas and discussion" has already been mentioned as an important individual and team skill.[34] Collaborative practice is actualized when all members of the interprofessional care team are willing to learn about, through, and with each other. In doing so they develop fluency in the language of each other's professions and cultures to understand their collective perspective and contributions. Being aware of what is relevant in any situation to help move the interprofessional teamwork in a positive direction is a key. In this case, where there was little communication on the part of Dr. Halamek with any other members of the interprofessional care team, it may have moved the situation along for him to have asked if there was an established protocol. At a minimum, he would know more about how situations such as this were handled, even though his view on the subject might not be shared by his new colleagues. He would also learn how his colleagues communicate about this topic and what skills they have to work toward the shared goal of protecting the Collins children and other children as well. For example, the daughter Mia was previously seen by an occupational therapist. Dr. Halamek might have taken advantage of that relationship with the family to revisit the vaccine question at a later visit rather than dismissing the family.

Autonomy

It might not seem that autonomy, the "ability to work independently," would be a key element of effective collaborative practice.[34] Interprofessional collaboration requires interdependence. However, autonomy does play a role. Members of the interprofessional care team may have less individual autonomy, but the team is more autonomous with all the members working together. Despite the focus on collective goals, individual members of the team may continue to hold to certain interests or duties unique to their role and maintaining a certain amount of autonomy.[36] Hence, when Dr. Halamek admits that he is not entirely convinced that this was a "team" decision regarding what is the best approach for vaccine-hesitant parents, he is expressing the tension between individual autonomy and the autonomy of the team.

Coordination

The final element for effective collaboration is coordination, defined as the "efficient organization of group tasks and assignments."[34] All members of a team need to possess the comprehension and communication skills to deliver patient-centered care. The discussion of vaccines in the ambulatory setting is but one example of a nearly inevitable challenge in pediatric practice that requires interprofessional coordination.[37] If the members of an interprofessional care team are coordinated in their efforts, they can avoid duplication and ensure that the most qualified person or persons on the team take care of the issue or problem that moves the team toward the goals of care.

Coordination today also requires that each member of the team be aware of guidelines, policies, and laws established by government, institutional, and professional specialty groups to further refine their individual and collective contributions. For example, referring to Dr. Halamek's situation, the American Academy of Pediatrics (APA) Clinical Report on responding to parental refusals of immunization provides useful strategies pediatricians should take advantage of in situations of vaccine refusals.[38]

Summary

As emphasized throughout this chapter the focus of the interprofessional care team is to realize the overarching goals of patient care. Our description of major challenges and opportunities of achieving collaborative practice highlight that these goals depend in part on the individual professional's preparation discussed in previous chapters. However, given today's health care structures and the complexity of patient care, it often also takes the members of a team exercising the elements of collaborative practice to fully realize the purpose of your work as a professional.

This chapter brings into center focus aspects of your professional identity and activity that so far have been addressed only in the background. Learning to be a collaborative member on an interprofessional care team relies on a solid foundation of individual preparation in your chosen field but adds components that help ensure you and others can meet the benchmarks of respect essential for high-quality care and patient safety. Specific competencies for interprofessional collaboration have been developed by professional organizations and are being implemented widely in health care. Personal attributes that are elements for ensuring your skillful participation on a team include trust, self-awareness, and flexibility. There are also several elements that the teams themselves must express, including mutual respect and strong communication skills. Our descriptions of barriers to collaboration and opportunities to successfully meet these challenges are resources that you can call on to help optimize your success.

References

1. Dean M, Gill R, Barbour JB. "Let's sit forward": Investigating interprofessional communication, collaboration, professional roles and physical space at EmergiCare. *Health Commun.* 2016;31(12):1506–1516.
2. Institute of Medicine Committee on Quality of Care in America. *Crossing the Quality Chasm: A New Health System for the 21st Century.* Washington, DC: National Academy of Sciences; 2001.
3. Institute of Medicine. *Who Will Keep the Public Healthy? Educating Public Health Professionals for the 21st Century.* Washington, DC: National Academy of Sciences; 2002.
4. Institute of Medicine. The future of nursing: leading change, advancing health. Retrieved from: http://www.nationalacademies.org/hmd/Reports/2010/The-Future-of-Nursing-Leading-Change-Advancing-Health.aspx; 2010.
5. Joint Commission. Sentinel Event Alert. Behaviors that undermine a culture of safety. Issue 40. Retrieved from: http://www.jointcommission.org/sentinel_event_alert_issue_40_behaviors_that_undermine_a_culture_of_safety/; 2008.
6. Joint Commission. Accreditation program hospitals: National patient safety goals. Retrieved from: www.jointcommision.org/assessts/1/6/2011_NPSGs_Hap.pdf; 2011.
7. World Health Organization. Framework for action on interprofessional education & collaborative practice. http://www.who.int/hrh/resources/framework_action/en/. WHO Reference Number: WHO/HRH/HPN/10.3, p. 13, 2010.
8. Hall P. Interprofessional teamwork: professional cultures as barriers. *J Interprof Care.* 2016;19(suppl 1):188–196.
9. Carnegie Foundation. Educating nurses and physicians: toward new horizons. Available from: http://www.macyfoundation.org/publications/educating-nurses-and-physicians-toward-new-horizons; 2010.
10. McCaffrey RG, Hayes R, Stuart W, et al. An education program to promote positive communication and collaboration between nurses and medical staff. *J Nurses Staff Dev.* 2011;27:121–127.
11. Zwarstein M, Rice K, Gotlib-Conn L, et al. Disengaged: a qualitative study of communication and collaboration between physicians and other professions on general internal medicine wards. *BMC Health Serv Res.* 2013;13:494.
12. *Interprofessional Education Collaborative: Core Competencies for Interprofessional Collaborative Practice.* Washington, DC: Interprofessional Education Collaborative; 2011.
13. *Interprofessional Education Collaborative: Core Competencies for Interprofessional Collaborative Practice.* Washington, DC: Interprofessional Education Collaborative; 2016.
14. Commission on Accreditation in Physical Therapy Education: Standards and required elements for accreditation of physical therapy education programs. http://www.capteonline.org/AccreditationHandbook.
15. Accreditation Council for Pharmacy Education. *Accreditation Standards and Key Elements for the Professional Program in Pharmacy Leading to the Doctor of Pharmacy Degree.* Chicago, IL; 2015. https://www.acpe-accredit.org/pdf/Standards2016FINAL.pdf.
16. Blechert TF, Christiansen MF, Kari N. Intraprofessional team building. *American J Occup Ther.* 1987;41(9):576–582.
17. Huynh T, Nadon M, Kershaw-Rousseau S. Voices that care: Licensed practical nurses and the emotional labour underpinning their collaborative interactions with registered nurses. *Nurs Res Pract.* 2011:6.

18. Maple G. Early intervention: some issues in co-operative team work. *Aust Occup Ther J.* 1987;34(4): 145–151.

19. Wackerhausen S. Collaboration, professional identity and reflection across boundaries. *J Interprof Care.* 2009;23(5):455–473.

20. Petrie HG. Do you see what I see? The epistemology of interdisciplinary inquiry. *J Aesthetic Educ.* 1976;10(1):29–43.

21. Mickam S, Rogers S. Characteristics of effective teams. *Aust Health Rev.* 2000;23(3):201–208; quote p. 204, 2000.

22. Gilbert JHV, Camp RD, Cole CD, et al. Preparing students for interprofessional teamwork in health care. *J Interprof Care.* 2016;14(3):223–235.

23. Dombeck MT. Professional personhood: training, territoriality and tolerance. *J Interprof Care.* 1997;11:9–21.

24. Glen S. Educating for interprofessional collaboration: teaching about values. *Nurs Ethics.* 1999;6(3):202–213.

25. Carnegie Foundation. *Educating Nurses and Physicians: Toward New Horizons.* Available from: http://www-.macyfoundation.org/publications/educating-nurses-and-physicians-toward-new-horizons; 2010.

26. Haig KM, Sutton S, Wittington J. SBAR: a shared mental model for improving communication between clinicians. *J Qual Patient Saf.* 2006;32(3):167–175.

27. Croker A, Grotowski M, Croker J. Interprofessional communication for interprofessional collaboration. In: Levett-Jones T, ed. *Critical Conversations for Patient Safety: An Essential Guide for Health Professionals.* Sydney: Pearson; 2014:55–61.

28. Salvatori P, Mahoney P, Delottinville C. An interprofessional communication skills lab: a pilot project. *Educ Health.* 2006;19(3):380–384.

29. Starmer AJ, Spector ND, West DC, et al. Integrating research, quality improvement, and medical education for better handoffs and safer care: disseminating, adapting, and implementing the I-PASS program. *Jt Comm J Qual Patient Saf.* 2017;43:319–329.

30. Leonard M, Graham S, Bonacum D. The human factor: the critical importance of effective teamwork and communication in providing safe care. *Qual Saf Health Care.* 2004;13(suppl 1):i85–i90.

31. Soskin P, Duong D. *Social Worker as SBIRT Instructor to Emergency Medicine Residents.* MedEdPORTAL Publications 2014;10:9840.

32. Corbally M, Timmins F. The 4S approach: a potential framework for supporting critical care nurses' patient assessment and interprofessional communication. *Critic Care Nurs.* 2016;21(2):64–67.

33. Coppard BM, Lohman HL. *Introduction to Orthotics: A Clinical Reasoning and Problem-Solving Approach.* St. Louis, MO: Elsevier; 2015:394.

34. Norsen L, Opladen J, Quinn J. Practice model: Collaborative Practice. *Crit Care Nurs Clin North Am.* 1995;7(1):43–52.

35. Leask J, Kinnersley P, Jackson C, et al. Communicating with parents about vaccination: a framework for health professionals. *BMC Pediatr.* 2012;12:154.

36. Rose L. Interprofessional collaboration in the ICU: how to define? *Nurs Crit Care.* 2011;16(1):5–10.

37. Opel DJ, Heritage J, Taylor JA, et al. The architecture of provider-patient vaccine discussions at health supervision visits. *Pediatrics.* 2013;132(6):1037–1046.

38. Diekema DS, and the Committee on Bioethics. Responding to parental refusals of immunization of children. *Pediatrics.* 2005;115:1428–1431.

CHAPTER 10

Respectful Communication in an Information Age

Prelude

After surgery last May, my first memory upon awakening in the ICU was a feeling as if I were choking on the ventilator, and of desperately wanting someone to help me. I could hear the nurse behind the curtain. I lifted my hand to summon her, only to realize I was in restraints, immobilized. I felt as if I were being buried alive. Lacking an alternative, I decided to kick my legs until someone came. This worked. The nurse came and suctioned me briefly, then disappeared behind the curtain. Still afraid and still feeling as if I needed more suctioning and the presence of another near me, I kicked again. She returned, this time to lecture me on how I mustn't kick my legs. And then she left.

S.G. JAQUETTE[1]

Patients rely on verbal and nonverbal communication to try to explain what is wrong or seek comfort or encouragement from health professionals. Yet they may have difficulty with language or with finding the right words, or they may literally be unable to speak and must resort to gestures, such as the patient in the opening scenario of this chapter. Unable to use words to convey her needs, she spoke the only way she could—she kicked her legs.

Talking Together

Understandably, a lot of health professional and patient interactions rely on verbal communication. The greater responsibility for respectful communication between you and a patient lies with you, although both must assume responsibility. By examining interdependent components of effective communication, you will gain insight into this critical area of human interaction. Health professionals rely on spoken, written, and electronic forms of communication to share information, plan and evaluate care, and collaborate with members of the interprofessional care team.

In your work as a health professional you will be required to communicate verbally with a patient to (1) establish rapport, (2) obtain information concerning his or her condition and progress, (3) confirm understanding (your own and that of the person with whom you are communicating), (4) relay pertinent information to other health professionals and support personnel, and (5) educate the patient and his or her family. Periodically, you are expected to offer encouragement and support, give rewards as incentives for further effort, convey bad news, report technical data to a patient or colleague, interpret information, and act as consultant or advocate. Naturally, you will be more comfortable with some activities than with others, per your own specific abilities and experiences. Nevertheless, all health professionals should be prepared to perform the entire gamut of communication activities.

Verbal communication is instrumental in creating better understanding between you and a patient. However, this is not always the result. You will often be able to trace the cause of a misunderstanding to something you said; it was probably the wrong thing to say, or it was said in the wrong way or at the wrong time. The way words travel back and forth between individuals has been the subject of considerable study in the communication field. Several models have been proposed to graphically describe what happens when two people exchange the simplest of words.

Models of Communication

Although the following quotation focuses on the exchange of information between a physician and patient, the same can be said of all health professionals as they communicate with patients. As you read the quote, recall the differences between how a patient tells his or her story that was elaborated in Chapter 7 and the traditional "interview" model of professional questioning to arrive at a diagnosis described here.

> *It is revealing to examine how this flow back and forth between physician and patient is shaped, what is revealed or requested, when, by whom, at whose request or command, and whether there is reciprocal revelation of reasons, doubts, and anxieties. When we look at the medical context, instead of a free exchange of speech acts we find a highly structured discourse situation in which the physician is very much in control. Some patients perceive this sharply. Others more vaguely sense time constraints and a sequence structured by physician questions and terminated by signals of closure, such as writing prescriptions.[2]*

Communication understood in this way involves the transfer of information from the patient to the health professional so a diagnosis or plan for treatment can be made. The focus is on the "facts" and generally begins with a question about what brought the patient to the health professional. However, once the initial complaint is stated, little time or attention appears to be devoted to other patient-centered concerns.[3]

Think of some reasons this model is problematic. For example, the first complaint that a patient mentions may not be the most significant. More important, the patient may take a health professional's hurried rush through a discussion as an overt sign of disinterest and disrespect. Most interactions with patients take the form of interviews rather than a conversation or dialogue.

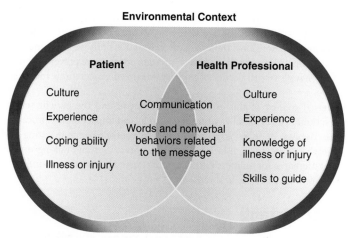

Fig. 10.1 Essential and influencing variables of the communication environment. (*From Keltner NL, Steele D. Psychiatric Nursing. 7th ed. St. Louis, MO: Elsevier; 2015.*)

Health professions students take great pains to learn interview techniques designed to reveal, by the process of data gathering and elimination, the patient's health problem. The interview becomes a means to an end, the end being a diagnosis, problem identification, and treatment plan. As was noted in Chapter 7, this end may not be the one the patient is seeking. Furthermore, by strictly following the interview model of communication, the health professional effectively controls the introduction and progression of topics. This pattern of communication involves the use of power and authority but remains largely hidden from awareness. Patients may literally be unable to get a word in edgewise during the time they have to speak.

Imagine yourself changing your view of communication to one of a dialogue or conversation so you can focus your attention on different aspects of the process such as minimizing the disparities in power and creating opportunities for true understanding between you and the patient. One such way to view the interaction between health professional and patient is to think of it as improvisation. For example, even though health professional and patient interactions are structured, they are not scripted in that "neither knows exactly what the other will say or do."[4] *Improvisation skills* can be effective tools in health professional and patient communication by "improving active listening, clear information delivery, and collaborative narrative building."[4] An underlying principle of improvisation is the "yes-and" response, which helps affirm what the speaker is saying. Including questions and prompts such as, "Tell me more about that," or "What have you tried that helps?" also offers greater opportunity for communication than mere "yes" and "no" types of questions that close off communication and create distance between those involved in the interaction. Also, keeping quiet and letting a patient tell his or her story is especially effective to build trust and gain a sense of what is most important to the patient. Fig. 10.1 conceptualizes communication, both verbal and nonverbal, as the bridge between you and a patient or the building blocks of the scene you and the patient are constructing as in the earlier examples from improvisation. The model also includes some of the primary and secondary cultural characteristics introduced in Chapter 5 that influence what each party brings to the dialogue. These factors (and others not listed in the figure) have an impact on the interaction.

The Context of Communication

Fig. 10.1 places the two parties who are communicating within an environmental context. Where, with whom, and under what circumstances the dialogue or conversation takes place also can have a profound influence on the process and outcomes of the interaction. Clinical encounters between you and your patients are, according to Arthur Frank, a form of dialogue: "Most of the particularities generate tensions: stakes are often high for both parties, time is often limited, intimate matters are being broached between comparative strangers, power differentials intrude, and—not last but enough—both parties often have idealized expectations for what should take place."[5]

Thus the internal context of this exchange between you and the patient sets it apart from everyday conversations. The external environment also has an impact on the process and outcome of your dialogue. Because of technology, you may find yourself communicating with the same patient in a variety of contexts (e.g., face-to-face in a clinical setting, talking on the telephone, participating in conferences for online, multidisciplinary assessments, corresponding via e-mail or in a patient's electronic chart or medical record).

In-Person or Distant

If someone is standing or sitting right in front of you, the type of interaction is different from what occurs on the telephone or through an e-mail message, text, discussion board, or video call or audio call on the Internet. What varies most between in-person interactions and those that occur across distances is proximity, messages portrayed through nonverbal communication, and the degree of relative anonymity. Direct personal contact with another person provides fewer places to hide fear, distaste, or discomfort for the person or about something in the interaction. In fact, knowing this, some health professionals specifically choose areas of practice in which they will have little direct contact with patients.

The value of direct contact is that when you can meet in person with a patient, all the possible ways of communicating can be engaged. Each sense can be a source of information about the other. This explains, in part, why the exchange is that much richer. During your career, there is a good chance you will use a variety of devices to communicate with patients. Perhaps in the future a holographic, computer-generated version of the patient and you will virtually "interact" with each other. In-person interactions with health professionals will continue but will be increasingly supplemented by forms of communication technology (Fig. 10.2).

For example, surveys show that patients want to be able to e-mail their clinicians to get test results and ask questions.[6] Online communication with patients has many positive attributes such as the verbatim record of the transaction between patient and health professional. However, electronic communication is not well suited to urgent problems, and it does not contain the nonverbal components of communication discussed later in this chapter that are crucial to understanding.

One-to-One or Group

Before you begin any type of interaction with a patient, whether one person or a group, you should make sure the patient knows who you are and what you do. This sounds so basic that it hardly seems worth mentioning. However, some health professionals are so focused on getting on with the clinical task that they forget the introductions. Many patients want to be greeted by a handshake or other means of personally "greeting" them in a culturally appropriate manner and verbal personalized contact with an explanation of your role.[7] If you have met before, but there has been some time between your interactions, it does not hurt to reintroduce yourself and explain your role. In addition, always wear your identification with your name and professional role clearly displayed.

If you are meeting a patient for the first time, be sure to use his or her full name. Do not presume to address a patient, unless the patient is a child, by his or her first name until the patient gives you explicit permission. Ask the patient how to pronounce his or her name if there is any

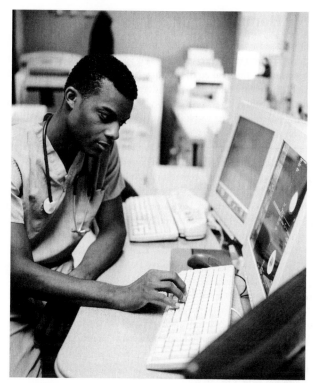

Fig. 10.2   Online communication with patients has both advantages and drawbacks. (© *NA/PHOTOS.com/ Thinkstock.com.*)

doubt about the correct pronunciation. A niece of one of the authors was highly insulted when her pediatrician continually mispronounced her first name after being corrected. The then six-year-old said, "How would the doctor like it if I kept saying her name the wrong way?" So even young children notice a lapse in common courtesy, discussed in Chapter 2, that reflects respect for the person.

After you introduce yourself, tell the patient what you do in a few sentences. It is helpful to practice this explanation with a sympathetic audience such as relatives or friends who will tell you if you are being too technical or confusing. Having established this initial rapport, you can now devote your attention to the patient before you and vice versa. We will address matters such as facial expression, gestures, and touch later in this chapter. All nonverbal forms of communication may override verbal messages, and this is especially obvious in face-to-face interactions.

Working with an individual patient is different in some significant ways from working with a group of patients. Because you will have opportunities to interact with groups of patients or patients and their families or friends, knowledge about group functioning is essential. Much of what you plan for and deliver, especially education about standard treatments, procedures, follow-up care, etc., may be best accomplished through a group process. To have a constructive effect in a group setting you must be familiar with how a group influences individual behavior and the forces that operate in any group. The groups you interact with as a health professional may be spontaneously formed for a short period, such as a group of patients who have diabetes being treated in an ambulatory clinic who come together for instruction about their disease management, or they may be groups that will interact for longer periods, such as a support or therapy group in a rehabilitation setting.

Institution or Home

In Chapter 6 we discussed a variety of settings in which patients receive care today. Whatever the environment in which you encounter patients, for social, psychological, and financial reasons, there is a strong tendency to medicalize the setting. So even in settings such as a skilled nursing facility or the patient's home, medical props and devices shape the atmosphere.

It is often evident to health professionals who work in patients' homes that they are viewed as guests at best or intrusive strangers at worst. Delivery of care in the home health setting places the health professional on the patient's turf. Communication in the home health care setting is shaped by that environment. Respect for the patient requires that health professionals are more deferential, more attuned to asking before doing. Other health care environments, such as intensive care units or emergency departments, do not even pretend to be "homelike" beyond the professional courtesies presented in Chapter 2 as a benchmark of respect in any setting. The sights, sounds, smells, and urgency of these high-tech environments have a profound impact on patients, particularly because these environments are often foreign and threatening. Consider this excerpt from a poem involving a mother who gets her first glimpse of her child in a critical care unit in a hospital.

Intensive Care

I am called.
     But nothing prepares me for what I see, my child

in her body of pain, hooked to machines. Grief
     comes up like floodwater. Her body floats on a sea

of air that is her bed, a force field of sorrow
     that pulls me to her side, I touch pain I know

I have never felt, move into a new land
     of nightmare. She is so still. Only one hand

moves, fingers oscillate like water plants risking
     the air. Machines line the desks,

the floor, the walls, confirm the deep pink
     of her skin in rapidly ascending numbers. One eye blinks . . .

L.C. GETSI[8]

REFLECTIONS

- If you were to enter this patient's room and come upon this mother, what would your first words to her be?
- How would this institutional environment affect communication?
- What might you do to minimize the strangeness of the surroundings?

Sensitive communication depends on an appreciation of the effect of the environment on what transpires between you and the patient.

Choosing the Right Words

The success of verbal communication depends on two important factors: (1) the way material is presented (i.e., the vocabulary used, the clarity of voice, and organization) and (2) the tone and volume of the voice.

VOCABULARY AND JARGON

As we note in Chapter 9, the descriptive vocabulary of the health professional is a two-edged sword. A student must learn to offer precise, accurate descriptions and must be able to communicate to other professionals in that mode.

Technical language is one of the bonds shared by health professionals among themselves. In contrast, highly technical professional jargon is almost never appropriate in direct conversation with the patient because it cuts off communication. It is imperative that you learn to translate technical jargon into terms understandable to patients when discussing their condition or conversing with their families. Only in the rarest instances are patients schooled in the technical language of health care sufficiently to understand its jargon, even in today's world of the Internet, various apps on smart phones, television, podcasts, and other health care–related media resources. Even when the patient happens to be a health professional, it is important to communicate in easily understandable language. Do not assume the therapist or nurse who is your patient is conversant in all areas of health care. The safest approach in working with another health professional who is your patient is to take a cue from the patient and use only the technical language he or she introduces.

Another common area for miscommunication is when the health professional and patient literally speak different languages. As was mentioned in Chapter 5, an increasing number of patients will require the assistance of medical interpreters because of the influx of a variety of refugees and immigrants into the United States. It is a rare health professional who does not routinely encounter language barriers with patients because approximately 8.6% of the total US population is considered to have limited English proficiency.[9] It is estimated that 20% of the US population speak a language other than English at home.[10] Patients, or families in the case of pediatric patients, who do not speak English or have limited English proficiency are sometimes seen as a burden by health professionals. As one health professional noted, "Non–English speaking patients take at least twice the time of others. Everything one says should be understood, and some of it jotted down, by the interpreter before being relayed to the patient. It is not the patient's fault, but I can already picture the irritated waiting room"[11]

Numerous options exist for bridging these language barriers, including interpreters (onsite and on the phone), bilingual health professionals, and trained volunteers. Some reasons to avoid the use of untrained volunteers or family members as medical interpreters include the following:

- Interpreters close to the patient may not be able to disregard their views regarding the situation, which can bias the information that is shared.[12]
- Family interpreters often speak as themselves rather than merely providing accurate information between parties.[13]
- Untrained interpreters often lack knowledge of medical terms, which can lead to miscommunication and misdiagnosis.
- Untrained interpreters may be emotionally harmed because of the stress of performing an essential activity for which they are not prepared.[14]

Formally trained interpreters should be used whenever informed consent for treatment is required. Patients may not initially trust formally trained interpreters, especially when they are on the phone rather than in person, for a variety of social and cultural reasons, but the risk for misunderstanding and errors without interpreter services is great enough to warrant their use.[15] If possible, a combination of the languages involved and nonverbal signs might be the best alternative when a patient refuses a trained interpreter. The main goal is to find a neutral and accurate means of communicating across language barriers in which both parties, patient and health professional, know what is being said.[16]

Choosing the right words is a special challenge when working with patients with changes in cognitive capacity, such as persons with Alzheimer's disease. In a study of caregivers who worked with this population of patients, a "yes/no" or forced choice type of question (e.g., "Do you want to go outside?") rather than an open-ended question (e.g., "What would you like to do?") resulted in more successful communication.[17] Family caregivers of patients with Alzheimer's disease also found that using simple sentences was more effective than other communication strategies, such as slow speech.[18]

As always, the general rule has exceptions, and you should assess what types of questions work best with each patient. Of course, the way to respectful communication is to try as much as possible to talk to patients as equals (because that is what most patients want) while remaining flexible in your style to meet individual patients' needs.

Inefficiencies from Miscommunication

Several problems arise when miscommunication occurs because the health professional is unable to communicate with the patient in terms understandable to him or her.

DESIRED RESULTS ARE LOST

In situations in which the health professional is having difficulty understanding the patient's attempts to explain his or her symptoms or problem because the explanation is vague or confusing, it could be tempting to turn to the objective criteria of laboratory and diagnostic findings or experience to plan a treatment program rather than continuing to try to understand what the patient is saying. This "miss" in communication all too often inhibits the results the health professional wished to achieve and could have achieved, had effective communication with the patient been established. Miscommunication can leave patients frustrated and anxious and so uncertain that it affects their ability to comply with treatment.[19]

MEANINGS ARE CONFUSED

Another common area for miscommunication is when the health professional and patient are both using the same word but ascribe different meanings to it. One example noted earlier in this chapter is the professionals' use of the word *complaint*. This ordinary clinical jargon can convey a different meaning to the patient than to a health professional. In the attempt to understand a patient's situation, the professional is searching for the complaint. If this term is used in the patient's presence it may carry an emotional content that makes the patient think he or she is a nuisance, when in fact the professional is simply searching for the relevant clinical signs, symptoms, or diagnosis.

In a qualitative study of patients with diabetes and their physicians, it was found that different conceptions of the term *control* affected the ability of patients and their physicians to communicate effectively.[20] Although the physicians in the study acknowledged the numerous physical, psychological, and social obstacles to treatment, they did not focus on these aspects of the disease when they interacted with patients. Rather, they focused almost entirely on managing blood glucose numbers. This led to a great degree of frustration on the part of the patients.

DOUBT ARISES ABOUT THE HEALTH PROFESSIONAL'S INTEREST

Another problem that can result from using technical language is that the person to whom you are speaking will not be convinced you really want to know how he or she feels. In addition, your choice of words can unintentionally hurt the patient. For example, after her first prenatal visit to the doctor, a pregnant teenager reported to her friends, "The doctor wanted to know about my 'menstrual history.' I didn't know what that was. Finally, I figured out she was talking about my periods. Why didn't she just say that? I felt so stupid."

When the health professional persists in using "big words" or technical language, the patient may interpret this as a sign that his or her problems are not important. The complexity and impersonality of a health facility will undoubtedly be communicated to the patient if health professionals are unwilling to explain carefully to the patient, in understandable terms, his or her condition and its treatment. What is accomplished within any allotted time, rather than the actual amount of time spent, will be the criterion that convinces the patient the health professional really cares. If the patient cannot understand what is being said, little will be accomplished, and poor health outcomes, including adverse events, can result.

The mastery of appropriate vocabulary, then, includes being able to communicate with your colleagues but at the same time being willing to converse with patients in words they can understand. You will need to become "bilingual," translating from professional terms to common, everyday language. When this is accomplished, the patient more likely will be able to do what is requested, respond accurately to your questions, and be convinced that you care about him or her. In a word, the person will feel respected.

Clarity

In addition to using words that are too technical for the patient to understand, a health professional may not speak with sufficient clarity to free the patient from uncertainty, doubt, or confusion about what is being said. What is the difference between the two? Lack of clarity can result if you launch into a lengthy, rambling description of treatment options (e.g., not realizing that the patient was lost at the outset). Even a highly organized, technically correct, and objectively meaningful sentence can be unclear if it is poorly articulated or spoken too softly or hurriedly. Lack of clarity also can result when patients become preoccupied with one facet of what you are saying and consequently interpret everything else considering that preoccupation.

It is surprising to some professionals that patients may be too embarrassed to ask them to repeat something, and so patients rely on what they think they heard. Patients are sometimes hesitant because they are a bit awed by you as the health professional and so try to act sophisticated instead of asking you to repeat what you said. Patients may be awed primarily because they realize that health professionals have skills that can determine their future welfare and that, regardless of their influence in the business or social world, they are at your mercy in this situation. Some ways to help enhance the clarity of your communication follow.

EXPLANATION OF THE PURPOSE AND PROCESS

Clarity begins with helping the patient understand why you are there and what you plan to do. As mentioned earlier in this chapter, you first establish the purpose of your interaction when you introduce yourself and explain your role. This general introduction should be followed by a statement of the purpose of this encounter (i.e., what is going to take place now and why). Thus you and the patient know what the goal of the interaction is from the start. Because the patient may be tired or uncomfortable, it is also helpful to state at the outset how long the interaction will take and what the patient will likely experience (e.g., "The head of this instrument may be a little cold at first when it touches your skin," "When you get up on the table we will ask you to roll onto your right side," and "Push this call button if you want to get out of bed or need assistance of any kind"). Questions the patient asks will then help you decide what more you need to say.

ORGANIZATION OF IDEAS

Think ahead about how you are going to present your information. You can quickly confuse a patient by jumping from one topic to the next, inserting last-minute ideas, and then failing to summarize or to ask the patient to do so. Failure to systematically progress from one step to the next toward a logical conclusion is usually caused by (1) your own lack of understanding of the subject or of the steps in the procedure or (2), ironically, a too thorough knowledge of the subject or procedure. The former causes the patient to have to figure out the relevant facts, whereas the latter causes the speaker to leave out points that are obvious to him or her but not to the listener. In either case, it is advisable to organize the description of a procedure or test into its component parts and then to practice describing it to a friend who is not familiar with the procedure. That person will be able to identify any obvious steps that have been omitted. Complicated information should be broken down into manageable chunks so that the patient is not overwhelmed by everything that follows. This is especially true when the information involves bad news.

AUGMENT VERBAL COMMUNICATION

Verbal information and instructions alone are not always adequate to ensure clarity. Written notes or instructions, diagrams, videotapes, and nonverbal demonstrations are highly desirable adjuncts to the spoken word because they may help the person organize the ideas and information more fully and can be used for future reference. The augmented instructions or follow-up information for patients should be written in clear, direct language in the order required such as telling a patient at the outset not to eat or drink any fluids after midnight when providing instructions for an upcoming surgery. The clarity of written exchanges is even more important when you are communicating with other members of the interprofessional care team because it "remains the most usual means of communication between healthcare professionals."[21] Beyond the specific words in written or spoken communication, there are factors that influence the meaning behind the words, which we examine next.

Tone and Volume

Paralinguistics is the study of all cues in verbal speech other than the content of the words spoken. Although paralinguistics is considered part of the realm of nonverbal communication, we will discuss tone and volume here because they are so closely connected to the content of speech. Sometimes a person's voice or volume belies his or her words. Any vocalized sound a person makes could be interpreted as verbal communication, so besides your words you will communicate "volumes" with the tone, inflection, speed, and loudness of the words you use.

TONE

Tone is a voice quality that can support or reverse the meaning of the spoken word. Each of us tries to communicate more than the literal content of our messages by using different tones of voice of the same spoken message. A low tone of voice sounds authoritative. Also, the rise in pitch at the end of a sentence indicates a question is being asked or approval is being sought. Listen to your own voice as you interact with others to catch any unconscious rise in pitch when you are not asking a question to decrease the uncertainty in your tone. Changing tone can thus change meaning. An expression as short as "oh" can be used to express anger, pity, disappointment, teasing, pleasure, gratitude, exuberance, terror, superiority, disbelief, uncertainty, compassion, insult, awe, and many more. Try this exercise with "no," "yes," and other simple words or phrases to fully grasp the rich variety of meanings a word can convey simply by varying the tone and inflection.

Tone can be reassuring or off-putting. When the patient's response is puzzling to the health professional, the latter should be alert to the tone in which the patient communicated a message or reacted to a statement. For example, if a seriously ill patient asks, "Am I going to get better?" the health professional can inadvertently confirm the patient's worst fears by hesitating and then answering in a not-too-convincing tone, "Why, of *course* you will."

VOLUME

Tone and volume are closely related voice qualities. An angry person may not only spit out the words indignantly but also may alter the volume of the message. For instance, it is possible to communicate anger either by whispering words through gritted teeth or by shouting them.

Voice volume controls interaction in subtle ways. For instance, if one person stands close to another and speaks in an inordinately loud voice, the listener invariably backs away. On the other hand, a soft whisper automatically causes the listener to move closer. Thus literally and symbolically the volume of the voice does control distance between people.

Whatever you say, you must make certain the patient can hear you. An easy way to assess if you are speaking loudly enough is to ask the patient to repeat instructions rather than just solicit "yes" or "no" responses. Make sure the patient can see your face when you speak because some patients need the physical cues of your expression and the movement of your lips to understand what is being said.

Choosing the Way to Say It

Your educational experience will provide you with the right words, but you will send many other messages to patients in addition to the spoken word. The most basic of nonverbal forms of communication is the way you think, feel, or act—your attitude. We will begin our discussion of attitudes by presuming inherent good intent in responding to one another. We presume an attitude of mutual trust and respect. Most health professionals maintain a caring attitude toward patients, and their way of speaking to them helps communicate this genuine concern and respect. On rare occasions, however, you may feel anger or disdain for a patient. In Chapter 16 we address some types of patients who present a challenge in this regard.

ATTITUDES AND EMOTIONS

One variable that is frequently overlooked and has considerable impact on the exchange of information is the patient's emotional and mental state and attitudes. Examples are anger or fear that complicate communication and the management of his or her condition. If you want to effectively communicate with a patient, you must be knowledgeable about his or her mental state. You do not have to perform an exhaustive mental status examination to determine a patient's ability to comprehend, orientation to the task at hand, or ability to follow directions. You can obtain this information as you interact with the patient. If there is any doubt as to the patient's general cognitive ability, you can use one of the many screening tools available to assess general mental functions.

The attitude or feeling that a health professional has toward the patient will help to determine the effectiveness of spoken interaction, too. Attitudes and emotions that are commonly encountered among health professionals are fear, grief, and a sense of humor.

Fear

Patients are often afraid for many reasons. Fear may manifest as stony silence, clenched fists, profuse sweating, or an angry outburst. Patients may not recognize the emotion they are experiencing as fear, so you must be watchful for the signs of fear and do your best to help reassure the patient.

The specific situations in which health professionals' fears arise are just as numerous as those for patients. How will your fear manifest itself during spoken communication? Fear can arise when the health professional is inexperienced or the patient is threatening in some way. Developing skills to de-escalate situations in which patients or family members are increasingly agitated is essential, especially if you work in high-stress areas such as emergency departments or psychiatric/mental health facilities.

Grief

Patients deal with grief in a variety of ways. It is likely that you will see some people at the worst time of their lives and come to witness many different reactions to profound loss. It is important to prepare yourself to comfort patients and family members who are grieving and to try to effectively address your own feelings. Some of the topics outlined as benchmarks of professional respect in Chapter 2 are useful at such a time. For instance, reacting with deep sorrow or tears to a patient's plight may at times be deemed "unprofessional" because it suggests pity or overidentification with the patient's or family's unique situation. However, if you remain stoic, patients may conclude you do not care. Striking the right balance between maintaining one's role as a professional in this situation (you are not a friend or family member) and conveying authentic human care for their situation warrants reflection every time you are faced with the other's suffering. That there is not a cut-and-dried formula for such a situation is evident in the following account of a struggle by a neurosurgical resident when she had to tell a patient he has a terminal brain tumor:

> I sat down and delivered the news. I hinted at the ultimate implications of his diagnosis, but I didn't want to hit this too hard too soon. I wanted to give him some time to digest the shock of the unexpected. I looked at his wife, his infant daughter, and at him. He nodded his head, slowly, calmly. I wanted to provide them with some hope so I started, reflexively, to enumerate all the treatments he could receive that would give him the best possible chance. I reassured him that he was young and healthy, which would put him in a more favorable category.

> I felt I had done enough talking at that point, so I stopped and sat in silence, a natural invitation for questions. I looked at the three of them. His wife was starting to cry, silently.

> Then, without warning, I started to cry, too, then sob, interrupting the silence. My usual calm professional demeanor had broken down. I was struck by a harsh paradox: the vision of this young vibrant family sitting with me in the present, clashing with my knowledge of biology and how this tumor was about to change their lives. I could see the future too clearly.

> The patient continued to look at me, stoically, nodding his head. He exhaled audibly and then thanked me. I didn't deserve much thanks, though. I worried that my unbridled outpouring of grief had wiped out any shred of hope.[22]

REFLECTIONS

- Because the prognosis was bleak, the message that the neurosurgeon related was accurate, but was it appropriate?
- Would the patient necessarily lose all hope as the surgeon feared?
- What might be another outcome of the neurosurgeon's expression of grief?
- What else might the neurosurgeon have said or done after her expression of grief?

Humor

A subtler, often effective way that both patients and health professionals deal with a problem or hide fear is using humor. Health care settings can be full of banter, laughter, and jokes, some of which serve useful purposes, whereas others are destructive. Humor can be used wisely to help patients cope with stress related to their illness and accompanying problems.

In communication between the patient and the health professional, joking and teasing can be used constructively to (1) allow the patient to express hostility and anxiety, (2) permit exploration of the humor and irony of the condition in which he or she is placed by illness or injury, and (3) reduce tension. Shared humor and a good laugh can often defuse anxiety in tense situations and open connections between you and the patient. The following story by a psychiatrist highlights the mutual benefits of humor:

> *I had one patient in therapy for a year who was completely bogged down in inappropriate guilt, always ready to take the blame for anything that happened to anybody anywhere in the world. She was, as usual, castigating herself, when I interrupted with, "You know, I don't mind the things you have done to the economy. I don't even mind the fact that you're responsible for high inflation. I don't even mind the taxes you cause me to pay. But I'm just madder than hell at you for causing it to rain the past three days."*

> *There had been a sharp intake of breath when I started. Her worst fears had been realized: I blamed her too! The seconds ticked by. First there was a small smile—just a twitch of the lips, really—then a grin, followed soon by a giggle, then a guffaw—which I joined. We literally laughed until we cried.[23]*

In the preceding situation, the psychiatrist was an experienced health professional and knew the patient well. Both components, experience and familiarity or a bond with the patient, and good timing need to be present for humor to be therapeutic and not destructive. The same psychiatrist compared humor to nitroglycerin: in the proper hands, it serves a useful purpose, but in the wrong hands it can cause great harm.

The inexperienced health professional and the layperson are often shocked by the openness with which patients joke about themselves. For instance, patients whose legs are paralyzed often joke about rubber crutches and icy surfaces, both of which are real threats in their present situations. Persons with disfiguring injuries may call themselves "freaks." Their joking helps to alleviate their anxiety about these problems. Patients with temporary or permanent sexual impotence also may joke a lot about sex. It is helpful to recognize their joking as one means of expressing difficult thoughts and emotions.

The use to which humor is put will determine whether it fosters respectful interaction or is a poor substitute for direct confrontation. "When used appropriately, humor can have positive psychological, communication, and social benefits, as well as positive physiological effects."[24] When used inappropriately, such as making fun of patients who are challenging or are perceived to be responsible for their own health problems, humor is hurtful and disrespectful. Although you may witness derogatory jokes about certain groups of patients, you should never join in because without exception it has no place in a professional role.

Communicating Beyond Words

In this section, we turn our attention beyond vocal utterances designed to engage us in dialogue and conversation to consider all the additional (or substitute) ways we enter into communication with patients and others. Collectively these means are often referred to as *nonverbal communication.* As important as effective verbal communication is, the majority of communication is nonverbal, with estimates of 7% of the message being verbal and the other 93% being nonverbal communication.[25] Supportive nonverbal behaviors such as leaning forward, making eye contact, nodding, smiling, gesturing, and using a warm tone of voice were positively associated with health outcomes and reducing distance between health professionals and patients.[26] Seriously ill patients in a study in Denmark noted that the health professionals' nonverbal communication was imperative for their experience of being confirmed or ignored and an inconvenience. Eye contact and tone of voice were key in confirming patients.[27] These nonverbal behaviors and others that follow are easy to adopt, so they become second nature when you interact with patients.

FACIAL EXPRESSION

Earlier in this chapter, you were asked to consider the variety of messages conveyed by altering the tone and volume of the spoken word "oh." It is possible to omit the word altogether and, with only a facial message, convey a variety of emotions.

Eye contact generally communicates a positive message. There is a powerful, immediate effect when we gaze directly at another person. If two people genuinely like each other, they will position themselves so that they look into each other's eyes. The distance between them as they face each other further communicates how they feel about each other. Distance as a form of nonverbal communication is discussed later in this chapter.

Even without eye contact, the rest of the face reveals many things. The presence or absence of a smile and the genuineness of a smile are all clues to a person's emotional state. Grimaces from pain, the vacant stare of a child with a fever, and the bland affect of a depressed patient provide important information that speaks volumes without the use of words. Your own facial expression can stimulate good feelings. For example, a genuine smile indicates that you are approachable, cooperative, and trustworthy.[28]

GESTURES AND BODY LANGUAGE

Gestures involving the extremities, even one finger, can suggest the meanings of a message. Consider the mother who folds her arms when a child begins to sputter an excuse for coming home late, the man who clenches his fist, or the adolescent girl twisting a lock of her hair. What unspoken messages are they sending? Refer to the patient scenario that opened this chapter. The patient would be considered "nonverbal" because she was intubated. Because the patient had no other way of communicating her fears and her need for the presence of the nurse, she kicked her legs. Gestures like this are often used by patients who cannot communicate verbally, and they are often misunderstood as anxiety. The patient may indeed be anxious but is often trying to convey a message. A common reaction to nonverbal gestures that are misinterpreted as anxiety or irritability is the administration of sedatives or restraints when other communication strategies would be more appropriate and less upsetting to the patient.[29]

Unlike the nurse in the opening scenario, many health professionals develop the skill of truly reading the meaning of the gestures and behaviors of patients. In more than one study, staff members in nursing home settings have demonstrated the predictive value of certain changes in nonverbal behavior in patients and the development of acute illness. One study found that the nursing assistants' documentation of nonverbal signs of illness preceded chart documentation of acute illness by an average of 5 days in a population of elderly patients.[30] Another study noted that the highest positive predictor values were for lethargy, weakness, and decreased appetite, each of which correctly predicted acute illness.[31] Understanding subtle and obvious gestures is an important component of learning respectful communication.

PROFESSIONAL DRESS

Stereotypes are commonly formed from outward appearances. In some instances, a person tries to adopt a stereotyped manner of dressing or speaking in the hope of being identified with a particular group.

Some health professionals adopt or are required to wear a stereotyped manner of dress (the uniform) to be identified easily within the world of health care. The "uniform" may include clothing such as scrubs, a patch, a pin, a lab coat, or a name tag or lanyard with a badge. Certain instruments also identify the person: the nurse's stethoscope dangling from the neck or the laboratory technologist's tray. Regardless of the symbols that can help patients identify health professionals, keep in mind that the first impression patients have of you will be how you look as you approach them.

REFLECTIONS

- What are the implications of wearing a white coat, scrubs, stethoscope, and other readily identifiable professional attire while engaging a patient in the admission process?
- In today's highly complex health settings with an increasing number of people caring for patients, do uniforms help patients identify who is caring for them, or do uniforms create greater distance?

TOUCH

In all societies, individuals come into physical contact with each other all the time, but the context is crucial (e.g., they tend not to put their hands on each other except in well-defined social and cultural rituals). However, on entering a health facility, regardless if they like or dislike physical contact, people may have to allow themselves to be palpated, punctured with needles, squeezed, rubbed, cut, examined, manipulated, and lifted.

These unusual touching privileges are granted to health professionals by society. Licensing of health professionals is primarily a protection against the charge of unconsented touching *(battery)*. In Chapter 3 we focused on boundaries, including physical ones, that must be maintained, even when legitimate touching is recognizable as part of the therapeutic encounter.

Fortunately, the comforting touch is usually regarded as legitimate, and you have in it a powerful tool for communicating caring (Fig. 10.3). Touching a patient on the arm, hand, or shoulder for less than a second can create a critical human bond.[28] The positive effects of a caring touch are sometimes observable in the patient. For example, you may observe one or more of the following: a lowering of the patient's voice, a slowing and deepening of the patient's breathing, or a spontaneous verbal response like a sigh or "I feel relaxed." A physician who was seriously ill commented on how much rubbing his back meant to him: "The nurse giving a back rub was so incredibly important to me. It was profoundly human—an act of caring. Even with painkillers, there's suffering and pain. Those back rubs were . . . somebody affirm[ing] that I mattered."[32]

People pick up signals conveyed by your manner of touching. This is often related to your appearance, the speed and ease with which you move, and the quality of your touch. The sensation received by the patient when his or her arm is lifted by the health professional's cold, clammy hand sends quite a different message from the gentle support of a warm, dry hand. Patients should be touched with respect for the person who lives inside the body being manipulated. Even if our touch is less than perfect, perhaps a bit clumsy, patients are generally deeply grateful for being handled with care by another.

Patients will be much more aware of this touching than the health professional, who has become used to touching, holding, and moving patients. The experienced health professional

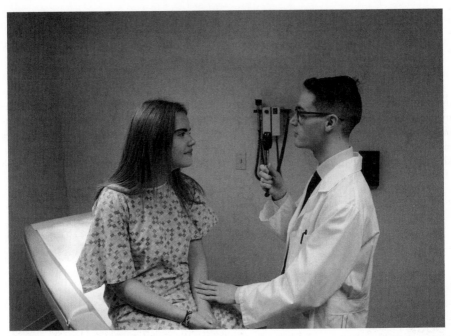

Fig. 10.3   A health professional who uses touch in an appropriate manner communicates caring to the patient. (*Courtesy Maren Haddad.*)

probably has so firm a concept of his or her good intentions that the question of inappropriateness or improper familiarity never arises. However, touch, as one form of nonverbal communication, does involve risk. It may be a threat because it invades an otherwise private space, or it may be misunderstood. So, an explanation before touching a patient is always in order. Speaking of space, we now turn our attention to the use of space in human interactions.

PROXEMICS

Proxemics is the study of how space is used in human interactions. For example, authority can be communicated by the height from which one person interacts with another. If one stands while the other sits or lies down, the person standing has placed himself or herself in a position of authority (Fig. 10.4).

Height is sometimes an unwitting message to a patient when the person is confined to a bed, a treatment table, or a wheelchair. In many instances, the relationship would be improved if the health professional would move down to the patient's level. An important rule for respectful interaction whenever you are talking to a patient is to sit down. This signals to the patient your willingness to listen and gives the impression, even if this is not true, that you are not going to rush through your time together.

Another aspect of proxemics is the distance maintained between people when they are communicating. In his now classic *The Hidden Dimension,* an intriguing book that explains the difference in distance awareness among many different cultural groups, anthropologist Edward T. Hall defines four distance zones maintained by healthy, adult, middle-class Americans.[33] In examining these zones, you may also be better able to understand how they differ from those of other cultural and socioeconomic groups. Dr. Hall stresses that "how people are feeling toward each other at the time is a decisive factor in the distance used." The four distance zones are as follows:

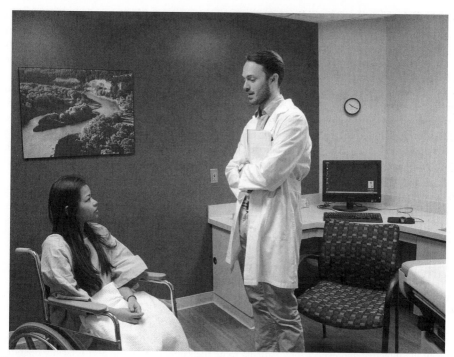

Fig. 10.4 Standing over a patient in a wheelchair is an example of inappropriate nonverbal behavior. (*Courtesy Maren Haddad.*)

1. Intimate distance, involving direct contact, such as that of lovemaking, comforting, protecting, and playing football or wrestling.
2. Personal distance, ranging from 1 to 4 feet. At arm's length, subjects of personal interest can be discussed while physical contact, such as holding hands or hitting the other person in the nose, is still possible.
3. Social distance, ranging from 4 to 12 feet. At this distance, more formal business and social discourse takes place.
4. Public distance, ranging from 12 to 25 feet or more. No physical contact and very little direct eye contact are possible. Shopping centers, airports, and city sidewalks are designed to maintain this type of distance.[34]

Health professionals perform many diagnostic or treatment procedures within the personal and intimate distance zones. You may have to invade the patient's culturally derived boundaries of interaction, sometimes with little warning. Consider, for instance, the weak or debilitated patient who comes for treatment and must be helped to a treatment table. To get the patient on the treatment table, you might have to "embrace" the patient and, in some cases, lift the patient to the table, deeply invading his or her intimate zone.

When you work with an ethnic or cultural subgroup outside of your own experience or travel to other parts of the world, culturally defined uses of space are clear. In addition, you may become aware of some things that you did not expect to be part of the interaction. For instance, body odors become more apparent when you are working at close range. In mainstream American society in which a man or woman is supposed to smell like a deodorant, a mouthwash, a hair spray, or a cologne, but not a body, it is not surprising that some health professionals find the patient's body odor offensive, sometimes nauseous; some admit that it so repulses them that they try to hurry through the test or treatment.

Patients will respond to the health professional's odors, too. An x-ray technologist confided to one of the authors that one of her biggest shocks while working in a mission hospital in India came when her assistant reluctantly admitted that patients were failing to keep their appointments because she "smelled funny," making them sick. The "funny" smell turned out to be that of the popular American soap she was using for her bath.

Bad breath is a problem. What constitutes "bad breath"? It is not necessarily the smell of garlic, onion, tobacco, or alcohol. Its definition depends on who is asked the question. The health professional who is unwilling to try to go beyond his or her own culturally derived bias will have difficulty in communicating with many patients. While working at close range, your reaction to body and breath odors will affect interaction. Most patients are far too ill or preoccupied with their problems to have sweet-smelling breath, and others are not aware that they are being hustled out quickly because of the garlic salami sandwich they had at noon.

Adhering to a patient's need to maintain an appropriate distance reinforces the patient's ability to feel secure in the strange new environment of health care institutions. By handling distance needs respectfully, you are helping patients to feel more secure in the sometimes-frightening vastness of the unknown health care setting into which they have been cast.

Differing Concepts of Time

A culturally derived difference that affects nonverbal communication is how people interpret time. The right time and the correct amount of time are relative, depending on one's cultural perspective. One aspect of the time dimension that directly affects the patient and health professional interaction is the scheduling and maintaining of appointments with patients. Most health professionals are punctual and expect their patients to be the same. In fact, the health facility operates each day on a strict schedule. Harrison points out that in mainstream Western societies "punctuality communicates respect while tardiness is an insult." However, "in some other cultures to arrive exactly on time is an insult (it says, "You are such an unimportant fellow that you can arrange your affairs easily; you really have nothing else to do."). Rather, an appropriate amount of tardiness is expected."[34] You may find that a patient is scheduled to arrive at "10 o'clock health-professional time" but arrives instead at "10 o'clock patient time," feeling no need at all to explain or apologize.

The amount of time spent in rendering professional service also may vary from one culture to another. How should a given amount of time be spent so that the patient benefits most? By majority middle-class American standards, you should greet the patient briefly and begin treatment or a test without delay. If you rush in setting up equipment, the patient may interpret it to mean you care enough to hurry. When the treatment is over, the patient usually leaves immediately.

However, in some cultures, if the treatment does not begin as soon as the patient arrives, it does not matter. Rather than rush into the procedure itself, you should first inquire about the weather, the family, and other things that may be important to the patient, sometimes spending several minutes in this way. During the actual treatment or test, you may hurry, but good-byes must not be short and rushed. One of the authors worked in an African village where she was expected to slowly enter the waiting area, then chat with the patient and other family members for a few minutes. The treatment or test could begin immediately after that, but at no time should she rush around the room or cut conversation short if the patient wanted to talk. To appear to be focusing only on the procedure was an unspeakable insult that meant the health professional believed herself more important than the patient.

Ways of operating within and indicating time, then, are highly relative. As mentioned in Chapter 5, you should always take possible differences into consideration when working with people whose cultural backgrounds are different from your own, recognizing that both distance and time awareness are deep seated and culturally derived. A person is usually not consciously aware of how he or she interprets time and distance, and so neither factor is easily identified as a cause of misunderstanding. This is another striking example of how culture influences the interpretation of verbal and nonverbal communication, warranting the professional's respect through the three aspects of respect mentioned in Chapter 1, appreciation, attention, and genuine care.

Communicating Across Distances

Much of the literature regarding communication between the patient and health professional has taken for granted that the two parties are within proximity of each other. In many cases, today, because of the mobility of society and technological developments, health professionals and patients can communicate across great distances. In addition, you may work with colleagues on the same complex patient problem and yet geographically be in two different physical sites, providing an expanded idea of the interprofessional care team. All the techniques to enhance communication in general apply to communication across distances, but they must be adapted to the special demands created by miles between a patient and health professional instead of inches.

Written Tools

Written communication includes information about diagnostic tests and evaluation observations, progress notes about patients, instructions to patients to perform activities, informed consent documents, and quality assurance surveys to obtain information from patients about services rendered. Whatever the reason for the written communication, there are distinct advantages to its use over verbal communication. Written communication has the advantage of visual cues, further enhanced when graphics are included. The reader has control over the pace of absorbing the information and can reread the information any number of times. However, written communication demands a high degree of accuracy. All written communication, whether it is a pamphlet explaining a diagnostic test, a formal letter indicating a change in office hours, an e-blast or a message in an electronic tool within a web-based patient portal, should clearly state and define the purpose of the communication. The content should be well organized. Clarity and brevity are also hallmarks of good written communication.

The vocabulary must be fitting for the recipient regardless of the mode of written communication. A good example of written communication is the consent form used for human research. Institutional review boards make judgments about research involving human participants. If the review shows that the proposed research design is ethically appropriate, it still relies heavily on a consent form signed by the participant for the research to take place. The form is supposed to be readable and understandable, outlining the purpose of the study, nature of the procedures used, and benefits and risks of the person's participation. However, study after study demonstrates that consent forms are often too long and complex. A recent review of the literature on consent forms for human participants in research reveals they are getting longer and that there is greater consistency in the description of risk.[35] The length of consent forms is certainly a problem because the more information that is given to people, the less likely it is for them to understand what is being proposed. In both research and health care environments, clear, concise written messages will be more easily understood and problems prevented if both spoken and written forms of communication can be used.

Health Literacy

Effective strategies for health care communication include health literacy. The Institute of Medicine (renamed the National Academy of Medicine) estimates that nearly half of all American adults (90 million people) have difficulty understanding and acting on health information.[36] *Health literacy* is "the degree to which individuals have the capacity to obtain, process, and understand basic health information and services."[36] Think of all the items a patient might need to read to manage their health, such as wording on medication bottles, food labels, appointment slips, medical forms, insurance applications, medical bills, and health education materials.[37] Not only do patients have to have a basic ability to read and comprehend what is written but "the increasing complexity of health care requires an understanding of digital communication, which may in turn require health, computer, numeric, computational and information literacy."[38] Older adults are less likely to be online than their younger counterparts and with the increasing use of digital health information, the divide will likely increase. Furthermore, vulnerable groups such as black Americans or those with low socioeconomic status are less likely to use electronic patient portals or other types of digital communication.[39,40]

Beyond the abilities of the patient, several other factors affect health literacy, including the quality of the information provided, the teaching method used, the context in which information is shared, the ability of the health professional to teach and communicate, and the patient's readiness to learn. Health professionals have a duty to teach patients effectively and evaluate their understanding and ability to use health information. Considerable attention has been dedicated to the research and development of various tools to screen patients for health literacy. Rather than spend time trying to determine each patient's health literacy abilities, organizations such as the American Medical Association and the Agency for Healthcare Research and Quality endorse adopting universal literacy precautions in much the same way as universal precautions for the protection of patients and health professionals from the spread of contagious disease.[41,42] In other words, health professionals should strive to communicate with all patients in simple, plain language, using lay language whenever possible to minimize the risk for any patient misunderstanding the information provided.

Voice and Electronic Tools

Because the telephone has become so much a part of our lives, you may not even notice how much you use it to communicate with patients. In an ambulatory setting, the phone may be your only contact with a patient between visits. It is best not to rely solely on this communication modality. It is especially important not to give bad news over the phone or try to explain a complicated evaluation finding or treatment plan. However, exchanging information or data such as blood glucose levels or electrocardiogram printouts electronically is an effective and efficient adjunct to other forms of communication. For example, telephones also can be used to triage patient care.

> Telephone triage is the process by which a health care provider communicates with a client via the telephone and, thereby, assesses the presenting concerns, develops a working diagnosis, and determines a suitable plan of management. Determination of the seriousness of the situation will dictate whether the client can be cared for at a distance or whether a more comprehensive in-person evaluation is in order.[43]

Of course, as we noted earlier, use of the telephone to render care must be done cautiously, particularly when you determine what follow-up is necessary.

E-mail and electronic patient records or patient portals to health records with messaging options (including apps and mobile text messages) are becoming more commonplace. Within such electronic communication platforms, patients can send nonurgent health-related messages to providers, ask follow-up questions about a treatment or prescriptions, view test results, and make appointments. Although these electronic forms of communication will not replace in-person visits, it can augment the health professional and patient relationship by providing a way to seek advice and follow up on tests or changes in prescriptions or a plan of care. Another advantage is that there is a written record of the exchange that both parties can refer to in the future.

Although electronic communication methods may assist in communication, their use depend on the availability of a personal computer or smart phone and a knowledgeable user on both ends.

Not everyone has access to such technology, but access is steadily increasing worldwide. In some cases, advanced communication technology may be the best solution to providing health care to people who would otherwise not be able to travel to places with the latest innovations in health care. The World Health Organization (WHO) views *telemedicine* as one of the most promising methods of health delivery to areas where the need for high-quality health care vastly outstrips the ability to deliver it. WHO defines telemedicine as, "The delivery of health care services, where distance is a critical factor, by all health care professionals using information and communication technologies for the exchange of valid information for diagnosis, treatment and prevention of disease and injuries, research and evaluation, and for the continuing education of health care providers, all in the interests of advancing the health of individuals and their communities."[44] As you will note, this use of information and communication technologies includes all members of the health care team, not just physicians, and for broader purposes than health delivery to patients who are at a distance. Additionally, social media offers yet another way to connect with patients also has opportunities along with challenges for you in your role as a student and eventually a health professional.

Social media is also called Web 2.0 or the read-write web because users of social media sites can create, share, edit, and interact with online content.[45] Patients use social media sites such as blogs or Facebook and reference sources, whether accurate or not, to access and share health information. Health professionals communicate with patients through social media because it can be used to share credible health information. Social media sites such as LinkedIn, professional websites with discussion boards, and Twitter can be used by health professionals to interact specifically with each other to share technical, clinical information. Although there are clear benefits of using social media, there are risks as well. The sheer reach of social media is enough to give one pause before using it in any situation that could be connected to one's professional role. Also, there is the problem of "content permanence" in that once something is posted or distributed, it is difficult, if not impossible, to remove entirely. Some of the consequences of misuse of social media include breached patient confidentiality, possible exposure to lawsuits by patients or others who are entitled to confidentiality, boundary issues in professional relationships and for students and faculty, and impairment of program integrity.[46] There are professional guidelines and standards for the use of social media developed by the American Nurses Association, the American Society of Health Systems Pharmacy, the American Medical Association, and the American Physical Therapy Association that all encourage members of each profession to adhere to ethical and legal standards with an emphasis on patient confidentiality, privacy, and appropriate boundary setting.[47-50] These standards serve as resources to both health professionals and patients as this communication technology continues to evolve.

Effective Listening

A considerable portion of a health professional's day is spent listening to patients and colleagues in person or over the telephone. Elizabeth Smith describes the following levels of listening and suggests that health professionals are usually involved in the more complex levels, cited first[51]:

1. Analytical listening for specific kinds of information and arranging them into categories
2. Directed listening to answer specific questions
3. Attentive listening for general information to get the overall picture
4. Exploratory listening because of one's own interest in the subject being discussed
5. Appreciative listening for aesthetic pleasure, such as listening to music
6. Courteous listening because one feels obligated to listen
7. Passive listening, as in overhearing something; not attentive to the matter being discussed[51]

Listening requires time that is free from interruptions, including phones, pagers, and e-mail. To listen well you need to set up the space for communicating so it is welcoming. Make sure that key attendees are there, and be prepared by knowing the patient's story and clinical details.[52]

In situations of high stress, it is important not to communicate alone to patients or family members. More than one member of the interprofessional care team should be present to ensure all elements are clearly discussed.

Most people lack the skills to listen effectively. If you are one of them, two goals for your further development are (1) to improve listening acuity so you hear the patient accurately and (2) ascertain how accurately a patient has heard you. The first step to achieving these goals is to examine the reasons messages get distorted by health professionals. Besides the often-overlooked but important possibility of a hearing deficit, there are at least three reasons a health professional distorts a verbal communication.

Distorted Meaning

First, a mind-set or frame of mind may distort meaning. It is the result of experience. In this case, a person fails to listen to the spoken words or to note subtle individual differences because he or she is sure of what the other person will say. A poignant example of people talking at and across each other and not really communicating in the health care environment is the following dialogue poem between members of an interprofessional care team and the mother of an infant in the neonatal intensive care unit. The mother speaks in stanzas 1, 4, and 7.

PATIENT CARE CONFERENCE

"I just want them to show some respect for me . . . to understand that I'm her mother."

"What she has to understand is these doctors are busy; they can't stand around waiting for her to come and besides, she doesn't always understand anyway."

"I'm leaving here and I'm glad of it. I've never been anywhere they let the nurses talk back like they do here. In Alabama, the attending is the only one allowed to talk to the family and he does, so it's all coordinated. This group of nurses sides with the family and sets us up to be the bad guys."

"I don't leave often. If I go to the store, the nurses know when I'll be back. Don't they have some legal thing that requires my permission before they do things to her?"

"What you have to understand is we have talked to her. I heard Dr. Smith on the phone with her just the other night. He went over each of the possible outcomes. We can't help it if she forgets. Maybe she should call us to see what's going on. That might fit her schedule better. I'm sure whoever is on call could deal with her."

"Well, so the pulmonary guys said the lung was blown. We didn't ask that. Why are we always blamed for not telling her? She didn't ask the right service."

"He said changing her trach wasn't considered a procedure. OK. So, what should I call those things I don't want them doing to her without me here?"

"What she has to understand is . . . ."[53]

REFLECTIONS

- Beneath the misunderstandings conveyed in the poem, what other communication issues are going on in the patient care conference?
- What are the attitudes of the health professionals described in the poem?
- What do you read "between the lines" in the poem about listening?

The patient's mother becomes just another mother in the neonatal intensive care unit, not a unique person with her own unique role, concerns, literacy level, and needs. Because the listeners, the health professionals, have made up their minds about what they will and will not hear, the mother's voice gets lost, and with it the care that would provide meaning for her in this situation.

SEARCH FOR FAMILIARITY

In addition to the risk that meaning becomes distorted, distortion can occur because most people tend to force an idea into a familiar context so that they can understand it quickly and ignore aspects of it that do not fit this context. Professionals are no exception. This tendency is, of course, related to their mind-set but is also a defense against possible change. It may be that a person's inability to accept new concepts is a result of a basic lack of self-understanding. Thus the weaker or more ill-defined a person's self-image, the greater the need to resist ideas that are more complex or ambiguous.

NEED TO PROCESS INFORMATION AT ONE'S OWN RATE

The rate at which incoming information can be processed varies significantly. This is partially but not entirely due to differences in innate ability to understand the information being conveyed by the patient. Overconfidence or too little confidence in predicting what will be said also determines whether you will cease to process incoming information. If you are overconfident, boredom settles in. If you have too little confidence the tendency for many people is to become overly anxious and tune out the message. Active listening also requires undivided attention. If distracted by too much sensory input, you will not be able to listen.

The rate and level of understanding at which you absorb communication will alter the ability to process the information. A listener's set and the need to defend existing precepts determine how accurately he or she will hear a message. Sometimes you will be the poor listener, and, as we discussed earlier, other times the patient will be.

Taking all these factors into account, you cannot control how effectively a patient listens, but you can become a more effective listener yourself. By simply restating what the patient has said, you can confirm part of a message before proceeding to the next portion of it. In addition, the following are some simple steps to more effective listening:

1. Be selective in what you listen to.
2. Concentrate on central themes rather than isolated statements. Listen in "paragraphs."
3. Judge content rather than style or delivery.
4. Listen with an open mind rather than focus on emotionally charged words.
5. Summarize in your own mind what you hear before speaking again.
6. Clarify before proceeding. Do not let vague or incomplete ideas go unattended.

The underlying theme in most discussions about listening is that it is a deliberate act. You must make a conscious decision to be fully present and engaged in the patient encounter to really understand what a patient is trying to tell you.[54]

Summary

The purpose of this chapter is to give you an overview of numerous components of respectful communication. You will communicate in many ways with your patients: in person and across the miles, individually and in groups, verbally and nonverbally. It may seem impossible to pay attention to the context of communication, the words you choose, your attitude, and the nonverbal messages you send all at the same time. However, communication designed for effective interaction in your professional relationships is a skill that can be learned and for that reason is included among the competencies of professionals. Effective communication takes practice and includes the ability both to convey clearly what you want to impart as well as actively listen, acknowledge a patient's concerns have been heard, and ensure their agenda is elicited and addressed. Effort to meet these challenges yields the reward of maintaining a relationship that honors professional respect for all persons involved.

See Section 4 Questions for Thought and Discussion on page 264 to apply what you've learned in this section to a variety of case scenarios.

References

1. Jaquette SG. The octopus and me: the nursing insight gleaned from a battle with cancer. *Am J Nurs.* 2000;100(4):24.
2. Smith JF. Communicative ethics in medicine: the physician-patient relationship. In: Wolf S, ed. *Feminism and Bioethics: Beyond Reproduction.* New York: Oxford University Press; 1996.
3. Byrne PS, Long BE. *Doctors Talking to Patients.* London: Her Majesty's Stationery Office; 1976.
4. Watson K. Serious play: teaching medical skills with improvisational theater techniques. *Acad Med.* 2011;86(10):1260–1265.
5. Frank A. From suspicion to dialogue: relations of storytelling in clinical encounters. *Med Humanit Rev.* 2000;14(1):24–34.
6. Grover Jr F, Wu HD, Blanford C, et al. Computer-using patients want Internet services from family physicians. *J Fam Pract.* 2002;51(6):570–572.
7. Wallace LS, Cassada DC, Ergen WF, et al. Setting the stage: surgery patients' expectations for greetings during routine office visits. *J Surg Res.* 2009;157:91–95.
8. Getsi LC. Intensive care. In: Getsi LC, ed. *Intensive Care—Poems by Lucia Cordell Getsi.* Minneapolis: New Rivers Press; 1992.
9. US Census Bureau. *Projected Population of the United States, by Race and Hispanic Origin: 2000-2050;* 2010. Available at: https://www.census.gov/programs-surveys/popproj.html.
10. Agency for Healthcare Research and Quality: Improving patient safety systems for patients with limited English proficiency: a guide for hospitals. Rockville, MD: U.S. Department of Health and Human Services.
11. Srivastava R. The interpreter. *N Engl J Med.* 2017;376(9):812–813.
12. Phelan M, Parkman S. How to work with an interpreter. *Br Med J.* 1995;311:555–557.
13. Schapira L, Vargas E, Hidalgo R, et al. Lost in translation: integrating medical interpreters into the multidisciplinary team. *Oncologist.* 2008;13:586–592.
14. Seidelman RD, Bachner YG. That I won't translate! experiences of a family medical interpreter in a multicultural environment. *Mt Sinai J Med.* 2010;77:389–393.
15. Garlock A. Professional interpretation services in health care. *Radiol Technol.* 2016;88(2):201–204.
16. Watermeyer J. She will hear me: how a flexible interpreting style enables patients to manage the inclusion of interpreters in mediated pharmacy interactions. *Health Commun.* 2011;26(1):71–81.
17. Ripich DN. Training Alzheimer's disease caregivers for successful communication. *Clin Gerontol.* 1999;21(1):37–56.
18. Small JA, et al. Effectiveness of communication strategies used by caregivers of persons with Alzheimer's disease during activities of daily living. *J Speech Lang Hear Res.* 2003;46(2):353–367.
19. Butow PN, Brown RF, Cogar S, et al. Oncologists' reactions to cancer patients verbal cues. *Psychooncology.* 2002;11:47–58.
20. Freeman J, Loewe R. Barriers to communication about diabetes mellitus: patients' and physicians' different view of the disease. *J Fam Pract.* 2000;49(6):513–542.
21. Vermeir P, Vandijck D, Degroote S, et al. Communication in healthcare: a narrative review of the literature and practical recommendations. *Int J Clinical Practice.* 2015;69(11):1257–1267.
22. Firlik K. *Another Day in the Frontal Lobe: A Brain Surgeon Exposes Life on the Inside.* New York: Random House; 2006.
23. Chance S. *A Voice of my Own: A Verbal Box of Chocolates.* Cleveland, SC: Bonne Chance Press; 1993.
24. Buxman K. Humor in critical care: no joke. *AACN Clin Issues Adv Pract Acute Crit Care.* 2000;11(1):120–127.
25. Argyle M. *Bodily Communication.* 2nd ed. London: Routledge; 1988.
26. Ruben MA, Blanch-Hartigan D, Hall JA. Nonverbal communication as a pain reliever: the impact of physician supportive nonverbal behavior on experimentally induced pain. *Health Commun.* 2017;32(8):970–976.

27. Timmerman C, Uhrenfeldt L, Birkelund R. Ethics in the communicative encounter: seriously ill patients' experiences of health professionals' nonverbal communication. *Scand J Caring Sci.* 2016;31:63–71.

28. Middaugh DJ. Watch your language! *Medsurg Nursing.* 2017;26(1):64–65.

29. Grossbach I, Stranberg S, Chlan L. Promoting effective communication for patients receiving mechanical ventilation. *Crit Care Nurse.* 2011;31(2):46–61.

30. Boockvar KS, Brodie HD, Lachs MS. Nursing assistants detect behavior changes in nursing home residents that precede acute illness: development and validation of an illness warning instrument. *J Am Geriatr Soc.* 2000;48(9):1086–1091.

31. Boockvar KS. Lachs MS: Predictive value of nonspecific symptoms for acute illness in nursing home residents. *J Am Geriatr Soc.* 2003;51:1111–1115.

32. Klitzman R. Improving education on doctor-patient relationships and communication: lessons from doctors who become patients. *Acad Med.* 2006;81(5):447–453.

33. Hall ET. *The Hidden Dimension.* New York: Doubleday; 1966.

34. Harrison R. Nonverbal communications: explorations into time, space, action and object. In: Campbell JH, Hepler HW, eds. *Dimensions in Communications: Readings.* 2nd ed. Belmont, CA: Wadsworth; 1970.

35. Albala I, Doyle M, Appelbaum PS. The evolution of consent forms for research: a quarter century of changes. *IRB: Ethics Human Res.* 2010:7–11.

36. Institute of Medicine. *Health Literacy: A Prescription to End Confusion.* Washington, DC: National Academies Press; 2004.

37. Hersh L, Salzman B, Synderman D. Health literacy in primary care practice. *Am Fam Physician.* 2015;92(2):118–124.

38. National Network of Libraries of Medicine: Health literacy [Internet]. Bethesda, MD, NNLM. Available from: https://nnlm.gov/initiatives/topics/health-literacy.

39. Levy H, Janke AT, Langa KM. Health literacy and the digital divide among older Americans. *J Gen Intern Med.* 2014;30(3):284–289.

40. Ancker JS, Barron Y, Rockoff ML. Use of an electronic patient portal among disadvantaged populations. *J Gen Internal Medicine.* 2011;26(10):1117–1123.

41. Weiss BD. *American Medical Association: Health Literacy and Patient Safety: Help Patients Understand.* Chicago, IL: American Medical Association Foundation; 2007.

42. Agency for Healthcare Research and Quality: Health literacy universal precautions toolkit. http://www.ahrq.gov/professionals/quality-patient-safety/quality-resources/tools/literacy-toolkit/index.htm.

43. DeVore NE. Telephone triage: a challenge for practicing midwives. *J Midwifery.* 1999;44(5):471–479.

44. World Health Organization. *Telemedicine: Opportunities and Developments in Members States, Report on the Second Global Survey on eHealth (Global Observatory for eHealth Series, 2).* Geneva, Switzerland: WHO Press; 2009.

45. Gagnon K, Sabus C. Professionalism in a digital age: opportunities and considerations for using social media in health care. *Phys Ther.* 2015;95(3):406–414.

46. Westrick S. Nursing students' use of electronic and social media: law, ethics and E-professionalism. *Nurs Educ Perspect.* 2016:16–22.

47. American Nurses Association. *Principles for Social Networking and the Nurse.* Silver Springs, MD: American Nurses Association; 2011.

48. American Society of Health System Pharmacists. ASHP statement on use of social media by pharmacy professionals developed through the ASHP Pharmacy Student Forum and the ASHP Section of Pharmacy Informatics and Technology and approved by the ASHP Board of Directors on April 13, 2012, and by the ASPH House of Delegates. *Am J Health Syst Pharm.* 2012;69:2095–2097.

49. Kind T. Professional guidelines for social media use: a starting point. *AMA Journal of Ethics.* 2015;17(5):441–447.

50. American Physical Therapy Association: Standards of Conduct in the Use of Social Media. *HOD P06-12-17-16.* 2012. Available at: http://www.apta.org/uploadedFiles/APTAorg/About_Us/Policies/Ethics/StandrdsConductSocialMedia.pdf.

51. Smith E. Improving listening effectiveness. *Tex Med.* 1975;71:98–100.

52. Warwillow S, Farley KJ, Jones D. Ten practical strategies for effective communication with relatives of ICU patients. *Intensive Care Med.* 2015;41:2173–2176.

53. Ogborn S. Patient care conference. In: Haddad A, Brown K, eds. *The Arduous Touch: Women's Voices in Health Care.* West Lafayette, IN: Purdue University Press; 1999.

54. Shipley SD. Listening: a concept analysis. *Nurs Forum.* 2010;45(2):125–134.

Respectful Interactions Across the Life Span

Having studied the basic foundations of respectful interaction, you now have an opportunity to apply your learning to several types of patients you will see throughout the course of your professional career. We have chosen to address them by age group, over the life span, being mindful that individual differences often outweigh the similarities we are emphasizing in these different cohorts.

Life span development encompasses constancy and change in an individual's behavior throughout the life span. Development is not bound by a single criterion—it is multidimensional and multidirectional. Any process of development entails aspects of growth (gain) and decline (loss), and these relate to an individual's adaptive capacity. Each lifetime also presents different paths. Often illness or disability takes patients and families down an unfamiliar path. Your role as a health professional and member of the interprofessional care team is to help these individuals navigate that path, adjusting and adapting along life's journey.

Section 5 begins with Chapter 11, highlighting the joys and challenges of working with newborns, infants, toddlers, and preschoolers. The family is a key element of consideration, and the principles of patient- and family-centered care serve as guideposts for the interprofessional care team working with this age group. Chapter 12 moves the focus of your attention to school-age children and adolescents. The evolving needs of the child and family as they mature are discussed, particularly as they relate to supporting health through transitions and adversity during these important developmental stages.

In Chapter 13 we discuss your interaction with people who become patients during young and middle adulthood. Only in recent times have these life periods been given more than a cursory glance, and we share some of the insights that researchers and others are finding. Identity development across cultures, expansion of caregiving roles, onset of chronic conditions, and stressors related to adult responsibilities are discussed.

Chapter 14 examines key issues related to working with older adults. Of all age groups, this one is increasing more in diversity and size worldwide than any other population. New research and theories on healthy aging are presented, given their importance in supporting older patients for optimal physical, cognitive, and mental health.

Throughout the life span, the person who becomes a patient is faced with many of the challenges we have been discussing so far. Injury and/or illness can disrupt a person's life patterns and development, challenging the acquisition of "normal" life skills. You have a substantial role in respectfully helping your patient meet these challenges.

CHAPTER 11

Respectful Interaction

Working With Newborns, Infants, and Children in the Early Years

The reader will be able to:

- Assess skills and activities that reflect respect toward newborns, infants, toddlers, and preschoolers
- Distinguish some basic developmental differences that need to be considered in one's approach to newborns, infants, toddlers, and preschoolers
- Discuss in general terms Erikson's sequential view of the psychological development of infants and toddlers
- List some everyday needs of the infant that may help explain an infant's response to the health professional
- Describe how a consistent approach builds trust in interactions with patients in early childhood
- Describe six types of play, and show how each can facilitate respectful interaction with a pediatric patient
- Describe how the young child's developing need for autonomy enters into the health professional and patient relationship
- Define early adversity and understand its impact on early childhood development

Prelude

Lou and I walked back to Alex's isolette. We peered in at the uncomfortable little being who was still pulling at his feeding tube and now making a faint mewing sound. I put my hands through the portholes in the side of the box and stroked his arms down away from the tube. I couldn't get myself to talk to him. I stared at him but could not make sense of what I was seeing. Who was this new person? "Spastic diplegia." Would he even walk? I couldn't picture anything. I left the hospital that day with an empty feeling.

V. FORMAN[1]

This is the first of several chapters that examine respectful interaction with patients across the life span. It begins with our smallest patients—neonates and newborns—and transitions to working with infants, toddlers, and children in the preschool years. The section on growth and development includes information that applies across childhood, although working with each age group has its own opportunities and challenges. Provided here is a wide range of relevant topics concerning interaction with young patients that provide a basis for more in-depth exploration in your other coursework and lifelong education.

Almost all health professionals interact at some point with newborns and children in the early years, including infants, toddlers, and preschoolers. Some health professionals work solely with these groups and others with their parents, grandparents, guardians, or siblings. These small patients must be treated with the respect they deserve as unique individuals like everyone else. Furthermore, the opportunity they are given to experience human dignity and support in their time of illness, injury, or other adversity can become a resource to help them and their families manage future difficulties. As the opening quote reminds us, we meet our youngest patients within the context of their families. It is through the loving care of family caregivers that infants bond, have their basic needs met, learn, and develop on their journey through early childhood.

Most of us take for granted that a newborn will live into his or her 7th or 8th decade of life. This has not always been so and is not the case in many countries. Today, the global average infant mortality rate is 32 infant deaths per 1000 live births.[2] In the United States, the infant mortality rate is 5.8 infant deaths per 1000 live births. Although US infant mortality rate is declining, it currently is higher than in other economically developed countries, with the United States ranking 169th among 225 countries.[3,4] The top five causes of infant mortality in the United States are birth defects, preterm birth, maternal complications of pregnancy, sudden infant death syndrome (SIDS), and injuries or accidents.[5,6]

Perhaps most significant to health professionals (and the public health sector) is that the overall infant mortality rate is not shared equally by all groups. Mortality is higher for infants and children living in poverty. The mortality rate for black infants is more than twice that for white infants. The causes of these disparities are multidimensional, including social determinants of health, maternal health and behaviors, economic status, structural racism, insurance, and health care access.[7]

Better opportunities for health education and overall longevity in white groups point to deep internal health disparities, the consequences of which must be reckoned with. As a health professional, you will need to call on your skills and knowledge to reach solutions that help close the disparities gap. As discussed in Section 2, being aware of unconscious biases and acting to decrease disparities can enhance high-quality, culturally informed, and nondiscriminatory health care delivery.[8]

Useful General Principles of Human Growth and Development

Growth and development occur in numerous ways—physical, emotional, intellectual (or cognitive), social, and moral—and all aspects of development affect one another. Some theories are hierarchical models of development, whereas others are dynamic. Although professionals often talk about growth and development simultaneously, *growth* can be thought of as quantitative (e.g., changes in height and weight) and *development* as qualitative (changes in performance influenced by the maturation process).

HUMAN GROWTH

Human growth proceeds in accordance with general principles of (1) orderliness, (2) discontinuity, (3) differentiation, (4) cephalocaudal, and (5) proximodistal and bilateral. Each is instrumental in helping you understand what occurs in the growth process, when, and why.

Orderliness

Growth and changes in behavior usually occur in an orderly fashion and in the same sequence. Thus infants can turn their heads before they can extend their hands. Almost every child sits before he or she stands, stands before walking, and draws a circle before drawing a square. Most babies babble before talking and pronounce certain sounds before others. Likewise, certain cognitive abilities precede the next. Preschoolers can categorize objects or put them into a series before they can think logically.

Discontinuity

Although growth is orderly, it is not always smooth and gradual. There are periods of rapid growth—growth spurts—and increases in psychological abilities. Parents sometimes speak of the summer that a child "shot up" 2 inches. Many adolescents experience a sudden growth spurt after years of being the ones with the smallest stature in their class.

Differentiation

Development proceeds from simple to complex and from general to specific. An example of differentiation in the infant is seen in an infant's ability to wave his or her arms first and later develop purposeful use of his or her fingers. Motor responses are diffuse and undifferentiated at birth and become more specific and controlled as the child grows. Beginning motor activity in the toddler involves haphazard and unsystematic actions, progressing to goal-directed actions and specific outcomes.[9]

Cephalocaudal

Cephalocaudal development means that the upper end of the organism develops earlier than the lower end. Increases in neuromuscular size and maturation of function begin in the head and proceed to the hands and feet. For example, after birth an infant will be able to hold his or her head erect before being able to sit or walk.

Proximodistal and Bilateral

Proximodistal development means that growth progresses from the central axis of the body (the trunk) toward the periphery or extremities. Thus the central nervous system develops before the peripheral nervous system. Bilateral development means that the capacity for growth and development of the child is symmetric—growth that occurs on one side of the body generally occurs on the other side of the body simultaneously. These principles apply throughout the life span, from infancy to old age.

HUMAN DEVELOPMENT

Development can be discussed in domains of human performance: cognitive, affective, and psychomotor or through standardized language/classification systems of human function and abilities such as the International Classification of Function, Disability and Health (ICF) developed by the World Health Organization.[10] The ICF dimensions of functioning and disability are body structure and function, activities and participation, and personal and environmental factors. We will focus primarily on cognitive development because it entails how a person perceives, thinks, and communicates thoughts and feelings. Time is also spent on psychosocial development because of the profound impact this has on the health professional's interactions with patients.

Cognitive Development

Cognitive development is a way of addressing the way a child learns to think, reason, and use language, which are vital to the child's overall growth and development.[11] Traditionally, health professionals have based their interventions with children on the stages of cognitive development described by Jean Piaget (1896–1980).[12] Piaget's theory is a logical, deductive explanation of how children think from infancy through adolescence. Piaget described the earliest stage of cognitive

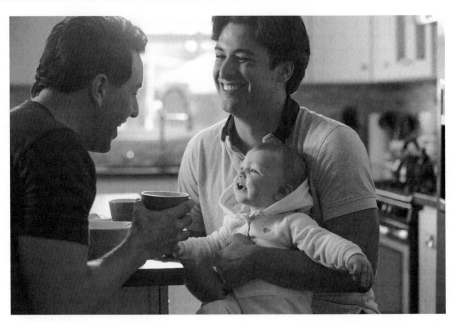

Fig. 11.1 Infants develop cognitive skills through verbal and nonverbal interactions with caring adults. (© monkeybusinessimages/iStock/Thinkstock.com.)

development as *sensorimotor*. At this stage, infants take in a great deal of information through their senses. Tactile and verbal stimulation and auditory and visual cues can have positive, long-range results. The early beginnings of cognitive development can be stimulated by talking to the infant and by face-to-face interactions (Fig. 11.1).

Piaget labeled the cognitive abilities of toddlers *preoperational*. Toddlers learn to think and understand by building each new experience upon previous experiences. Miller[13] summarized Piaget's depiction of the cognitive stage of toddlers in terms of egocentrism (seeing the world from a "me-only" viewpoint), rigidity of thought ("Mom is always right"), and semilogical reasoning ("My dog died because I was a bad boy"). Children in this stage are confused about cause and effect, even when it is explained to them, and think in terms of magic (e.g., wishing something makes it so). However, more current researchers refute Piaget's beliefs and claim that he may have underestimated the cognitive abilities of toddlers. These researchers suggest that children have far more potential to understand complex illness concepts than they have previously been given credit for.[14] Thus some toddlers can appreciate the perspective of another and adapt their behavior accordingly. Others propose that, rather than viewing the toddler as incapable of thinking a certain way, one should view him or her as a novice. Children have much less life experience than adults. Thus, when children gain experience through chronic illness, for example, or perform tasks involving their own expertise, they can demonstrate adult-like performance and more sophisticated thinking and reasoning.[15] The debate in cognitive development is ongoing. For example, researchers in the field of evolutionary developmental psychology consider genetic and ecological mechanisms, as well as the effect of cultural contexts. They have recently added their voices to discussions regarding early childhood brain development.[16-18] The insights of various developmental theorists are important to explore because they have direct implications for how best to work with young children.

As with cognitive development, there are numerous stage/phase theories about *psychological and social development*. Development, seen this way, is a process or movement. "Movement from potentiality to actuality occurs over time and in the direction of growth and progress. It is not surprising, then, that most conceptualizations of development incorporate the notion of improvement—of 'better' more integrated ways of functioning."[19]

Almost all theories stress the importance of bonding or forming attachments as the primary developmental task. No one has done more to promote this idea than Erik Erikson, a psychologist who, in the 1950s and 1960s, proposed eight stages of psychosocial development.[20] According to his theory, the development of trust introduced in Chapter 2 as fundamental to the effective patient and health professional relationship is one of the tasks facing the child in all relationships. He or she is engaged in a process that will affect the ability to engage in respectful interaction with everyone. During infancy, the child is introduced to trust and begins to experience (or to not experience) its power.

The psychosocial development of the toddler involves acquiring a clearer sense of himself or herself that is separate from that of the primary caregiver, becoming involved in wider social relationships, gaining self-control and mastery over motor and verbal skills, and developing independence and a self-concept. Later in this chapter, we consider specific examples of how you can effectively interact with infants, toddlers, and preschoolers by anticipating the developmental tasks specific to their age group. However, a caveat about relying on developmental stages is that it is difficult to place a child in a specific stage solely based on chronological age. Behaviors occur in context, and the environment or task-specific demands can alter function during that process.

Early Development: From Newborn to Preschooler

Between the first day of life and the first day of kindergarten, development proceeds at a lightning pace like no other. Consider just a few of the transformations that occur during this 5-year period:

- The newborn's avid interest in staring at other babies turns into the capacity for cooperation, empathy, and friendship.
- The 1-year-old's tentative first steps become the 4-year-old's pirouettes and slam dunks.
- The completely un-self-conscious baby becomes a preschooler who can describe herself in detail. Her behavior is partially motivated by how she wants others to view and judge her.
- The first adamant "no!" turns into the capacity for elaborate arguments about why the parent is wrong and the preschooler is right.
- The infant, who has no conception that his blanket came off because he kicked his feet, becomes the 4-year-old who can explain the elaborate (if messy) causal sequence by which he can turn flour, water, salt, and food coloring into play dough.

It is no surprise that the early childhood years are portrayed as formative. The supporting structures of virtually every system of the human organism, from the tiniest cell to the capacity for intimate relationships, are constructed during this age period.[21]

NORMAL NEWBORN

The anticipation of the birth of a child is fraught with emotions ranging from joy to fear. In economically developed countries the birth process has largely moved from the home to the hospital. Many hospitals attempt to duplicate the comforts and familiarities of home by designing birthing suites complete with wifi and comfy seating. With the move to shorter lengths of stay for a normal delivery, it is unlikely that you will have much opportunity to work directly with these tiniest of patients unless you choose to work in labor and delivery or neonatology. At the same time as noted earlier, many family members may be involved in one way or another with the birth event, and all health professionals should be prepared for a respectful response to the whole family.

Normal newborns experience relationships through their senses.[22] They are highly vulnerable but also amazingly adaptable to the new environment outside the womb. The newborn period ends at the first month of life. After that, newborns are called *infants*. Newborns have many needs, especially when health problems are present at birth. They are human beings worthy of full respect.

LIFE-THREATENING CIRCUMSTANCES

New technology is changing the possibility for survival in neonates and newborns. A full-term pregnancy lasts for 40 weeks. Some full-term newborns along with increasingly smaller neonates who have had gestations as short as 23 weeks in the womb are seen in neonatal intensive care units (NICUs). In the clinical setting, you may hear these patients referred to as *fragile neonates* or *preemies*. Many variables impact survival for these tiny patients.

Newborns in these settings range from those with high-intensity care needs (such as mechanical ventilation) to those with lower intensity care needs (such as monitoring of oxygen levels or postoperative support for corrective neonatal surgery). Sometimes a neonate who weighs more than the fragile neonate in the next isolette is the one who does not survive. Each year tens of thousands of babies end up in a NICU. In each case, parents and health professions share a common goal—to make each baby healthy. New medical technologies are saving babies who until only recently would not have survived. For some of these families, however, the result may be a baby whose future involves lifelong chronic health conditions. With little or no preparation, parents often find themselves in times of great uncertainty and are asked to decide when the technology is doing more harm than good. It is interesting to note that in retrospect, many parents do not identify involvement in decision-making. In Pinch's longitudinal study of parents' experiences in the NICU, "parents recalled that possibilities or alternatives were seldom offered to them. They were simply told what the professionals were required to do, what the baby needed, or what was suggested as the best treatment."[23] The NICU can be an overwhelming environment for many families. Thus respectful interaction with parents of these fragile newborns requires that you take extra care to inform them about the status and progress of their children. More generally speaking, one essential key to respectful interaction with parents is your understanding and empathy for the complex stresses and, for some, losses they are experiencing as they cope with their new roles as parents.[24]

MOVING INTO INFANCY

When working with an infant, you, along with other members of the interprofessional care team, will be able to make key clinical judgments about the patient's best interests and observe the interaction between parents and their new baby. Happily, the parents almost always provide the primary supportive bridge between you and the infant patient, interpreting the baby's expressions, babbles, and postures and providing insight into how continuity of approach to the infant can be maximized. During this time, parents must learn cues from their infants, and sometimes you can teach the parents, as well as learn from the parents' comments and behavior. The needs of infants are sometimes difficult to determine because these small patients are vulnerable and lack sufficient verbal skills to express their wants and needs. Professionals who rely solely on a patient's ability to ask for what he or she needs take a narrow view of needs assessment. As with any nonverbal patient, the health professional must learn to read the infant's signals and collaborate with the family caregivers to determine the infant's needs.

INFANT NEEDS: RESPECT AND CONSISTENCY

There are two contexts by which to view the infant's needs. The first focuses on the stage of psychosocial development that we have already discussed and the second on immediate concrete needs such as the need for a drink of water, food, pain relief, or a diaper change. You have an opportunity to demonstrate respect for the infant by responding effectively to each type of need.

Remember that parents often have explicit ways of doing things for their infant that can help, too. For example, parents may hold the infant in a certain way or play a favorite game such as pretending to sneeze or rubbing the baby's back that will, at a minimum, help calm the infant while you look for other reasons for the infant's distress.

A primary approach is characterized by the three "Cs": consistency in approach, constancy of presence, and continuity of treatment. Consistency is especially important because it builds trust (infant self-confidence) through the following steps:[25]

1. An infant's need exists.
2. The infant exhibits generalized behavior.
3. The caregiver responds.
4. The need is satisfied.
5. The need recurs.
6. The infant predicts the caregiver's response.
7. The infant repeats previous behavior.
8. The caregiver responds in a consistent manner.
9. The need is satisfied.
10. The infant's trust toward the caregiver develops.
11. The need recurs.
12. The infant is confident that the caregiver will respond appropriately.

Of course, all infants have different temperaments, which will create differences in responses to you, the health professional. These individual differences are welcomed by health professionals because they support the belief that humans are unique, each deserving of unique respect.

EVERYDAY NEEDS OF INFANTS

By now you have discovered in this book that the "solutions" to challenges during interaction with patients are sometimes concrete and dictated by common sense. Fussy, irritable, crying infants are in the vulnerable position of becoming the least liked (and potentially least cared for) patients on the pediatrics unit. Crying is one way infants try to communicate distress.

More likely than not, because of the infant's age and stage of development, this distress is related to a concrete, immediate need. Respectful interaction with infants in distress requires careful attention to several types of details.

Attention to the Comfort Details of Care

Small children most often become irritable when they experience physical discomfort. Careful attention to comfort is key to their sense of well-being. This becomes even more reason to check for factors that could lead to discomfort whenever possible. It is too easy to assume that a baby's crying or other belligerence is because he or she is a fussy or cranky baby. Examine the onesie, diaper, and crib sheets.

REFLECTIONS

Which of these comfort detail questions should health professionals ask themselves?
- Is the onesie, diaper, or crib sheet wet from urine, sweat, or a spilled medication?
- Are they wrinkled and creating pressure spots?
- Does the baby have abrasions, punctures, or other bodily tenderness that causes contact pain? Is tape pinching the baby, or has an intravenous line infiltrated?
- Are the infant's throat and mouth dry?
- What did the baby eat and when? Is he or she taking fluids?
- Is a bowel movement creating skin irritation?
- Is the infant hungry or thirsty?
- Is the infant having some predictable side effect from a medication?
- What is the environment like? Is it too noisy? Too bright? Too dark?

What other comfort questions can you name?

Health Professional Detail. Discomfort also can be caused by what you are wearing or doing. Think about the kind of clothing and adornments such as name tags that you wear in clinical practice.

- Is your uniform scratching the baby? Is the color or design too complex?
- Are you wearing jewelry that scratches, pokes, or pinches?
- Are your hands clammy and cold?

Think about the number of providers evaluating or treating the infant.

- Is the baby constantly being dressed and undressed?
- Has the baby been assessed by several different members of the interprofessional health team without the opportunity to rest?
- Is the baby overstimulated by machines and mechanical or procedural-based handling (vs. skin contact and loving touch to facilitate bonding with providers)?

Your conduct is like a mirror to the baby. If you are anxious or uncomfortable with caring for an infant, the infant will sense it. In addition to the immediate discomfort you may cause an infant by inattention to these details, a more persistent negative response could be a sign of deeper discomfort. A good general rule is to remain consistent, approaching the infant similarly in each interaction in hope that the familiarity itself will be a comfort. Also, watch how the infant interacts with others, especially those who appear to be successful in calming him or her. Try altering your approach to match those that seem to calm the infant. Always orient the infant to your presence, and provide comforting touch when procedural touch is also required.

Environmental Detail. Like all of us, infants have various comfort zones, which include temperature, space, noise, and other environmental factors.

REFLECTIONS

Look around the room that you are currently occupying, and imagine it is one that includes an ill infant.

- Is the room too warm or is there a source of cold air that is directed on you?
- Have you adjusted your clothing because you were sweaty or chilled?
- Are there distracting noises in the area from nearby construction, an open window, or a piece of electronic equipment?
- Are there different smells in the air such as the fumes from painting in the hallway, a disinfectant, or food preparation nearby?
- What else do you notice about the environment that could have an impact on an infant's well-being?

In short, this section is a reminder of ways you should be attentive to the behavior of the young patient and to the people who are associated with his or her care. One of the primary developmental goals of infancy is social attachment. Attention to comfort of the infant, the family care providers, and the environment is essential so that the infant can trustingly engage with others.[26]

Case Study

Lucy Bahal is a 2-month-old infant referred to Bayside Early Intervention for an interprofessional developmental evaluation because of failure to thrive. Lucy was born at 38 weeks of gestation and transitioned home from the hospital with her family on her fifth day of life. Lucy was a little "slow to eat," so the care team recommended that she be bottle fed until the mother, Lydia, and Lucy could get into a routine. Lydia is a 29-year-old operating room nurse who breastfed her other two children without any difficulties. Lucy, however, is just "not taking to it," which is frustrating Lydia. You arrive at the Bahal home for the intake visit. Lucy is in a portable crib on her back. She is fussy and the two other

Case Study—cont'd

children (age 28 months and 4 years old) are arguing over which cartoon show they would like to watch. Lydia greets you by saying "just another day in paradise." You talk with Lydia about your role and start to take a developmental history on Lucy. Lydia reports that Lucy is her "hardest baby." She has not been able breastfeed and reports that she is "very fussy." You ask Lydia what a typical day is like, and she reports that she is so overwhelmed by it all and there is no typical. Lydia says all she really wants to do is sleep and that she does not feel like eating or playing with Lucy.

- What additional questions do you have for this postpartum mother? Besides the infant's failure to thrive, what other health issues might be going on in this family?
- How might you show respect and consistency for Lucy, while attending to the principles of patient- and family-centered care presented in Chapter 8?

Early Development: The Toddler and Preschool Child

Much of the material related to respectful interaction with the infant patient and his or her family can be applied to the child past the stage of infancy into other stages of early childhood. As a child grows, however, new challenges confront both parents and health professionals. This is especially true of the toddler and preschooler. These years are ones of rapid physical, social, emotional, and cognitive growth. Children begin to walk, run, and climb. They have increased control over feeding and toileting habits and start learning about limits.

All children develop at their own pace, and some, like Lucy in the case study, may experience delays in reaching a milestone in a select area of growth and development. You often hear this reflected in the comments of parents who recall how one of their children did not talk until almost 3 but has not stopped talking since. Variations in the growth and development trajectory are not atypical but do require close monitoring. When children fail to reach multiple milestones over key developmental periods, and parents and health professionals have concerns about the child's day-to-day functioning, developmental testing is indicated. Early monitoring and developmental testing are vitally important because developmental disabilities are typically diagnosed in the early years.[27] Given their effect on early childhood functioning, developmental disabilities such as autism spectrum disorder (ASD) are being diagnosed much earlier than in years past. It is not uncommon for diagnosis to occur in the 18-month-old to 2-year-old child. The median age of ASD diagnosis is 4.2 years, yet most parents report seeing signs and symptoms of it as early as 6 months to 1 year of age.

A review of Erikson's stages shows that the young patient's psychosocial tasks in moving from infancy to becoming a toddler and then an older child focus on becoming one's own "self," separate from others. Unique personalities develop, and at this early age respect for a toddler and preschool age child can be enhanced when the child asks for what he or she wants. Of course, sometimes the toddler will have difficulty making himself or herself understood and may be embarrassed by his or her own awkward attempts to act grown up. Especially important to the child is the need to succeed at "adult" tasks (which include anything new, from the early tasks of learning how to walk and to feed oneself, to everything that mimics the behavior of older children and adults).

PLAY

Play is an important vehicle through which a toddler patient's sense of worth can be fostered. According to developmental psychologists, play may be the child's richest opportunity for physical, cognitive, social, and emotional development. Play is the primary tool through which the child learns social and cultural roles and norms. Freiberg describes several types of play, any of which can be encouraged as part of treatment or other aspects of interaction with the child. These include the following:

- *symbolic play*, which children use to make something stand for something else, such as when the young patient "becomes" the more powerful health professional by wearing the health professional's stethoscope or donning her parents' shoes or scarf;

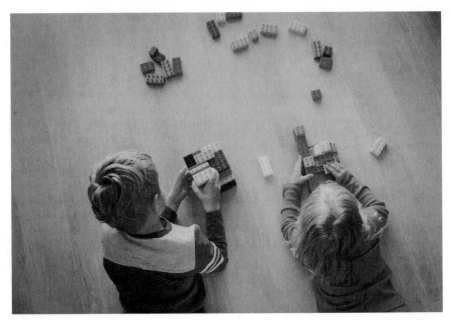

Fig. 11.2 Parallel play can be encouraged as part of treatment or other aspects of interaction with a young child. (© Nadezhda1906/iStock/Thinkstock.com.)

- *onlooker play,* which involves intently watching others, such as when the health professional entertains the child or when the child observes others at play but does not actively participate;
- *parallel play,* which is side-by-side play characterized by activity that is interactive only by virtue of another's presence. (Participation by observation and side-by-side types of play may help decrease a young patient's loneliness, even though he or she cannot fully interact with others) (Fig. 11.2);
- *associative play,* which involves shared activity and communication but little organized activity;
- *constructive play,* which involves the making or building of things; and
- *cooperative play,* which requires following group rules and achieving agreed-on goals. (Associative play and cooperative play are generally beyond the capabilities of the toddler but emerge in preschoolers).[30]

Toddler and Preschooler Needs: Respect and Security

Attention to personal detail outlined in the section on infants applies to interaction with the toddler as well. Fortunately, in most cases, toddlers can verbalize their basic needs ("Me hungry," "Me go?" "More," or "No") and express their curiosity by pointing to something and asking, "Dis?" Their illness, the intimidating surroundings, or their shyness, however, may make young children even more reticent than most patients to make their needs known in this direct manner. They often show their feelings of insecurity about what is happening to them by being cranky or acting overly fearful and demanding.

Children, like all patients, tend to regress when they become ill. Having so recently moved out of infancy, toddlers sometimes return to infant-like behavior. This is a normal tendency and should not be cause to condemn young patients who do not "act their age."

One of the authors recalls hearing a health professional tell a pediatric patient the patient was acting "like a baby," to which the patient confidently responded, "Well, I may not be a baby, but I am only 3!" Remember, even the smallest patients need care providers to validate their emotions. Tone and cadence of speech matter greatly in respectful interactions with children. In the following story, a nurse tells of a toddler with Burkitt's lymphoma, a particularly fast-growing cancer, who was not doing well and was essentially silent:

> *I don't know how I knew this, but something said to me that he needed to be held right then. I asked him if he would like to rock in the rocking chair, and of course he didn't answer but he did not resist when I picked him up. We sat in that rocking chair for an hour and a half, and I could feel him settling in. I had on this knit sweater with a print, and when he finally sat up I laughed and said, "Jason, you've got waffles on your face!" He said, "I know, I've got them on my knees, too." That was the first time he spoke, and after that we couldn't shut him up.*[31]

A combination of gentle support for age-appropriate behaviors and tender care, such as holding and rocking, can encourage the young child to feel nurtured and secure. As they age, predictable routines, respectful responses, and consistent guidance allow young children to explore, learn, and develop a sense of who they are as individuals.

School Readiness

Because the early years are a such a critical period in learning and development, it is during this stage that school preparedness begins. Children 3 to 5 years of age understand rules, share, begin to navigate conflict, initiate separation from their caregivers, explore social relationships, play, listen, and take turns. They begin to develop preliteracy skills (alphabet) and prenumeracy skills (counting) and are categorized as "preschoolers." Research shows that children who participate in high-quality preschool programs have better health, social-emotional, and cognitive outcomes than those who do not.[32] Despite this, participation in preschool activities varies greatly. Some children start preschool at 2.9 months of age, yet others may not enter until the start of kindergarten at age 5 or 6. In the United States, public funding for preschool varies from state to state. In fact, 6 of every 10 children are not enrolled in publicly funded preschool or Head Start programs.[33] According to the US Department of Education, in 2015, 38% of 3-year-olds, 67% of 4-year-olds, and 87% of 5-year-olds were enrolled in preprimary programs (preschool or kindergarten).[34] For health professionals who practice in the school and early childhood education settings, this means that the school setting may be the first time a child meets a health professional or has a developmental need identified. Positive parenting and following principles of patient- and family-centered care, as described in Chapter 8, will help support respectful interaction with children and their families in the early years.

Early Adversity

Participation in typical childhood activities may be disrupted as a result of environmental factors such as deprivation, isolation, abuse, or exposure to violence.[35] *Early adversity,* or an *adverse childhood experience,* is the personal experience of abuse, neglect, or trauma associated with proximity to an unstable family member (i.e., a close family member who has a substance abuse problem or mental health illness, is incarcerated, and/or is a victim of domestic violence) or a suddenly departed family member (i.e., divorce, death, abandonment).[36] Advances in biology are providing deeper insights into how early experiences are "built into the body" and the lasting effects of these stressful experiences on learning, behavior, and health.[37] Just as each personal or environmental situation is unique, so is each child's response to early adversity. Children who have experienced early adversity commonly develop insecure attachments, and research has shown that these experiences are biologically linked to an increased risk for cardiovascular disease, type 2 diabetes, addictions, and depression in adulthood.[38] For these reasons it is essential that health professionals attend to the impact of early adversity and work to support at-risk children, families, and communities. Approaching children who have experienced adversity with consistency and reassurance helps garner their trust. Building resilience through the development of early coping skills is also a key intervention because young children carry these skills through childhood into the adult years.

Abuse and Neglect

Legally, the parents or another formally appointed guardian are the voice of the young child, except in rare instances in which government agencies intervene to protect the child from care-givers whom the state deems are not acting in the child's best interest. The most grievous situation results when there is growing suspicion or knowledge that the patient is a victim of *child abuse* or *neglect*. In the case of a dysfunctional family in which abuse is suspected, however much you may empathize with the family's suffering, you must turn your attention to the protection of the victimized child. The Child Abuse Prevention and Treatment Act (CAPTA), originally enacted in 1974, has been amended several times. It was most recently amended and reautho-rized under the CAPTA Reauthorization Act of 2010 (Public Law 111-320). CAPTA is the key federal legislation addressing child abuse and neglect. It mandates reporting and provides support for community-based grants to prevent child abuse and neglect.[39] CAPTA defines child abuse and neglect as "any recent act of failure to act on the part of a parent or caretaker, which results in death, serious physical or emotional harm, sexual abuse, or exploitation, or an act or failure to act which presents an imminent risk of serious harm."[40] Younger children are more frequently maltreated than older children, with those younger than the age of 1 being at the greatest risk. A good general rule is to be suspicious of maltreatment when reports of the history of the child's injuries do not coincide with physical findings. Furthermore, you must be-come acquainted with appropriate reporting procedures for persons in your chosen profession. Most health professionals and educators are mandated reporters, although reporting procedures vary from state to state. Parents and other caregivers who maltreat children are deeply troubled. Your support of policies and practices that address maltreatment of children as a family affair is a valuable contribution to society.

In summary, despite the occasional problematic family situation, the family is usually a sound and reliable bridge to building better understanding of the needs of infants, toddlers, and young children. Involving family systems in care is critical because families are the primary social context in which children live and receive care and nurturing.

Summary

This chapter beamed attention on the ways respectful interaction applies to the youngest patients and their families. To help highlight some unique and special characteristics of such relationships this chapter presented an overview of a variety of theories that seek to explain how human beings develop biologically, psychologically, and socially over the life span. The progression from birth to infancy to early childhood is shaped by the environment, the most important element of which is the family. As an infant develops into a toddler, then a preschooler, they start taking steps, literally and figuratively, toward a lifelong journey that is unique to each child. Recognizing the unique-ness of the child as an individual, as well as being a product of a developmental phase, will help readers to better understand the many dimensions in which respect can be conveyed, and how the success of patient- and family-centered care will be maximized.

References

1. Forman V. *This Lovely Life: A Memoir of Premature Motherhood.* Boston: Houghton Mifflin Harcourt; 2009:109.
2. WHO Global Health Observatory (GHO) data: *Infant Mortality.* At: http://www.who.int/gho/child_health/mortality/neonatal_infant_text/en/.
3. Central Intelligence Agency: *The World Factbook.* Washington, DC; 2016. At: https://www.cia.gov/library/publications/the-world-factbook/rankorder/2091rank.html.
4. MacDorman MF, Mathews TJ, Mohangoo AD, et al. *International Comparisons of Infant Mortality and Related Factors: United States and Europe, 2010,* National vital statistics reports. Vol. 63, no 5. Hyattsville, MD: National Center for Health Statistics; 2014.
5. Centers for Disease Control and Prevention: *Division of Reproductive Health. Infant Mortality.* https://www.cdc.gov/reproductivehealth/maternalinfanthealth/infantmortality.htm.
6. Jacoba J. US infant mortality rate declines but still exceeds other developed countries. *JAMA.* 2016;315(5):451–452.
7. Speights JSB, Goldfarb SS, Wells BA, et al. State-level progress in reducing the black-white infant mortality gap, United States, 1999-2013. *Am J Public Health.* 2017;107(5):775–782.
8. White AA. *Seeing Patients: Unconscious Bias in Healthcare.* Boston: Harvard University; 2012.
9. Puskar KR, D'Antonio IJ. Tots and teens: similarities in behavior and interventions for pediatric and psychiatric nurses. *J Child Adolesc Psychiatr Ment Health Nurs.* 1993;6(2):18–28.
10. World Health Organization: *International Classification of Functioning, Disability and Health.* Geneva: ICF; 2002. http://www.who.int/classifications/icf/training/icfbeginnersguide.pdf.
11. Mott S, James S, Sperhac A. *Nursing Care of Children and Families.* 2nd ed. Reading, MA: Addison-Wesley; 1990.
12. Piaget J. *Six Psychological Studies.* New York: Vintage; 1964.
13. Miller SA. *Developmental Research Methods.* Englewood Cliffs, NJ: Prentice Hall; 1987.
14. Myant K, Williams J. Children's concepts of health and illness: understanding of contagious illnesses, non-contagious illnesses and injuries. *J Health Psychol.* 2005;10(6):805–819.
15. Yoos HL. Children's illness concepts: old and new paradigms. *Pediatr Nurs.* 1994;20(2):134–140, 145.
16. Geary DC, Bjorklund DF. Evolutionary developmental psychology. *Child Dev.* 2000;71(1):57–65.
17. Suizzo MA. The social-emotional and cultural contexts of cognitive development: neo-Piagetian perspectives. *Child Dev.* 2000;71(4):846–849.
18. Lally JR, Mangione P. Caring relationships: the heart of early brain development. *Young Children.* 2017;72(2):17–24.
19. Clark MC, Caffarella RS, eds. *An Update on Adult Development Theory: New Ways of Thinking About the Life Course: New Directions for Adult and Continuing Education.* San Francisco: Jossey-Bass; 1999.
20. Erikson EH. *Identity and the Life Cycle.* New York: WW Norton; 1959.
21. Shonkoff JP, Phillips DA, eds. *From Neurons to Neighborhoods: The Science of Early Childhood Development.* Washington, DC: National Academy of Sciences Press; 2000.
22. Dosman C, Andrews D. Anticipatory guidance for cognitive and social-emotional development: birth to five years. *Paediatrics & Child Health* (1205-7088). 2012;17(2):75–80.
23. Pinch WE. *When the Bough Breaks: Parental Perceptions of Ethical Decision-Making in NICU.* Lanham, MD: University of America Press; 2002.
24. Sweeney J, Heriza C, Blanchard Y, Dusing S. Neonatal physical therapy. Part II: practice frameworks and evidence-based practice guidelines…second article of a 2-part series [corrected] [published erratum appears in PEDIATR PHYS THER 2010 Winter;22(4):377]. *Pediatr Phys Ther.* 2010;22(1):2–16.
25. Schuster CS, Ashburn SS. *The Process of Human Development.* Boston: Little, Brown; 1986.
26. Cronin A, Mandich MB. *Human Development and Performance Throughout the Lifespan.* 2nd ed. Clifton Park, NY: Thomson Delmar Learning; 2015.
27. Boulet SL, Boyle CA, Schieve LA. Health care use and health and functional impact of developmental disabilities among US children, 1997–2005. *Arch Pediatr Adolesc Med.* 2009;163(1):19–26.
28. CDC. Autism Spectrum Disorder. Data and Statistics. 2017. https://www.cdc.gov/ncbddd/autism/data.html.
29. Christensen DL, Baio J, Braun KV, et al. Prevalence and characteristics of autism spectrum disorder among children aged 8 years — Autism and Developmental Disabilities Monitoring Network, 11 Sites, United States, 2012. *MMWR Surveill Summ.* 2016;65(No. SS-3):1–23.

30. Freiberg KL. *Human Development, A Life Span Approach*. 4th ed. Boston: Jones and Bartlett; 1992.
31. Montgomery CL. *Healing Through Communication*. Newbury Park, CA: Sage; 1993.
32. U.S. Department of Education. *A Matter of Equity: Preschool in America*. 2015. https://www2.ed.gov/doc uments/early-learning/matter-equity-preschool-america.pdf.
33. National Institute for Early Education Research (NIEER). *2016 State Preschool Yearbook*; 2016. http://nieer .org/state-preschool-yearbooks/yearbook2016.
34. U.S. Department of Education, National Center for Education Statistics. *The Condition of Education 2017 (NCES 2017-144), Preschool and Kindergarten Enrollment*.
35. Whitcomb DA, Carrasco RC, Neuman A, et al. Correlational research to examine the relation between attachment and sensory modulation in young children. *Am J Occup Ther*. 2015;69:6904220020.
36. Lynch A, Ashcraft R, Tekell LM. Understanding children who have experienced early adversity: implications for practitioners practicing sensory integration. *SIS Quarterly OT Practice Connections*. 2017;2(3):5–7.
37. Shonkoff JP. Capitalizing on advances in science to reduce the health consequences of early childhood adversity. *JAMA Pediat*. 2016;170(10):1003.
38. Shonkoff JP, Boyce WT, McEwen BS. Neuroscience, molecular biology, and the childhood roots of health disparities: building a new framework for health promotion and disease prevention. *JAMA*. 2009;301(21):2252–2259.
39. CAPTA Reauthorization Act of 2010 Public Law 108-36, 111th Cong., 2010. http://www.gpo.gov/fdsys/ pkg/PLAW-111publ320/pdf/PLAW-111publ320.pdf.
40. Child Welfare Information Gateway: *Definition of Child Abuse and Neglect, State Statutes Series*. Washington, DC: U.S. Department of Health and Human Services: Children's Bureau/ACYF; 2016.

CHAPTER 12

Respectful Interaction

Working With School-Age Children and Adolescents

The reader will be able to:

- Discuss the key developmental tasks of children and adolescents
- Distinguish some developmental challenges that require consideration in the health professional's approach to school-age children and adolescents
- Describe how the six types of play introduced in Chapter 11 are relevant—or not relevant—to respectful interaction with older children
- Describe how a child's developing need for successful relatedness enters into the health professional and patient relationship
- Make several suggestions that will help minimize the disequilibrium of the family during a child's illness
- List some compelling reasons for giving respectful attention to an adolescent's desire to exercise authority in regard to health care decisions, and describe legitimate limits on that authority
- Understand the impact of social media on identity development in school-age children and adolescents
- Describe high-risk behaviors in adolescence that can lead to long-term health problems

Prelude

The important thing about you is that you are you. It is true that you were a baby, and you grew, and now you are a child, and you will grow, into a man, or into a woman. But the important thing about you is that you are you.

M.W. BROWN[1]

Much of the material related to respectful interaction with the infant or toddler and his or her family can be applied to older children. As a child grows, however, some new challenges confront the child, parents, families, and interprofessional care team. Therefore, in this chapter we add to the groundwork we laid in Chapter 11 to highlight some of the most important differences, as well as focus on the distinct needs of adolescent patients.

The Child Becomes a Self

A young child's psychosocial tasks of moving from early to middle childhood focus on the need to recognize that one has a "self," separate from others, but also that ultimately many aspects of that self must survive and thrive in relationships with others. Therefore much activity and energy are focused on being different from others at the same time that much is invested in learning how to be accepted by others and having some say in relationships. As we address later in this chapter, these tasks become paramount during the adolescent years, but the fundamental building blocks begin much earlier.

Needs: Respect and Relating

A major part of the child's developmental task is that of becoming a "self" different from others. Children, in general, want to make it alone and have learned not to accept the full dependence of infancy. The toddler and preschool years are not yet independent either. Just as in earlier stages of development discussed in Chapter 11, when children become patients, the dependence side of the scales tips, and the good fit of selfhood that the child is slipping into suddenly escapes. In this confusing never-never land of being neither fully child nor fully adult, children must try to reestablish some sense of equanimity and self-identity during their time of being patients. This situation increases the health professional's challenge of finding means to convey respect for the young patient.

Most children beyond the preschool years have learned to communicate verbally and have many more experiences upon which to rely compared with an infant or a toddler. Thus their resources for effective relating are greater than those in their earlier years. The school-age years open up the child's world to interactions with many new and different people. These are mainly authority figures, such as teachers, coaches, and other role models, as well as peers, playmates, and older children.

Health professionals often present types of authority that are unfamiliar to the child. Family and school authority figures usually do little to prepare him or her for the health professions setting and its unique challenges and choices.

THE IMPORTANCE OF PLAY

Play is a child's primary occupation.[3] Play appropriate to the child's age and social development is an important vehicle to help ease the tension a child is feeling about relating to people in the health care setting. In Chapter 11 we introduced six types of play and noted that as children develop new motor, cognitive, and social-emotional skills, their play changes. Gender is an important contributor to play, as are age, peer group, and play opportunities. In their study of 7- to 11-year-old children, Miller and Kuhaneck[3] found that friends, siblings, and even pets figured prominently in children's descriptions of play and fun. This and other studies remind us that regardless of environment (hospital, school, or home), children *need* to play. Some older children who become patients may regress to an earlier stage of play, but many will be able to assume roles at the higher levels of play, which will allow them to act out their predicament of being in such a new situation. For example, associative play can involve playing "hospital" with a health professional or family member and assuming the powerful role of the nurse or someone else in charge, thereby revealing children's own anxieties and how they perceive their situation. Clues to how they think their tension could be eased may be expressed in their attempts to minister to the play partner who has now become the patient. Cooperative play can involve table games, card games, or sports, using their participation and mastery as an effective way of relating.

Young patients often play with toys, too, so a truck, doll, puzzle, or other object may be an effective means of helping to establish a relationship. At the same time, children can be sensitive about being "too old" for certain types of toys, so health professionals and others must think carefully about which toys to offer and how to best integrate family and siblings into their sessions. Health professionals also must be sensitive to the fact that some children may not have access to toys and books. Of children ages 0 to 17 in the United States, 20 percent live in families with incomes below the poverty level ($24,036 a year for a family of four).[4] These children are often vulnerable to environmental, health, educational, and safety risks. They are also at particular risk for developmental challenges. Thoughtful considerations on how to help families modify environments and maximize access can bring about meaningful change in the number of opportunities for children to engage in play (e.g., repurposing everyday items as toys, accessing library services).

REFLECTIONS

- When was the last time you engaged in "play"?
- How did you feel during the activity? After the activity?
- How did it contribute to your mood?

TRANSITIONS IN SCHOOLING

Starting school is a rite of passage and a major transition for children and families. As discussed in Chapter 11, some children start the transition to school as early as age 2.9 when they begin preschool. Others transition at the start of kindergarten or first grade. Regardless of the age in which they transition, every child goes through both the challenge and excitement of new roles, routines, and learning experiences. Each school-based transition brings with it a period of adjustment to new rules, teachers, friends, and environments. Emotions related to school transitions include excitement, happiness, sadness, and worry.[5] When school-age children become patients, health professionals are faced with additional challenges. Even a short illness or injury may disrupt school attendance and may not only put the child behind in schoolwork but also have devastating consequences socially. During the school years, children organize most of their relational activity around family and school; therefore they are at risk for being "out of the action" in every way when removed from the educational environment. At the very least, patient-centered respect for the child requires you to be aware of this loss and show interest in any school-related activity being carried on at the moment.

Most children with chronic illnesses or long-term disabilities will receive special attention regarding education through the school system itself. Over the past 30 years, the definition of disability has changed. In the 1970s and 1980s, the concept of a disability referred to an underlying physical or mental condition that reduced one's abilities. Today, disability is seen as a complex interaction between a person and his or her environment. The development of the international classification of functioning, disability, and health by the World Health Organization (introduced in Chapter 4) reflects this new perspective. In this classification, *disability* is an umbrella term for impairments, activity limitations, and participation restrictions. This perspective acknowledges that any individual can experience a decline in health at various points in his or her life span, hence experiencing disability. It is a biological, individual, and social perspective of health rather than a diagnosis or label.[6] In the United States a significant portion of children, estimated to be 7.94% of all those 18 years or younger, have experienced some degree of disability.[7] The number of US children with developmental disabilities and mental health conditions is on the rise. The prevalence of developmental disability in school-age children ages 3 to 17 is 15%.[8] Children living in poverty consistently experience the highest overall rates of disability; however, recent findings show an interesting trend, with a documented 28.4% rise in disability rates among children living in households greater than 400% of the poverty level.[7] Regardless of sociodemographic trends, these statistics have a direct bearing on the need for health, educational, and social services for school-age children and their families.

The Individuals with Disabilities Education Act (IDEA) (formerly called *Public Law 94-142* or the *Education for all Handicapped Children Act of 1975*) is the federal law that governs the provision of special education services. It requires public schools to make available to all eligible children with disabilities a free, appropriate public education in the least restrictive environment appropriate to their individual needs.[9] However laudatory this is, the law does little to address the accompanying problems that sometimes arise, such as able-bodied children being cruel toward peers who have disabilities, parents thinking their child is not getting adequate care or disagreeing with the individualized education program that has been developed for their child, teachers thinking they do not have enough time to devote to the needs of all the children in their classrooms, and children with serious but not permanent conditions not qualifying for servies.[10] When you come into contact with families who are trying to work through some of these issues, you can often encourage them and direct them to the appropriate resources when problems arise. For example, if parents disagree with the individualized education program, they can request a due process hearing and a review from the state educational agency if their state provides for this type of input and parent participation.

In short, during the school-age years a child's feelings of self-worth and experiences of relatedness usually are tied to school. Any means by which you can convey empathy for the child's predicament and respect for his or her capacities will enhance the child's self-esteem and help ensure success in the relationship. It will also serve him or her well beyond the immediate relationship you have helped to develop.

FAMILY: A BRIDGE TO RESPECTFUL INTERACTION

All of the family dynamics described in Chapter 8 apply as the child grows older. The growing child, however, does present some additional challenges to the family and health professional working with the family. The needs of the school-age child revolve around tasks, hobbies, and activities. It is during this stage that 7- to 12-year-olds develop a sense of values to guide decision-making and interests.

A child's desire to become more independent is one of the major developmental tasks of this growth period, while at the same time he or she may feel extremely lonely and insecure when illness strikes. The family is often torn between wanting to support the child as an independent "big girl" or "big boy" while being attentive to his or her needs. They also may be dismayed by the child's obvious regression or respond to their own feelings of guilt for the child's illness with overprotectiveness. Your awareness of, and caring professional attention to, their struggles and needs are essential ingredients for success. Family members warrant your due respect. They are the people who are most knowledgeable about the child and are key collaborators in clinical decision-making. Lawlor and Mattingly[11] put this best when they stated: "Collaboration is much more than being nice. It involves complex interpretive acts in which the practitioner must understand the meanings of illness or disability in a person and family's life and the feelings that accompany these experiences."

CHILDREN AS ACTIVE PARTICIPANTS IN CARE

Respect for the child's input, especially when his or her opinions seem to differ from those of parents, is essential. Although developmental psychology has often used age as an indicator of reliable decision-making capacity (i.e., in clinical terms, patient *competency*, with decisions based on the patient's informed consent), this view is being challenged and replaced by the principle that maturity and experience are more reliable markers of the ability to participate in decisions related to the child's health care.[12,13] Although the legal age of consent is 18 in the United States, many policies now acknowledge the importance of listening to children and having them *assent* to care decisions. Assent in children honors respect for persons and should be sought from the age of 7 upward. It ensures that children have the opportunity to understand their condition, share their views, and participate in decisions regarding their care.[13] Assenting to decisions allows

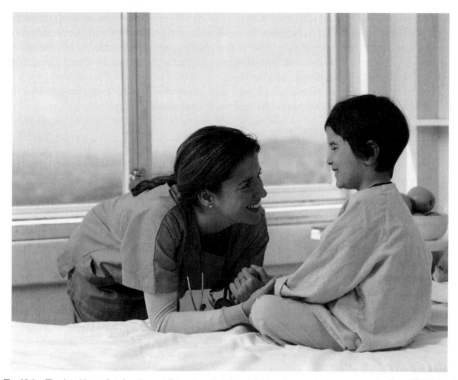

Fig. 12.1 The health professional must listen to what the child has to say during an examination. (© *Michael Blann/Digital Vision/Thinkstock.com.*)

children to communicate a choice and have a say in what happens.[14] Children often express their preferences through body language and actions. However difficult the discussion may be, many children should be invited to be active participants in the care planning process. It is through this participation that they learn the life skills necessary for decision-making and illness management. Children often are aware of their parent's anxiety, opposition, or denial, and they try to act as referees among family members or between health professionals and family. Children can participate in a meaningful way in discussions about their health care (Fig. 12.1).

In studies in which children themselves are asked to identify the characteristics of a good health care provider, the following themes present[15,16]:

1. *Good communication:* Using terms of endearment, sitting down to meet children at their eye level, having good body language (e.g., hands visible), being cheerful
2. *Professional competence:* Being capable, organized, knowledgeable, skilled (including performing painless procedures), and prompt
3. *Safety and appearance:* Following good hygiene practices, wearing a hospital identification badge
4. *Virtues:* Being honest, trustworthy, polite (particularly toward family and visitors)
5. *Fun:* Someone who does not forget that kids still need to play, laughing or using humor when performing care activities, playing games together

In addition, brothers and sisters of the ill child are affected by the stress that illness creates in the family. In a study of the siblings of hospitalized children, the brothers and sisters noted stress that included feelings of loneliness, resentment, and fear and positive feelings of resilience, such as lessons learned and independence.[17] You can help siblings cope by providing support and information. Anything the health professional can do to keep the supportive context for siblings alive is well worth the effort. It is through the application of the principles of patient and family-centered care, supportive participation, information sharing, and collaboration that siblings feel engaged and supported. You also can help by trying to keep family disequilibrium at a minimum while acting primarily as an advocate for the child.

This balancing act is sometimes easier said than accomplished. For example, consider the below case study regarding John, his family, and the interprofessional care team.

Case Study

When John was 9, he fell from a swing, had some joint pain of the lower left extremity, and was unable to fully extend his knee. Numerous radiographic studies were completed, and results were largely normal. However, John could still not play soccer and continued to complain of tenderness. Finally, a magnetic resonance image (MRI) revealed a lesion that turned out to be non-Hodgkin's lymphoma (NHL). John received combination chemotherapy and has been in remission for 2 and a half years. His mother has been his primary in-home caregiver. When the physician asked about John's father, John replied, "He can't deal with having a wimp for a kid." His mother said that she "had everything under control" and that John's dad was "a very busy man who spends a lot of time on out-of-town business." As John has gotten older the team who has followed John and his family has grown somewhat concerned about his mother's overprotectiveness. Although it was less noticeable when he was first diagnosed, it has been the topic of conversation among the interprofessional care team when he and his mother have come to the clinic. For instance, she mentioned that she still will not let John go on a sleepover and accompanies him almost everywhere. She also is very aware of symptoms that she notes in him even though John tries to protest that they either did not occur or were just in passing. You believe he is becoming more withdrawn on visits and that she increasingly overrides questions the team members try to pose to him directly.

REFLECTIONS

- If you were a member of the interprofessional care team following John and his family, what would you do at this point?
- How might you respect both the mother and John in their attempt to be heard?
- What are some key considerations given John's developmental stage and age?

Several suggestions may help you decide what to do when you are faced with dilemmas concerning how much information to share with patients:

1. *Make your own position clear* to yourself and to the patient's parents. Do you think the child is able to handle information about his or her condition? Why or why not? What is in the best interests of the child? Of the family as a unit? Under what conditions would you feel morally bound to disclose relevant health information to this child? Under what conditions would you withhold such information, even if you believed that doing so could increase the child's distrust in you?

2. *Explore the resources available in your health care setting* to support families as they work out their anxieties and difficulties. As one author notes, "The purpose is ... to support, not supplant, the family. An atmosphere of acceptance and assurance allows each family to manage their own lives and to arrive at a solution most adequate for them."[18] Social workers and ethics committees are two examples of the many supports available to families and teams of care providers in these types of situations.

3. *Present information in a way the child can understand* with ample opportunity for questions and explanations from the child in his or her own words about what has been discussed. Present opportunities for alternative questions by asking "is there a reason that you were curious about x? Assent in children should help the pediatric patient achieve a developmentally appropriate awareness of the nature of his or her condition, while informing them about what to expect in the future.[19]

4. *Implement strategies to lower family stress.* Two major tasks can help lower family stress and ensure that they are involved. The first is providing information. As collaborators in the care process, families need ongoing information. Structured communication such as a intermittent phone calls, frequent family meetings, or simply involvement in team rounds can help the family understand and cope with their child's prognosis.[20] The second is involving families in the care of their family member. Family involvement in various patient care tasks may help reduce the sense of powerlessness.

In summary, a child brings to the health care interaction hopes, fears, and dreams that reflect his or her need to establish autonomy and initiative as a "self" while maintaining the security of relationships with family, friends, and others. The delicate balance between being an individual and being part of relationships that are difficult under the best of circumstances is further challenged by illness or other incapacity. The efforts of health professionals and family alike are required for successful adaptation or recovery. The benefit is that within a context of respect for the child as a unique individual, the health professional and family will be able to work together to meet the patient's best interests.

Adolescent Self

The word *adolescent* means literally "to grow into maturity or adulthood." During the later stages of child development, all children are thrust into the difficult position of having to show industry and individuality in the larger world, to assert who they are, to command authority in some areas, and to explore the mysteries of developing sexuality. "Adolescence typically is defined as beginning at puberty, a physiological transformation that gives boys and girls adult bodies and alters how they are perceived and treated by others, as well as how they view themselves."[21] It is a time of rapid biological, cognitive, and social-emotional growth and development and lays the foundation for adult health.

EARLY AND LATE ADOLESCENCE

Most psychologists and others writing about adolescence divide it into two stages: early and late, each with developmental tasks. Early adolescence lasts for about 2 years and is characterized by growth spurts, maturing of reproductive functions and sex organs, increased weight, and changes in body proportions. These profound changes understandably may have profound psychological results.

Teenagers are often described as irrational, impulsive, oversensitive, and at times oppositional. Anyone who is around early teens knows that their self-images govern much of what they do. The teen years are a time of intensely seeking one's "self." In its extreme form, the self is the way the body looks and nothing more. However, for many teens the absorption with the self goes beyond bodily appearance alone. Adolescents are generally concerned with fitting in with their peers. They will try various roles in an attempt to integrate their developing social skills with goals and dreams.

This early period of adolescence is so unsettling that psychologists and others have described it as a period of adolescent turmoil. However, other researchers indicate that adolescence may not be as fraught with emotional issues as has been previously thought. In an ethnographic study of early adolescent girls, both popular and not so popular, the findings revealed a close relationship with parents and certainly not the trauma and stress suggested by common discourses (or myths) about adolescence. Teachers, parents, and health care professionals may expect trouble from adolescents because of, or attributed to, "raging hormones," but in this study the trauma did not materialize.[22] At a minimum, there is clearly a disconnect between physical development and psychosocial maturation that may be the source of some conflict and also in part offers an explanation for the number of teen pregnancies and instances of sexually transmitted diseases.

REFLECTIONS

You walk into your co-worker's office, and she is distracted and teary. You ask her what is wrong, and she says, "I am so upset. I found a bag of marijuana in Emma's (her daughter's) backpack this morning. She is only 13. I don't understand what she could be thinking!"
- What advice would you give your colleague?
- Are there resources you would recommend?
- How would you feel if this was your daughter?
- How does your knowledge as a health care provider inform this scenario?

After this period of rapid and profound change, young people move into late adolescence. Here self-identity fully emerges as they practice the various roles and responsibilities they will assume as adults. Some adolescents do not move on to this stage of development because they literally do not survive. Teens 12 to 17 years old were, on average, more than twice as likely as adults (18 years and older) to be victims of violent crimes. Among this group, blacks were five times as likely as whites to be homicide victims.[23] In the United States, the fourth leading cause of death for all juveniles aged 7 to 17 from 1990 to 2010 was suicide, trailing only unintentional injury, homicide, and cancer.[23] These differences in causes of death between adults and teens, and teens by racial or ethnic group, is an indication of the profound impact disparities and health behaviors can have on an adolescent mortality. Globally, adolescent health has increased from 1990 to 2015.[24] Adolescents in developing countries have to contend with poverty, starvation, and infectious diseases. Those in developed countries contend with obesity, gun violence, and eating disorders. Attending to these statistics guides health professionals in effective care interventions and health policy for the teenage population.

FRIENDS AND PEER GROUPS

Adolescents tend to spend less time with family and more time in new environments such as work settings, peer relationships, and romantic relationships. They move toward a more mature sense of themselves and start to question old values without losing their identity. Friendships are an important part of adolescent development. The impact of a peer's behavior on an adolescent is significant (Fig. 12.2). Research supports the biological science behind the influence of peers on teenage behavior and decision-making. Substance use (cigarette, marijuana, and alcohol use), violence (weapons and physical fighting), and suicidal behavior (suicidal ideation and attempts) have been shown to relate to a teen's friends' substance use, deviance, and suicidal behaviors, respectively. Although the stereotypical negative effects are often highlighted, there are also positive effects. Peers help teens learn social norms and provide the support needed during the challenging time of adolescence. Prosocial behavior in friends has been shown to negatively correlate with violence and have a positive influence on academic performance, skill, and personality development.[25,26] Other factors, such as family function, depression, and social acceptance, influence adolescents' health-risk behavior as well, but parents continue to be the most influential people in teen's lives. Supporting parents to keep communication open with teens during this rapid time of change (and sometimes conflict) is of prime importance in the context of supporting family health.

To highlight some challenges of showing respect for and working with adolescents and their families we return to the story of John and his mother introduced earlier.

Case Study

John is now 15, and during a follow-up visit to the oncologist, it is discovered that he has a recurrence of NHL. Everyone is concerned; however, the prognosis for children with NHL has greatly improved, with nearly an 80% survival rate.[27]

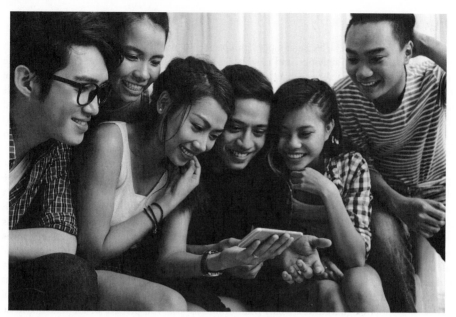

Fig. 12.2 An adolescent's behavior is influenced by that of his or her peers. (© *DragonImages/iStock/Thinkstock.com.*)

Case Study—cont'd

John is readmitted to the hospital for treatment. His mother visits for a minimum of 6 hours every day and remains steadfast at the bedside. In a recent conversation with the interprofessional care team during early morning rounds and before his mother arrives, John says, "Hey since you guys are going to knock me out with all those killer chemo drugs again, what do you say we talk about saving my sperm? I talked with my buddies about sperm banking after reading about it in a survivor's blog and we think it's a good idea. I mean, I want to have kids someday, too."

The physician approached John's mother about the team's desire to follow up with John regarding his recent question. She was shocked and enraged, stating: "John is just being provocative. He is too young to talk about such things. I bet he got this crazy idea from the girl he met at the cancer support group. And hard as I try, he is hanging out with boys I don't like. They are having a bad influence on him. This is not to be discussed with him under any circumstances." Although the team knows she is the legal decision maker for John, many of them think she is limiting his participation in care planning and not making decisions in his best interests. Their opinions on whether he should be allowed to sperm bank are divided.

REFLECTIONS

- What should you and the interprofessional care team do differently from your interactions with John and his family when John was younger?
- What questions do you personally want to raise with John and the care team about the most caring way to proceed in expressing respect toward John and his mother?

Whether you follow a patient from childhood through to adolescence, the opportunity to express respect continues to be a major factor in respectful interaction. The rule of thumb is always to take into account that the child's evolution of self-identity, independence of expression, and authority to speak on his or her own behalf is somewhere on the continuum toward full adulthood. At the same time, family and other authority figures continue to exert a major influence on the patient's decision.

Digital Media

In today's digital world, a teenager's peer group extends beyond the individuals they interact with in school, sporting activities, and neighborhoods, to include those in their digital life. The Internet and social media apps such as Instagram, Twitter, Snapchat, and Facebook have become a place of social connection for many teenagers (Fig. 12.3). Gone are the days of calling friends to see if they want to get together at the mall—today's teens post, participate in group chats, and send text messages through their cell phone or other web-enabled device. Eighty-nine percent of adolescents use social media, and a recent study found teens spend an average of 9 hours on these sites a day.[28]

Teens are digitally connected behaviorally and biochemically. Electronic distractions such as social media apps and gaming can influence the brain's reward circuitry, leading to a rush of the chemical dopamine being released, influencing adolescent brain development.[29] Electronic media have both positive and negative effects on adolescents.[30,31] Among the positives are access to health information, social connections, and expanded learning opportunities. For example, John mentions that his request for sperm banking initiated with his researching the topic online. The negatives include high-risk behaviors, sexting, cyber aggression, social isolation, Internet addiction, and digital invasions of privacy. Misuse of digital media is common for teenagers, and health professionals and parents alike must educate teens on the impact of digital media on health and development. Health professionals must be aware of the influence of social media on their teenage patients and discuss appropriate digital health. Many health professionals who practice in the school system, such as school psychologists, teachers, school nurses, and occupational therapists, have turned their attention to helping school-age children and adolescents critically evaluate which apps to choose, what information to share, and how to safely participate in social media platforms.

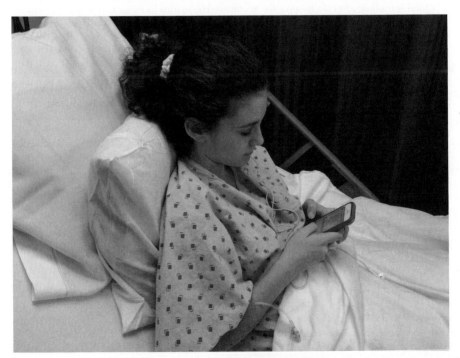

Fig. 12.3 Digital lives and social media influences in adolescent and school-age children. Photo courtesy of R.F. Doherty

Needs: Respect, Autonomy, and Relating

Autonomous decision-making raises some delicate questions for health professionals who work with adolescent patients because adolescents often want to aggressively assert their authority in decisions. Only in recent years has there been an attempt to address the legal rights of adolescents. The most prominent view, referred to as the *Mature Minors Doctrine,* allows for parents or the state to speak on behalf of a minor's interests only as long as the minor is unable to represent himself or herself. Thus the level of the young person's development emerges as a decisive factor. In keeping with the legality of the Mature Minors Doctrine, you can try to assess the maturity of an adolescent patient in regard to his or her ability to cope effectively with illness or injury. The question whether an adolescent is a "mature minor" must be decided by health care professionals independent of parental judgment.[32]

There are some compelling reasons to give decision-making authority to mature adolescents. Some adolescents would never consult a health care provider with a problem if they knew it would require parental consent before treatment. Also, in their developing autonomy, they would never share delicate information with the provider if they thought confidentiality would be violated. Coupled with the reluctance of adolescents to speak about risky behavior or other health issues, they often do not receive recommended and preventive counseling or screening services appropriate to their age group.[33]

Adolescence was often viewed as a relatively healthy time in a person's life. However, behavior patterns can change rapidly in adolescence and can include irregular dietary habits, lack of sleep, inactivity, experimentation with drugs, alcohol and tobacco use, sexual activity, and reckless driving. The connection between these behaviors and long-term consequences for health is being increasingly recognized:

> *[A] degree of experimentation and risk taking seem [s] to be an integral part of the transition from childhood to adulthood, and most young people come through this phase of life relatively unscathed. So the challenge to researchers and clinicians alike is to be able to identify those at most risk of adverse consequences, without interfering with normal development, and to evaluate possible interventions that will result in improved long-term outcomes.[34]*

Programs to promote healthy lifestyles for adolescents should include information on nutrition, activity, stress management, family planning, prevention of smoking, alcohol and substance abuse, safety (particularly digital and motor vehicle safety), and the spread of sexually transmitted diseases. Adolescents should be involved in the design of such health promotion programs so that they are both age and culturally relevant.

FAMILY AND PEERS: BRIDGES TO RESPECTFUL INTERACTION

Families and friends should not be excluded from the health care interaction process for adolescent patients. The emphasis on the importance of the adolescent's autonomy and authority should in no way be seen as undermining the importance of treating the patient as a part of a family unit and a peer group. Most adolescents like to argue about adult rules, even those they accept. Listening to family exchanges about rules that the adolescent disagrees with often will provide insight into the conduct of the adolescent toward you, too. In addition, the health professional should not assume that the adolescent's attitude toward parents means there is not a deep dependence on them or heartfelt caring from the family. Although adolescents always challenge authority figures, they need or want limits. Limits provide a safe boundary for teens to grow and function.[35]

REFLECTIONS

- What does it mean to "set limits"?
- Is limit-setting easy or hard for you?
- How do you envision setting limits with clients and families in your professional practice?
- Do you anticipate that limit-setting will be an easy or hard task for you?

It is important to note that families, like individuals, also develop over time. The family system changes as children and parents age. Normal life events such as job changes, relocations, changes in schools, changes in the family structure (e.g., loss of a grandparent), and changes in support systems all have an impact on family function. Contemporary trends in family systems, such as divorce and remarriage, also may require additional developmental tasks to reestablish family cohesion. These types of families may exhibit higher levels of conflict during a child's illness because individuals who typically do not interact with each other may need to come together around care.[21] Illness and disability are in no one's life plan or aspiration for their children. Many adolescents who experience injury, illness, or disability find themselves halted in their progression to adulthood. The quote below by a parent sums this up nicely.

> *Jeffery's accident struck him like a bomb as he was crossing the bridge to manhood. He was approaching independence .... Quadriplegic paralysis steals legs, arms, hands, fingers—and the future. Jeffery's paralysis stole our future ... because no dream included paralysis. Not one.*[36]

Health professionals often benefit from including an adolescent patient's close friends and peers in interactions. Peer group activity is essential for identity formation, and all illnesses or injuries are jolts to the adolescent's identity. Getting to know an adolescent patient's friends by name, seeking their support, and trying to understand their feelings about the patient's condition can be helpful to all. We did not discuss the function John's friends played in his decision, but you can reflect on it yourself as to whether the opportunity to bring them into your discussion with John should be considered.

Principles of patient- and family-centered care serve as continuing guides for family and health professionals during adolescence. The interprofessional care team will find the following suggestions helpful when caring for teenage patients and families[29,37]:

■ *Stay involved.* When communication begins to break down, make extra efforts to let the teen know that you care and are a steadfast resource.
■ *Stay calm.* Argumentative teens can fluster even the best of us. Try not to lose your temper or express undue anger. Talking to teens calmly regarding their positions and mistakes can help their brains process the information and learn.
■ *Set limits.* Teens need limits and enforcement of limits. Limits help teens maintain safety and learn effective life skills and health habits.
■ *Encourage self-awareness.* Teens are always asking adults why. Flip the question, and help the teen reason through decisions and/or actions. Doing so helps encourage new ways of thinking and mindfulness.
■ *Emphasize the positive.* The adolescent years come with many ups and downs, for which the teenage patient may not have any perspective given their stage of development. Help teens see the positives of life events, reinforcing effective health coping strategies and positive adaptation.

Summary

In this brief overview of school-age children and adolescents, the theme of respect revolves around at least two ideas—patient autonomy and effective relatedness. There are numerous ways in which the young patient will try to exert autonomy and find a way of relating with you effectively. By showing imagination—and at times, patience—you will have an opportunity to build a close and rewarding relationship.

One of the greatest challenges for you as a health professional is to think of the development of people from birth to adulthood as a continuum, with some moving along it faster than others and with large areas of overlap. We have provided some guidelines that will help you think generally about people as they pause—then continue to pass through—older childhood and adolescence. The individual patient will present themself as a unique individual still in the process of forming and refining an identity. You have a responsibility to be sure that, in the midst of activities such patients may engage you in, their health care needs are met. Having said that, we move ahead to the next chapter and the unique challenges associated with treating people in the adult years.

References

1. Brown MW. *The Important Book*. New York: HarperCollins Publishers; 1949.
2. Deleted in review.
3. Miller E, Kuhaneck H. Children's perceptions of play experiences and play preferences: a qualitative study. *Am J Occup Ther*. 2008;62:407–415.
4. Federal Interagency Forum on Child and Family Statistics. *America's Children: Key National Indicators of Well-Being, 2017*. Washington, DC: U.S. Government Printing Office; 2017. https://www.childstats.gov /pdf/ac2017/ac_17.pdf.
5. Caspe M, Lopez E, Chattrabhuti C: Four Important Things to Know About the Transition to School. *Family Involvement Network of Educators (FINE) Newsletter*, 7(1), 2015. Harvard Family Research Project. http://www.hfrp.org/publications-resources/browse-our-publications/four-important-things-research-tells-us-about-the-transition-to-school.
6. World Health Organization. *International Classification of Functioning, Disability and Health (ICF)*. Geneva: WHO; 2002. http://www.who.int/classifications/icf/training/icfbeginnersguide.pdf.
7. Houtrow AJ, Larson K, Olson LM, et al. Changing trends of childhood disability, 2001–2011. *Pediatrics* 134(3):530–538.
8. Centers for Disease Control and Prevention: Developmental disability, https://www.cdc.gov/ncbddd/dev elopmentaldisabilities/about.html#ref.
9. U.S. Department of Education: Office of Special Education Programs: IDEA 04. *Building the Legacy*. https://sites.ed.gov/idea/.
10. Sullivan PM, Knutson JF. Maltreatment and disabilities: a population-based epidemiological study. *Child Abuse Negl*. 2000;24(10):1257–1273.
11. Lawlor MC, Mattingly C. Family perspectives on occupation, health and disability. In: Cohn ES, Gillen G, Scaffa ME, Schell BA, eds. *Willard and Spackman's Occupational Therapy*. 12th ed. Philadelphia: Wolters Kluwer / Lippincot Williams & Wilkins; 2014:154.
12. Ruhe KM, Wangmo T, Badarau DO, Elger BS, Niggli F. Decision-making capacity of children and adolescents—suggestions for advancing the concept's implementation in pediatric healthcare. *Eur J Pediatr*. 2015;174(6):775–782.
13. Koller D. 'Kids need to talk too': inclusive practices for children's healthcare education and participation. *J Clin Nurs*. 2017;26(17/18):2657–2668.
14. Doherty RF, Purtilo RB. *Ethical Dimensions in the Health Professions*. 6th ed. St. Louis: Elsevier; 2016.
15. Brady M. Hospitalized children's views of the good nurse. *Nurs Ethics*. 2009;16:543–560.
16. Boztepe H, Çınar S, Ay A. School-age children's perception of the hospital experience. *J Child Health Care*. 2017;21(2):162.
17. Fleitas J. When Jack fell down Jill came tumbling after: siblings in the web of illness and disability. *MCN Am J Matern Child Nurs*. 2000;25(5):267–273.
18. Fleming SJ. Children's grief: individual and family dynamics. In: Corr CA, Corr DM, eds. *Hospice Approaches to Pediatric Care*. New York: Springer; 1985.
19. Committee on Bioethics. Informed consent, parental permission, and assent in pediatric practice. *Pediatrics*. 1995;95(314):314–317.
20. Leon AM, Knapp S. Involving family systems in critical care nursing: challenges and opportunities. *Dimens Crit Care Nurs*. 2008;27(6):255–262.
21. Call KT, Riedel AA, Hein K, McLoyd V, Petersen A, Kipke M. Adolescent health and well-being in the twenty-first century: a global perspective. *J Res Adolesc*. 2002;12(1):69–98.
22. Finders MJ. *Just Girls: The Hidden Literacies and Life in Junior High*. New York: Teachers College Press; 1997.
23. Sickmund M, Puzzanchera C, eds. *Juvenile Offenders and Victims: 2014 National Report*. Pittsburgh, PA: National Center for Juvenile Justice; 2014.
24. Kassebaum N, Kyu H, Vos T, et al. Child and adolescent health from 1990 to 2015: Findings from the global burden of diseases, injuries, and risk factors 2015 Study. *JAMA Pediatr [serial online]*. 2017;171(6):573–592.

25. Prinstein MJ, Boergers J, Spirito A. Adolescents' and their friends' health-risk behavior: factors that alter or add to peer influence. *J Pediatr Psychol.* 2001;26(5):287–298.

26. Khan A, Jain M, Budhwani C. An analytical cross-sectional study of peer pressure on adolescents. *Int J Reprod, Contracept, Obstet Gynecol [serial online].* 2015;3:606–610.

27. Minard-Colin V, Brugières L, Reiter A, et al. Non-Hodgkin lymphoma in children and adolescents: progress through effective collaboration, current knowledge, and challenges ahead. *J Clinic Oncol.* 2015;33(27):2963–2974.

28. Argo T, Lowery L. The effects of social media on adolescent health and well-being. *J Adolesc Health [serial online].* 2017;2:75–76.

29. Jensen FE, Nutt AE. *The Teenage Brain: A Neuroscientist's Survival Guide to Raising Adolescents and Young Adults.* New York: HarperCollins Publishers; 2015.

30. Concerns regarding social media and health issues in adolescents and young adults. *Obstet & Gynecol [serial online].* 2016;127(2):e62–e65.

31. Primack BA, Shensa A, Sidani JE, et al. Social media use and perceived social isolation among young adults in the U.S. *Am J Prev Med.* 2017;53(1):1–8.

32. Sean Reynolds, Grant-Kels Jane M, Bercovitch Lionel. How issues of autonomy and consent differ between children and adults: kids are not just little people. *Clin Dermatol.* 2017.

33. Alderman E. Original study: confidentiality in pediatric and adolescent gynecology: when we can, when we can't, and when we're challenged. *J Pediatr Adolesc Gynecol.* 2017;30:176–183.

34. Churchill D. The growing pains of adolescent health research in general practice. *Prim Health Care Res Dev.* 2003;4:277–278.

35. U.S. National Library of Medicine, National Institutes of Health: Adolescent development: MedlinePlus medical encyclopedia. http://www.nlm.nih.gov/medlineplus/ency/article/002003.htm.

36. Galli R. *Rescuing Jeffery: A Memoir.* New York: St. Martin's Griffin. 2000;48.

37. Damour L: *Untangled: Guiding Teenage Girls Through the Seven Transitions Into Adulthood.* New York: Ballantine Books.

Respectful Interaction

Working With Adults

The reader will be able to:
- Compare the unique challenges of development in young and middle adulthood
- Discuss "responsibility" as it applies to the middle years of life and how it may affect the patient's trust that health professionals are showing due respect for the person's situation
- Discuss the meaning of work for adults
- Describe at least three social roles that characterize life for most middle-age persons and ways in which showing respect for a patient requires attention to those roles
- Discuss how stress enters into attempts to carry out the responsibilities of each of the roles and some health-related consequences of negative responses to stress
- List basic challenges facing health professionals who are working with an adult going through a midlife transition
- Describe some opportunities for growth and enrichment that arise through continued development during the adult years

Prelude

From a young 30- or 40-year-old, I turned into an old 30- or 40-year-old. But once I was 59 I wasn't too certain that the same magic as had been wreaked once I became a novice in other decades would continue to exert its power once I reached 60. Like Doris Day, I thought that the really frightening thing about middle age is the knowledge that you'll grow out of it.

V. IRONSIDE[1]

Who Is the Adult?

It may be true that of all the life periods, adulthood has been the least understood and least studied. A stereotype about adult life is that it is only a waiting period or holding place made up of work, establishing a family, or dealing with menopause or other physical changes on the way to retirement and old age. There is a wide variation in the types and timing of transitions and activities in adult life that is far richer than this stereotype suggests. For these reasons, it is important to examine some vital issues concerning life as an adult today.

Adulthood can be legally defined by chronological age or at the time a person begins to assume responsibility for himself or herself and others.[2] In the majority of the United States, the legal adult age of capacity is 18.[3] It also can be defined by achievement of certain developmental tasks such as being independent; establishing long-term relationships; establishing a personal identity in a reflective way; finding a meaningful occupation; contributing to the welfare of others or making a contribution to family, faith community, or society at large; and gaining recognition for one's accomplishments. Finally, adulthood can be defined in psychological terms—that is, by the level of maturity exhibited by a person. Mature persons can take responsibility, make logical decisions, appreciate the position of others, control emotional outbursts, and accept social roles. What it means to be an "adult" is a combination of many factors, the most important of which you will be introduced to in these pages.

Needs: Respect, Identity, and Intimacy

Adult development is not marked by definitive physical and psychomotor changes such as those seen in early childhood (e.g., learning how to walk) or adolescence, but it is full of challenging and largely unpredictable experiences. The health professional's understanding of this difference is essential as an orienting position for entering a professional relationship that conveys genuine respect for the adult patient. Adult life is marked by concepts such as independent life choices, midlife physical and emotional challenges and changes, and generativity. For many it includes raising a family, facing the empty nest, the return of adult children, and the addition of grandchildren. In addition, there may be differences in the way adulthood is experienced by men and women. Also, the specific point in history that a person enters adulthood may have profound implications for adult life. For example, many women in Western societies who entered adulthood during the women's movement of the 1960s and 1970s faced more opportunities regarding work and sexual freedom than the previous generation of women. Finally, development also may differ because of sexual orientation, race, ethnicity, socioeconomic status, culture, and education, to name a few.

BIOLOGICAL DEVELOPMENT DURING THE ADULT YEARS

Biological development sometimes is treated as complete when a person shows the result of changes that occur during adolescence, but human beings continue to grow and mature throughout their life span. *Aging* can be defined as "the sum of all the changes that normally occur in an organism with the passage of time."[4] Demographers, social scientists, and developmental psychologists consider young adulthood to be roughly between the ages of 21 and 40 and middle adulthood to be between the ages of 40 and 65.[5] Aging, like adulthood itself, is complex and varies from one person to another. The rate at which individuals age is highly variable, but so is the way they adapt to age-related changes and illness. Aging also gives rise to feelings of anxiety in a way no other area of human development does. Failing intellectual or biological functions in the middle years can become a preoccupation for patients in your care. For example, during this period the pure joy of physical activity experienced in younger years may acquire a sober edge. One of us overheard a man who for years has enjoyed running just for the sport of it tell his friend, "Yeah, my running will probably guarantee that I live 5 years longer, but I will have spent that 5 years running!"

Adults also may worry about the age-related changes that begin to take place in their mental functions and body structure and function. Suddenly, forgetfulness is no longer something to be taken lightly but could portend more serious problems generally associated with age. Perhaps the anxiety that aging provokes is due to the close relationship most of us think exists between biological development and illness, decline, and death.[6] Rather than view aging in this way, gerontologists have proposed the concept of *compressed morbidity*, which suggests that people may live longer, healthier lives and have shorter periods of disability at the end of their lives. The focus of health care then becomes one of prevention, maintenance of quality of life, health promotion, and postponement of chronic conditions and disability or death rather than cure.[7,8] In Chapter 14, we discuss different views of aging and their impact on your interactions with older patients.

The human life span is thought to be about 110 to 120 years. In the United States, the average life expectancy is said to be 78.8 years, although this varies according to race and other variables (black females, 78.4 years; black males, 72.3 years; white females, 81.4 years; white males, 76.7; Hispanic

TABLE 13.1 ■ Leading Causes of Death in the United States

Causes of Death	Total Number of Deaths in the U.S. Population
1. Diseases of the heart	633,842
2. Malignant neoplasms	595,930
3. Chronic lower respiratory diseases	155,041
4. Unintentional injuries	146,571
5. Cerebrovascular diseases	140,323
6. Alzheimer's disease	110,561
7. Diabetes mellitus	79, 535
8. Influenza and pneumonia	57,062
9. Nephritis, nephrotic syndrome, and nephrosis	49,959
10. Suicide	44,193

From the U.S. Department of Health and Human Services, Centers for Disease Control and Prevention, National Center for Health Statistics. (2017). *Health, United States, 2016: With Chartbook on Long-Term Trends in Health*. DHHS Publication No. 2017-1232. Available at: https://www.cdc.gov/nchs/data/hus/hu s16.pdf#019.

females, 84.2; and Hispanic males, 79.2).[9] The 10 leading causes of death for all age groups in the United States are listed in Table 13.1.[10] Cause of death varies according to race and gender but this table provides a general idea of the types of illnesses you will encounter most often with adult patients. This of course does not consider that some entire populations within the United States and Western societies are refugees or immigrants from countries with a variety of stresses that affect their health and life course. Table 13.2 highlights the 10 leading causes of death globally.[11] As you compare these two tables, you will likely note some similarities and differences. Depending on your worksite, the challenge is to become sensitive to each patient's situation to express due respect to them.

Many causes of death among all adult populations are the result of chronic diseases. One in four Americans has multiple (two plus) chronic diseases,[12] and the burden and treatment of chronic disease among race and socioeconomic status is notably disproportionate.[13] Fortunately, conditions such as diabetes, depression, and cardiovascular disease are being diagnosed and treated earlier in adulthood than ever before; however, chronic disease management remains a key health concern in the United States. Given these observations, you can see why the interprofessional care team has become the norm for diagnosis and treatment interventions.

As science progresses, we learn more about how individual genes, biology, and behaviors interact with the social, cultural, and physical environment to influence health outcomes. Targeting prevention, illness management, and lifestyle modification in young and middle adulthood can increase quality of life and prevent the development and severity of chronic disease in older adulthood. Young adulthood is often referred to as the *healthy years and the hidden hazards*. Individuals in early and middle adulthood tend to underestimate the impact over time that poor lifestyle choices or unpreventable environmental situations may have on their overall health quality and life span.

EMERGING AND EARLY ADULTHOOD

As discussed in Chapter 12, it is during late adolescence that self-identity begins to form. These processes of identity exploration and consolidation continue in the beginning of emerging or early

TABLE 13.2 ■ Leading Causes of Death Globally

Causes of Death	Total Number of Deaths Globally
1. Ischemic heart disease	8.76 million
2. Stroke	6.24 million
3. Lower respiratory tract infections	3.19 million
4. Chronic obstructive pulmonary disease	17.17 million
5. Trachea, bronchus, lung cancers	69.69 million
6. Diabetes mellitus	59.59 million
7. Alzheimer's disease	1.54 million
8. Diarrheal diseases	1.39 million
9. Tuberculosis	37.37 million
10. Road injury	1.34 million

From World Health Organization. The Top Ten Causes of Death Worldwide Fact Sheet, January 2017. Available at: http://www.who.int/mediacentre/factsheets/fs310/en/index2.html.

adulthood (generally between the ages of 18 and 25). Adulthood is not defined by a single factor, rather an integration of cognitive development, physical development, reflective judgment, and societal experience. The way an individual transitions through adulthood is heavily influenced by experiences in previous stages of life.

REFLECTIONS

The transition from adolescence to adulthood is a process.
- Can you identify two or three factors that influenced your own transition to adulthood?
- How did your family or peers influence your transition?
- If you could go back in time, would you do anything differently? If so, why?

In the span of a few generations, the path to adulthood has changed dramatically. In his extensive research with young adults ages 18 to 29 in the United States, Arnett[14] identified several distinguishing features of emerging adulthood. These five main features are (1) identity exploration, (2) instability, (3) self-focus, (4) feeling in-between, and (5) possibilities. In general, today's young people are taking longer to leave home, attain economic independence, marry, and form families than did their peers half a century ago.[15] These longer transitions put strains on families and institutions (such as health care systems) that work with young adults. For example, adults who have children might think that they have moved through an adult developmental task of parenting, only to find their children returning home after a divorce or unemployment. Therefore a parent or parents who might have been rejoicing in an empty nest and time for each other may find their adult children under their roof once again and with grandchildren in tow. In mainstream Western societies delayed acquisition of independence, earlier physical maturation characteristic of modern cultures, pressures on young people to take on appearances of being grown up, return of adult children to their parents' home, and delayed childbearing all complicate traditional views held about progression through adulthood. Even if we hold several variables constant (e.g., age, gender), it is still difficult to predict how two adult patients might react to the same diagnosis. Consider the example of Ms. McLean and Mrs. Jeon, both of whom have just learned that they have in situ cancer of the cervix.

Case Study

Sara McLean, age 34, has a family history positive for cervical cancer. Her maternal aunt and older sister both died of cervical cancer. Ms. McLean has recently become engaged and plans to be married in 6 months. She put off committing to a permanent relationship and starting a family until she completed graduate work in clinical psychology. With the support of her husband-to-be, she had planned on balancing a career as a private therapist with raising a family. She is devastated when the oncologist presents information about the treatment of choice for her condition—a total hysterectomy.

Eunice Jeon, age 33, also has in situ cancer of the cervix. She has no family history of cancer and has always prided herself on her "hearty" family stock. All her grandparents are alive and well. Mrs. Jeon married her high school sweetheart the weekend after graduation. The Jeons have four children aged 5, 8, 10, and 12. Mr. Jeon is an emergency medical technician and plans someday to enroll in medical school after he finishes his bachelor's degree. Mrs. Jeon works as a secretary/receptionist at the Catholic grade school her children attend. She is troubled by the diagnosis but is relieved when her husband explains that "in situ" means that the cancer has not spread and the hysterectomy would remove the cancer. So, when presented with treatment options she merely asks, "When can we schedule the surgery? I want to get this taken care of as soon as possible."

Both women's feelings and reactions are the result of their life experiences to this point, which in turn are influenced by their roles and familial contexts. In Ms. McLean's case, her response to the diagnosis is influenced by her roles as daughter, sister, niece, fiancée, and psychologist. Mrs. Jeon's response is influenced by her roles as mother, wife, daughter, granddaughter, and receptionist. These life roles are only a few that we can ascertain based on the information presented in the brief cases. It is highly probable that both women have many more roles. Ms. McLean planned her life around finishing her education. Mrs. Jeon's has revolved largely around her family. In short, just looking at their ages, it would be impossible to predict how Ms. McLean and Mrs. Jeon would interpret this crisis.

Along the life span, illness and injury invariably result in changes in the patient's *identity*. Identity is an understanding of the basic self that provides continuity over time and across problems and changes that arise in life. Thus there is a sense of maintenance of one's self through identity and yet room for change to accommodate the vicissitudes of life. Adult patients are generally more capable of entering a patient-centered professional relationship as an equal partner than younger people. Even though most adult patients are better able to protect their own interests and make their wishes known, they are still worthy of the respect that we accord to younger, generally more vulnerable, patients. Respect, in its three expressions of appreciation of the other, attention to specific characteristics, and individualized care, introduced in Chapter 1, continue to be the benchmarks of effective interaction in this period, as well as all the others through the life span.

Intimacy is another developmental task of the adult. According to Erikson, adult development is marked by the ability to experience open, supportive, and loving relationships with others without the fear of losing one's own identity in the process of growing close to another.[2] You were introduced to the difference between personal and intimate relationships in Chapter 4 illustrating that the type of intimacy a patient will experience with family members, lovers, and friends is deeper and more involving than the professional, care-based relationships in which the patient and you will engage. It is that deeper intimacy that Erikson is talking about. The major developmental facets of adult life are referred to repeatedly as we explore the social roles, meaning of work, and challenges of midlife.

PSYCHOSOCIAL DEVELOPMENT AND NEEDS

Maturity requires the acceptance of responsibility and empathy for others. The concept of achievement central to adult life can be defined in many ways. Some midlife challenges discussed later in this chapter seem to stem from a person's having adequately assumed responsibility and realized his or her achievement potential, whereas others arise when the individual has failed to do so.

A profile of a person in the adult years of life will necessarily involve a consideration of his or her sense of "responsibility." Underlying the idea of responsibility is an assumption that the individual is a free agent (i.e., one who is willing and able to act autonomously). Thus a person coerced into performing an act is not considered to have accepted responsibility for it. Given these conditions of ability and agreement, we want to know whether the person can be trusted to carry out the acts, regardless of whether the agreement was explicit (i.e., a promise to abide by the terms of a contract) or implicit (i.e., a promise to provide for one's own children or parents).

REFLECTIONS

Describe an activity you currently participate in and enjoy or feel a sense of responsibility for the outcome.
- What are the environmental, personal, and family or societal factors that facilitate your participation?
- How has this activity helped you find purpose/meaning in your life?
- How does this activity relate to those you were exposed to as a child or young adult?
- Do you project that you will still be doing this activity in later stages of your adulthood? Why or why not?

During adulthood, another aspect to acting responsibly involves having a high regard for the welfare of others. The adult must find a way to support the next generation by redirecting attention from him- or herself to others. In other words, the adult learns to care.[16] This involves empathy for the predicaments that befall others in life. The acts may flow from a free will, but the will must operate in accordance with reasonable claims and justifiable expectations of other people. The claims of society on a person peak during the middle years, so "acting responsibly" must be interpreted in terms of how completely the person fulfills the conditions of those claims. For instance, in Hindu culture, one stage of acting out one's karma involves active engagement in the affairs of family and business. Only when an individual has successfully completed these tasks may he or she move on to higher, more contemplative levels of existence.

One way to view the matter in our culture is to review the concept of self-respect. During the adult years, most people perceive their self-respect as being vulnerable to the judgments of others. One's self-respect at least partially depends on the extent to which he or she commands the respect of employer, family, and friends. This idea is related to our concept of "reputation": One commands respect by giving due consideration to society's claims. Hiltner[17] notes, correctly we think, that to a large extent even the personal values of the middle years must include a regard for others. For most, it is a highly social period when interdependencies are complex and pervasive.

Adulthood sometimes involves people going back to previous developmental tasks such as establishing a basic identity if they did not resolve these issues previously in late adolescence or early adulthood. Researchers have begun to move away from the linear perspective of identity development, recognizing the importance these milestones hold over the life span. For example, some LGBTQ (lesbian, gay, bisexual, transgender, queer/questioning) adults may experience difficulties with self-identity and sexual identity development given the high levels of stigma and low levels of social support they experience.[18] As health professionals, being aware of the isolation that sexual or other minority groups often encounter provides one avenue of professional respect that must be expressed. Attentiveness to this difference also is essential given that LGBTQ adults taken together experience health challenges at higher rates, including mental illness, substance use, heart disease, HIV, and physical violence than their heterosexual peers.[19] Positive outcomes of reaching sexual identity milestones and adopting an identity include improved self-esteem, sense of community, sense of living authentically, and improved relationships with romantic partners and parents.[20]

SOCIAL ROLES IN ADULTHOOD

Several social roles most fully characterize this period involving primary relationships, parenting, care of older family members, and involvement in the community in the form of political, religious, or other social or service organizations and groups.

Primary Relationships

It is almost always during adulthood that a person decides with whom lasting relationships will be developed. Fortunately, an increasing number of older people are also developing new relationships, but they are usually people who could sustain deep and lasting relationships in the middle years as well.

The primary relationship takes priority over all others, the most common type being the relationship with a spouse. Choosing a spouse or other permanent companion and becoming better acquainted (i.e., learning to know the person, discovering potentials and limits, similarities and differences, and compatibilities and incompatibilities) are processes interwoven with the more basic activities of eating, sleeping, acquiring possessions, working, worshipping, relaxing, and playing together.

Those who do not enter a marriage relationship sometimes develop a deep and lasting involvement with a partner, often a friend or sibling. One of your first tasks of respectful interaction with an adult patient is to find out if there is a key person in his or her life and, if so, who that person is. This can be accomplished without unnecessary probing into the person's private life. Particularly in times of crisis the patient looks to that key person for comfort, sustenance, and guidance. However, sometimes the person you assume would be the most supportive is not. Consider the case of Mary Ogden and Pam Carlisle.

Case Study

Mary Ogden, age 52, is a single teacher who is hospitalized for treatment related to severe diabetes. The entire small community where she has resided and taught for 25 years adores her. Through the years she has received numerous awards for community service. She is a cheerful person, who, despite her illness, continues to be an inspiration to everyone. She is especially fond of Pam Carlisle, the head nurse on the unit where Mary is being treated.

On the afternoon before Mary's planned hospital discharge, an unscheduled visitor comes to the nursing desk insisting to speak to Pam about a highly personal matter. The visitor is Agnes Ogden, an elderly woman who informs Pam that she is the older sister (and only living relative) of Mary. The visitor seems sincere and asks that Pam provide details of her sister's condition so that Agnes might be better prepared to aid Mary with both her physical illness and personal affairs. Pam complies with her request, feeling relieved that there is someone to share this burden with her. The following morning Pam visits Mary's room and finds her profoundly irate for the first time. She informs Pam that she has not been on speaking terms with her sister for many years, that she considers her sister to be untrustworthy, and that she thoroughly resents her sister having the knowledge of her personal affairs and illness. Mary feels betrayed and expresses her distrust of Pam as her health care provider. She becomes withdrawn, agitated, and uncooperative.

We can assume that Pam shared the information with Agnes Ogden believing that she was doing so with Mary's well-being their shared goal. Still, what could Pam have done differently to foster Mary's trust rather than to destroy it? What would you have done when Agnes came to you requesting information?

Besides violating the federal Health Information Portability and Accountability Act (HIPAA) regulations, discussed in Chapter 6, that are designed to legally protect Mary's privacy and confidentiality, Pam has also broken the trust that is so fundamental to a respectful health professional and patient relationship. How might you rebuild the trust that once existed between you and a patient should such a breakdown occur?

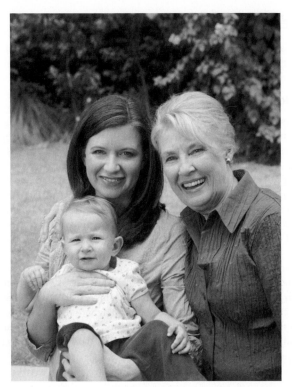

Fig. 13.1   Parenting relationships are among the most enduring and complex of human interactions. (© *David Woolley/Digital Vision/Thinkstock.com.*)

PARENTING OF CHILDREN

Caring for children is often a part of adult life. Gender role stereotypes traditionally assigned to mothering, fathering, and co-parenting are breaking down in many families so that both parents share the whole range of parenting skills. The concept of parenting is being expanded, too. There are married parents, divorced parents, single parents, same-sex parents, foster parents, and children who live within extended family situations in which parenting is shared by several persons.

REFLECTIONS

Parenting is often a part of adult life.
- What are some of the advantages and disadvantages of parenting children today?
- Is it one of your life goals to be a parent? Why or why not?
- If you are already a parent, how did you transition into this role?

Whatever the challenges of each model, all share the assumption that the child's welfare depends on the quality of parenting. The age-old recognition that a child's physical and emotional well-being depends on adult care is now buttressed by more recent assertions that the child's potential for fulfillment and satisfaction in later years is also determined in the earliest years of life that are strongly influenced by the parent. The least that can be said of parenting relationships is that they are among the most enduring and complex of human interactions (Fig. 13.1). We saw in earlier chapters that parents play a key role in the delivery of patient- and family-centered care. The health professional who fails to consider parents respectfully neglects an integral part of the patient's identity.

Care of Older Family Members

Not only do many adults care for children as a part of their daily responsibilities, they also care for their parents, parents-in-law, and other older friends and relatives. Middle-age adults are often referred to as the "sandwich" generation because they are responsible for care of both young (children) and old (aging parents/family members). They are "sandwiched" between these two generations. The move toward supporting the older adult to age in place often increases the demands placed on adult children. There are an estimated 43.5 million adult caregivers in the United States, with 6.5 million nonprofessional caregivers caring for both adults and children simultaneously.[21] The average caregiver in the United States is a female in her late 40s. Six in 10 caregivers report being employed at some point while caregiving, with 56% working full time.[21] Caregivers often put the needs of their care recipients ahead of their own, placing themselves at high risk for poor physical and emotional health, as well as decreased quality of life as described in Chapter 8. The responsibilities of caregiving can disrupt employment, health maintenance, leisure, and social participation during adulthood.[22]

It is important to remember that just as family structure and functions differ from culture to culture, so do caregiving roles and expectations. A recent systematic review of the multicultural experiences of caregiving highlights some general themes that emerge in caregiving roles and expectations. The authors found that Latino caregivers valued family decision-making regarding care; Asian-American caregivers experienced strained interpersonal relationships and shame asking for help; African American caregivers reported a reliance on community and striving to maintain cohesion of their family; and Native American caregivers reported feeling pressure to provide care despite limited resources and a lack of formal resources.[23] This and other research highlights that the cultural lens is essential for accurately viewing this role of adult life.

Political and Other Service Activities

Involvement in political and social organizations has traditionally been at a peak during the adult years. Responsibilities stemming from membership in such organizations are often second only to those of work if measured in terms of energy consumption and personal commitments beyond those toward family. A sense of identity in adulthood depends heavily on belonging to such groups whether they be a political party, religious group, or service or arts organizations. These service activities are not only a source of identity but also a vehicle for contributing to one's profession or community.

In summary, there are many sources of claims on adults, but attending to primary relationships such as spouses or significant others, children, and parents while contributing to public initiatives constitutes highly significant ones.

WORK AS MEANINGFUL ACTIVITY

Work, like family and adulthood, is a concept that can be variably defined. Work as meaningful activity can occur in a variety of settings and assumes many patterns. Therefore the meaning of work and the responsibilities it requires will depend on the person's value system, expectations, and aspirations, as well as the specific environment, job title, and position within a hierarchy. For some, work is performed primarily in the home; for a great many others, it entails a significant amount of time away from home. Adults are judged to spend about half of their waking hours engaged in work, and it is during middle adulthood that career consolidation typically occurs. The average U.S. employee works 7.9 hours a day. Women have a greater likelihood of working part time compared with men.[24] The kind of work they do largely determines their income, lifestyle, social status, and place of residence. Because of the amount of time and energy expended, the type of information one acquires over a lifetime is often influenced by the working situation (Fig. 13.2). Studies of professional socialization suggest that the kind of work one does also contributes to one's worldview.

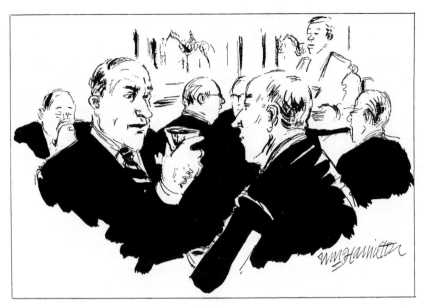

Fig. 13.2 "I've learned a lot in 63 years. But, unfortunately, almost all of it is about aluminum." (*From The New Yorker, November 11, 1977, p. 27. © The New Yorker Collection 1977 William Hamilton from cartoonbank.com. All Rights Reserved.*)

Work-related responsibilities still differ generally for men and women. You have undoubtedly observed what most women experience in their work roles: expectations on them include not only doing a job in the labor force but also maintaining the quality and amount of work performed in the home. Women respond to these various needs or demands by trying to balance their impulse to care and the level of personal support available.[25] When the limits of caregiving are reached, something else must give. Expectations of caregiving responsibilities for women often result in women working fewer hours and getting paid less in comparison to men.[26]

Two types of responsibilities are associated with the work role: (1) to do one's job well and (2) to fulfill the reasonable expectations of others (e.g., employer, peers, family members). The professional relationship has the added dimension of caregiving that one is expected to help those who seek professional services.

Work relationships are different from simple friendships in several ways, although the former can be lasting, deep, and complex. Moreover, there is not always clear separation of the two. The carpool phenomenon is an intriguing combination of how work and friendship roles become intermingled; here people who are grouped together for getting to and from their workplace also usually engage in camaraderie over minutes or hours each week and sometimes more regularly than with their own family members. We have known some carpool members who interact as friends or acquaintances during the commute, then assume their "proper" workplace role with each other when work begins.

Your task as a health professional is to assess how the patient views his or her work situation, what work means, and particularly the responsibilities and relationships in it. Whether a patient's work involves providing quality child care, laboring on the section crew to replace railroad ties, or presiding over a meeting in the executive suite, the work entails responsibility toward both a job to be done and other human beings. Treatment goals must be tailored to help the patient carry out these responsibilities, modify them, or accept that work may no longer be possible.

Those who work with adult patients in the areas of occupational health are keenly aware of the relationship among health, injury, or illness and the worker's role. Consider the following case:

Case Study

Masie Baldwin has worked as a certified nursing assistant in a skilled nursing facility for the past 15 years. She is the sole provider for her three children, one of whom has just started college. Although Ms. Baldwin has attended the mandatory in-service sessions on proper body mechanics and lifting of patients, she has not always followed the proper procedure. Ms. Baldwin stated to her fellow workers more than once, "I'm big and strong. I don't like waiting for help or lugging out the lift to get patients up. I can get them up and out of bed without help." Unfortunately, while getting Mr. Collins out of bed, Ms. Baldwin injured her lower back and neck. Ms. Baldwin has been on workers' compensation leave for the past month and is now involved in a "work-hardening" program to determine if she can return to work in the nursing home. The health professionals working with Ms. Baldwin observe that she is highly motivated to return to work but frightened of reinjury. Her confidence in her strength and sense of invulnerability have been badly shaken. During a particularly trying day in the work-hardening program, she tells her therapist, "If I can't work in the nursing home, I don't know what I'll do. It's the only kind of work I've ever done. All my friends are there."

REFLECTIONS

- What "meanings" do you think Ms. Baldwin gives to her work?
- How does her identity tie to her work roles?
- What are some of the challenges you might face in working with Ms. Baldwin?

We have emphasized responsibility in terms of relationships and work roles in the adult years and that self-respect during this period is determined in large part by meeting the justifiable expectations of others. However, self-respect unquestionably also depends somewhat on believing in and being true to oneself. Thus adults who meet all of society's expectations can still be unfulfilled.[27] That, in fact, is precisely the plight of many people today who have not pursued personal interests and goals at all or minimally. This situation can be viewed as an inability or unwillingness to assume responsibility toward oneself, and it contributes to the challenges of midlife that are discussed in this chapter. Accepting the consequences of one's own behavior is vital; all of us share, to some extent, the problem expressed by the motto on President Truman's desk, "The buck stops here." The sense of "being somebody," such an integral part of adolescent development, must become more fully defined in the young and middle adult years. By middle adulthood, individuals are expected to be able to show more clearly who they are and what they can contribute to the welfare of loved ones and to society.

STRESSES AND CHALLENGES OF ADULTHOOD

"In terms of social roles, adulthood is described generally as a time when the individual is a responsible member of society under pressure to coordinate multiple roles (e.g., spouse, worker, parent, caregiver)."[28] The more responsibilities a person assumes, the more vulnerable he or she becomes to the symptoms associated with stress. Stress is recognized as a potential threat to well-being, and its negative effects will increase if steps are not taken to respond positively. Major problems associated with negative responses to stress in adult life are finally gaining the attention of researchers, health professionals, workplace counselors, and religious groups. Given the associated negative health behaviors and outcomes of work and life stress, identification of protective factors such as physical activity, mindfulness, and sleep for adult patients is essential.[29]

Chapter 4 addresses some sources of stress in professionals as they move through their student years and into becoming a professional, and Chapter 8 suggests some types of challenges patients face that are likely to produce stress at any age. The specific sources differ, but how a young person has learned to cope and deal with stress will be carried into adulthood. One significant difference is that, in the middle years, no clearly defined end to some sources of stress—no "gracious exit" from an impossible situation—may be in sight. The stress attending next week's examination can be more easily managed than that arising from the realization that one has a stressful lifestyle in general.

Some stresses result from personal life choices. The responsibilities assumed in marriage and other primary relationships (e.g., childrearing, parent care, work) all create stress, as do unemployment and some factors in the social structure itself. Each is discussed separately.

Primary Relationship Stresses

Marriage relationships during the middle years have been studied more extensively than other types of primary relationships, but it is reasonable to think that all such intimate relationships produce stressful situations. Common sources of stress in the marriage relationship include nonfulfillment of role obligations by a spouse, lack of reciprocity between marital partners, a feeling of not being accepted by one's spouse, and strain related to co-parenting. Research supports that sources of stress that are damaging to the marital relationship are those of an ongoing nature instead of those of a discrete event.[30-32] Illfeld[33] maintains that common, mundane stressors in everyday life take more of a toll in suffering than does the impact of a dramatic life crisis. Couples with children often experience stress around the departure of their children, leaving both (and not only the woman, as is often thought) with the "empty nest syndrome." In addition to the empty nest, women's middle age is often discussed in terms of menopause and new opportunities for activity and self-expression. Although a positive relationship has been established between successful aging and positive self-esteem in postmenopausal women, menopause can be perceived negatively among cultures that value fertility.[34,35]

A more violent expression of stress, the primary source of which may not arise from the relationship itself but is acted out within it, is domestic violence, or intimate partner abuse. Domestic violence is defined as "willful intimidation, physical assault, battery, sexual assault, and/or other abusive behavior as part of a systematic pattern of power and control perpetrated by one intimate partner against another. It includes physical violence, sexual violence, threats, and emotional/psychological abuse."[36] Some persons involved in situations of domestic violence receive attention from self-help groups and other organizations, but not all do. They will be present among your patients, exhibiting both overt and covert symptoms that deserve attention. It is important to note that domestic violence occurs across the socioeconomic spectrum and among all ethnic and other demographic groups. For many generations, abuse survivors have remained largely hidden and silent, victimized by the fear of stigmatization, shame, and having no place to go for safety and support. For many, financial dependence is a common reason to return to an abusive partner. Increasingly the inhumane situation abuse leaves victims in has prompted health professionals, lawmakers, volunteers, and others to try to help provide an antidote to this devastating state of affairs. Currently more educational and legal mechanisms are being put in place to provide professional caregivers with the tools to recognize, assess, and report certain or suspected domestic violence in a patient. The professional who treats adult patients must be aware of clinical guidelines that express deep respect through the discovery of symptoms or behaviors, institutional policies regarding suspected or obvious abuse, local sources of support available to patients, and legal requirements to report domestic abuse. For example, any health professional can become familiar with the location of refuges, or safe houses, that are in many cities and sometimes in rural areas. In addition, an increasing number of health professionals are becoming involved more directly in the treatment and rehabilitation of vulnerable women and men and the perpetrators of their abuse.

Parenting Stresses

The tremendous responsibility associated with parenting also leads to stress situations in young and middle adulthood. Parenting is socially constructed, and there are both burdens and benefits to parenting. Because there is no "instructor's manual" on how to manage the twists and turns of parenthood, patients in your care may turn to you for advice. As a health professional, you may be the first to recognize the signs of parental stress. Providing a listening ear and care for the caregivers are key first steps in helping parents cope with stress. This supports the health of the family as a unit. Child abuse and neglect (discussed in Chapter 11), which are increasing (or, perhaps, are being reported more systematically), are tragic examples of what can happen when stress is not controlled. Most stress related to childrearing leads to less deplorable results, but nonetheless it does take an immense toll on both parent and child.

Stress in Care of Elderly Family Members

Growing numbers of baby boomers will experience the struggles of an aging parent. Assuming the parents of baby boomers bore an average of two children, there are about 76 million parents of baby boomers who are dealing with the acute and chronic disabilities of old age.[37] As previously mentioned, most of the burden for parent care falls on adult women. Many quit their jobs to fulfill the responsibility of caring for one or more elderly family members. The stress is often borne with considerable grace as adult children express the desire to care for their parents and the satisfaction and joy it brings them in concert with the burdens.

Work Stress

For many individuals in the middle years, stress related to work is their primary stress, manifesting itself in a wide range of disorders. Chronically elevated work-related stress is a risk factor for numerous physical and mental health outcomes, including depression and cardiovascular disease. Interestingly, work-related stress in the form of low job control, low social support at work, and high job strain is associated with an increased risk for cognitive decline and dementia later in life.[38] Some jobs are in themselves highly stressful. One of the highest stress jobs is an enlisted soldier. Others are working in an airport control tower or a medical intensive care unit. Studies have demonstrated that a job with high responsibility in which the consequences for a mistake are dire creates the highest stress. Boredom and repetition also create stress. Work-related stress can be a key factor in the development of serious health problems such as cardiovascular disease and alcoholism or other substance abuse.

A form of stress related to the work role is caused by the inability to find or to hold a job. In a society that rewards its members for paid work and in which adult responsibility is tied to societal contribution, the stress of working can be less threatening to health and well-being than the stress of being unemployed.

Thus it becomes evident that the middle years, in which a person is in many ways at his or her prime, are also years of responsibility and stress. The burdens, although each taken alone may be a small constraint, sometimes have the overall effect of making the middle-age person feel exhausted and overwhelmed. Although these years are sometimes characterized as a plateau or holding pattern, they are much more intense and varied than that. They are filled, instead, with alpine meadows, treacherous cliffs, cool blue pools, and swift undercurrents.

REFLECTIONS

Think about all your current major life roles.
- Did you choose these roles, or were they assigned to you?
- What are the behaviors expected by you in these individual roles?
- How do your roles influence your use of time? Do they conflict?
- How have you shaped this role? How has the culture in which you live shaped the role?
- What are the stressors associated with this role?

DOUBT AT THE CROSSROADS AND MIDLIFE CHALLENGES

The task of assuming responsibility and its attendant stresses, the great desire to achieve, or transitions in career, family life, and health condition may at some critical moment trigger an opportunity to take stock. The feeling accompanying the experience is most clearly expressed as doubt. It differs from the vacuous zero point of boredom and lacks the volcanic fervor of other types of stress. Doubt allows no rest; indeed, it is a relentless churning that nakedly reveals almost all the dimensions of one's life. The masks that have allowed the masquerade to go on, the clatter that has accompanied the parade, and the walls that have kept fearful monsters from view all suddenly evaporate and leave a pregnant silence. The self stands alone. Middle-age adults may wonder "Is this all there is?" and feel that "something is missing." Also, the focus on worldly aspirations may start to shift to more spiritual aspects of life and their place in the bigger scheme of things. Middle-age adults make more informed decisions about their futures.

The various transitions that are a part of adult life allow people to come to terms with new situations. Bridges[39] conceptualizes a transition as a three-phase psychological process people go through: ending, neutral zone, and new beginning. A transition begins with an ending. Something must be left behind to move to the next phase. A transition may be sought or thrust upon a person.

Case Study

Consider the case of Tanya Zorski, who has worked as a claims processor at an insurance company for the past 10 years. Recently, Tanya's employer merged with another company, resulting in "downsizing," or firing of many people in the claims department, including Tanya. Tanya's transition begins with the ending of her job. The next phase of transition is the neutral zone. After letting go, willingly or unwillingly, she must examine old habits that are no longer adaptive.[33] As Tanya begins to look for another position, she will discover that the computer skills that had been adequate at her old job are not marketable. Employers want people with experience in leading-edge computer programs, and Tanya does not possess these skills. During the neutral zone phase, people start to look for new, better adapted skills or habits. People may take this opportunity to pursue a long-held dream. The final phase is the new beginning. Tanya decides to move into a new beginning in her life by pursuing a degree in nursing. She reasons that if she is going to invest the energy, time, and financial resources in learning new skills, she might as well do it in a profession that she has wanted to join since she was young.

REFLECTIONS

- Do you anticipate working in the same job for your entire career?
- What would lead you to "shift gears" in your work, living arrangements, or location?

Although changes in midlife have often been labeled as a "crisis," perhaps the language is too strong for most people. "Instead, perhaps, many individuals make modest 'corrections' in their life trajectories—literally, 'midcourse' corrections."[40] These corrections to one's life course are often the opportunity for growth and learning along the life span. As is the case with Tanya Zorski, the more life-changing an event, the more likely it is to be associated with learning opportunities. In the face of stress, adults with a strong learning goal orientation develop more effective, problem-focused coping styles.[41]

Regardless of whether a vision is being claimed or reclaimed, the adult's task is to prepare for the adjustments and challenges still to come.

Working With the Adult Patient

This chapter deals primarily with the physical and especially the psychosocial processes people face in their young and middle adult years. Some suggestions for maintaining respectful interaction have been offered, and we turn more fully to the relationship in this last section.

The patient you encounter in the adult years who arrives at the health facility may be working to maintain health or may be experiencing an illness-related symptom. Because these years are not "supposed to be" characterized by painful or other troubling physical symptoms, patients may feel especially angered or confused by this physical intrusion into their work of being a responsible person and pursuing goals. A woman of middle years who was being interviewed recently in a seminar reported that "being an adult was overrated!" Her father was in hospice for end-of-life cancer care, two of her three sons required special education services for attention deficit/hyper-activity disorder and learning disorders, and she was just told by her primary care physician that she needed to follow up with an oncologist for a positive mammogram. The ideas of being struck down in one's prime and that of the "untimely" accident or death are often applied to this age group. The denial, hostility, and depression that patients feel about being so attacked are factors to which you should give your attention, whether your interaction occurs only once or extends over a long period.

Because psychological and social well-being are preeminent for adults, treatment must be attuned to both. Of all the challenges presented by illness, injury, or disability, the loss of inde-pendence most epitomizes the overall loss experienced by the great majority of adult patients. Of course, the person's former self-image is threatened, too, but this is almost a direct outgrowth of the loss of independence. Patients who can no longer go about meeting the responsibilities expected of them and pursuing the numerous life roles and established goals may feel trapped, vul-nerable, and frustrated. The primacy of these concerns in middle life should help you understand why a patient seems overly concerned about having to get a babysitter for an hour, or having to be home at a given time, or why he or she is willing to forego treatment rather than to take time from work for a trip to the health facility.

Furthermore, an adult patient experiencing acute stress poses special problems and challenges. Each one must be treated according to the manifestations of the stress. Part of the respect you must express is to assess physical or psychological symptoms that may be arising from stress. This, of course, often must be done with a psychiatrist or psychologist, but not always. As you learned in Chapter 7, the skills of listening to the patient's narrative are tools to help you discern what is on a patient's mind. Listening may not only help decrease their anxiety at the moment but also may enable you to make adjustments in schedule, routine, or approach that will further diminish it.

Many of the suggestions given throughout this book apply to all age groups. However, if you are alert to some of the central concerns and roles of young and middle adulthood, you may well find that your success in achieving respectful interaction with the adult patient is heightened. In the next chapter, you have an opportunity to examine some changes that are faced by the person who has successfully lived through the middle years. As you will see, these changes involve some of life's greatest challenges, both positive and negative.

Summary

Even though biological capacities peak and begin to diminish in adulthood, adults have sufficient capacity for personally satisfying and socially valuable participation in life with all that it offers. The major life tasks for adults are to establish personal identity, develop intimate relationships, and feel and act on the desire to make a lasting contribution to the next generation. A key claim on adults is to accept responsibility through parenting, work, and public service activities. Although some people never resolve the issues that are brought into focus during the transitions of midlife, fortunately most do. Some emerge from the process with a new job, a new mate, or a new life view. The various aspects of adult development that were presented in this chapter are a sampling of the ways you can look at the complex process of how people grow and develop as adults, with an eye to how these observations can help you be respectful in your relationships with adult patients and their families.

References

1. Ironside V. *You're old, I'm old … Get used to it! Twenty Reasons Why Growing Old Is Great*. New York: Plume—The Penguin Group; 2012.
2. Erikson EH. *Childhood and Society*. 2nd ed. New York: WW Norton; 1963.
3. *Black's Online Law Dictionary*. 2017. http://thelawdictionary.org/adulthood/.
4. Matteson ES, McConnell ES, Linton AD, eds. *Biological Theories of Aging in Gerontological Nursing: Concepts and Practice*. 2nd ed. Philadelphia: WB Saunders; 1996.
5. Cronin A. Mandich MB: *Human Development and Performance Throughout the Lifespan*. 2nd ed. Boston, MA: Delmar Cengage Learning; 2015.
6. Cannon M. What is aging? *Dis-A-Mon [Serial Online]*. 2015;61:454–459. Issues on Aging.
7. *U.S. Department of Health and Human Services Healthy People (Website)*. 2017. https://www.healthypeople.gov.
8. Luyten W, Antal P, Rattan S, et al. Ageing with elegance: a research proposal to map healthspan pathways. *Biogerontology [serial online]*. 2016;17(4):771–782.
9. U.S. Department of Health and Human Services. Centers for Disease Control and Prevention, National Center for Health Statistics: United States Life Tables, 2013 (DHHS Publication No. 2017-1120). *Natl Vital Stat Rep*. 2017;66(3):1–63.
10. U.S. Department of Health and Human Services, Centers for Disease Control and Prevention, National Center for Health Statistics: Health. United States: 2016: With chartbook on long-term trends in health (DHHS Publication No. 2017-1232), 2017. Retrieved from https://www.cdc.gov/nchs/data/hus/hus16.pdf#019.
11. World Health Organization. *The Top Ten Causes of Death Worldwide Fact Sheet*. 2017. http://www.who.int/mediacentre/factsheets/fs310/en/index2.html.
12. Institute of Medicine. *Living Well with Chronic Illness: A Call for Public Health Action*. Washington, DC: National Academies Press; 2012.
13. Assari S. Number of chronic medical conditions fully mediates the effects of race on mortality; 25-year follow-up of a nationally representative sample of Americans. *J Racial Ethn Health Disparities [serial online]*. 2017;4(4):623–631.
14. Arnett JJ. *Emerging Adulthood: The Winding Road from Late Teens Through Early Twenties*. 2nd ed. New York: Oxford University Press; 2015.
15. U.S. Department of Commerce, Economics and Statistics Administration, U.S. Census Bureau: America's families and living arrangements: 2012, Current population reports (P20-570), 2013 Retrieved from https://www.census.gov/prod/2013pubs/p20-570.pdf.
16. Malone J, Liu S, Vaillant G, et al. Midlife eriksonian psychosocial development: setting the stage for late-life cognitive and emotional health. *Dev Psychol*. 2016;52(3):496–508.
17. Hiltner S. Personal values in the middle years. In: Ellis EO, ed. *The Middle Years*. Acton, MA: Publishing Sciences Group; 1974.
18. Dirkes J, Hughes T, Ramirez-Valles J, et al. Sexual identity development: relationship with lifetime suicidal ideation in sexual minority women. *J Clin Nurs*. 2016;25(23/24):3545–3556.
19. The LGBT. Resident in Long-Term Care, CNA Training Advisor: Lesson Plans for Busy Staff Trainers. 2017;25(5):1–8.
20. Riggle ED, Whitman JS, Olson A, et al. The positive aspects of being a lesbian or gay man. *Prof Psychol, Res Pr*. 2008;39:210–217.
21. American Association of Retired Persons Public Policy Institute, & National Alliance of Caregiving: Caregiving in the U.S. 2015, 2015. Retrieved from http://www.caregiving.org/wp-content/uploads/2015/05/2015_CaregivingintheUS_Final-Report-June-4_WEB.pdf.
22. Piersol CV, Earland VT, Herge EA. *Meeting the Needs of Caregivers of Persons with Dementia: An Important Role for Occupational Therapy*, OT Practice. Bethesda, MD: AOTA Press; 2012:8–12.

23. Apesoa-Varano EC, Tang-Feldman Y, Reinhard SC, et al. Multi-cultural caregiving and caregiver interventions: a look back and a call for future action. *J Am Soc Aging*. 2015;39(4):39–49.
24. U.S. Department of Labor Bureau of Labor Statistics. American time use survey summary. *News Release*. 2017. Retrieved from https://www.bls.gov/charts/american-time-use/emp-by-ftpt-job-edu-h.htm.
25. McGrew KB. Daughters' caregiving decisions: from an impulse to a balancing point of care. *J Women Aging*. 1998;10(2):49–65.
26. Gender differences in employment and why they matter. *World Development Report 2012: Gender Equality and Development*. Washington, DC: World Bank; 2011:198–253. Retrieved from https://siteresources.worldbank.org/INTWDR2012/Resources/7778105-1299699968583/7786210-1315936222006/Complete-Report.pdf.
27. Moos RH, Billings A. Conceptualizing and measuring coping resources and processes. In: Goldberger L, Breznitz S, eds. *Handbook of Stress: Theoretical and Clinical Aspects*. New York: Free Press; 1982.
28. Helson R, Sato CJ. Up and down in middle-age: monotonic and nonmonotonic changes in role, status and personality. *J Pers Soc Psychol*. 2005;89(2):194–204.
29. Williams N, Grandner M, Jean-Louis G, et al. Social and behavioral predictors of insufficient sleep among African Americans and Caucasians. *Sleep Medicine*. 2016;18:103–107.
30. Elam K, Chassin L, Eisenberg N, Spinrad T. Marital stress and children's externalizing behavior as predictors of mothers' and fathers' parenting. *Dev Psychopathol [serial online]*. 2017;29.
31. Sampasa-Kanyinga H, Chaput J. Associations among self-perceived work and life stress, trouble sleeping, physical activity, and body weight among Canadian adults. *Prev Med*. 2017;96:16–20.
32. Timmons A, Arbel R, Margolin G. Daily patterns of stress and conflict in couples: associations with marital aggression and family-of-origin aggression. *J Fam Psychol*. 2017;31(1):93–104.
33. Illfeld FW. Marital stressors, coping styles and symptoms of depression. In: Goldberger L, Breznitz S, eds. *Handbook of Stress: Theoretical and Clinical Aspects*. New York: Free Press; 1982.
34. White AJ, Taliaferro D. Relationship between postmenopausal women's successful aging, global self-esteem, and sexual quality of life. *Int J Hum Caring*. 2016;20(2):102–106.
35. Sievert LL. Menopause across cultures: clinical considerations. *Menopause*. 2014;21(4):241–423.
36. National coalition against domestic violence. *Domestic Violence National Statistics*. 2015. Retrieved from https://ncadv.org/assets/2497/domestic_violence.pdf.
37. Sherman FT. This geriatrician's greatest challenge: caregiving. *Geriatrics*. 2006;61(3):8–9.
38. Sindi S, Kareholt I, Solomon A, et al. Midlife work-related stress is associated with late-life cognition. *J Neurol*. 2017;9:1996–2002.
39. Bridges W. *Managing Transitions: Making the Most of Change*. Reading, MA: Addison-Wesley; 1991.
40. Stewart AJ, Ostrove JM. Women's personality in middle age: gender, history, and midcourse corrections. *Am Psychol*. 1998;53(11):1185–1194.
41. Delahaij R, van Dam K. Coping style development: the role of learning goal orientation and metacognitive awareness. *Personal Individ Differ*. 2016;92:57–62.

CHAPTER 14

Respectful Interaction

Working With Older Adults

Prelude

John Quincy Adams is well. But the house in which he lives at present is becoming dilapidated. It is tottering upon its foundation. Time and the seasons have nearly destroyed it. Its roof is pretty well worn out. Its walls are much shattered and it trembles with every wind. I think John Quincy Adams will have to move out of it soon. But he himself is quite well, quite well.

JOHN QUINCY ADAMS IN A RESPONSE TO A QUERY REGARDING HIS WELL-BEING
ON HIS 80TH BIRTHDAY[1]

One of the challenges confronting anyone who attempts to speak of the older adult is to earmark exactly when old age begins, even though it is a phase of life everyone enters if he or she is fortunate enough to live past middle age. According to many social policies, eligibility for financial and other support benefits for the older adult begins at age 65, but the usefulness of this age as a distinguishing line largely ends there. In fact, many people's feelings that they are "old" are determined by the presence (or absence) of sickness, disability, or other limiting factors rather than simply by their chronological age. For the purposes of this chapter, terms such as "elder," "old," and "aged" will refer to individuals in later adulthood—age 65 or older. Late adulthood can be divided into the young old, age 65 to 75; the middle old, age 75 to 85; and the old old, age 85 and older.

The older population in the United States numbers 44.9 million, representing 14.4% of the US population.[2] By 2060, there will be about 98.2 million older adults, and the US Census Bureau projects that the population age 85 and over could grow from 6 million in 2014 to 20 million by 2060.[3,4] The baby boomer generation is largely responsible for this increase in the older adult population. A *baby boomer* is an individual born between 1946 and 1964. Boomers comprise one of the largest generations in US history. The boomers began crossing into the older adult (65+) category in 2011, and they will continue to do so until 2030, shifting the US age structure and the face of health care and society. Geographically, the South contains the greatest number of people age 65 and older, and the Northeast has the largest percentage of people reaching the older ages.[5] Even though not all in this population are sick, the average patient in a US inpatient health care facility is likely to be older than 75 years of age. Additionally, the older population—the heaviest users of the health care system—will be far more diverse and will be women, especially among the oldest old—that is, people older than 85.[5]

Most of us have stereotypes of old age. But almost every generality advanced about the older person is quickly countered by personal experience with a chronologically older man or woman. Many processes that take place in a person as he or she advances in years are similar in broad strokes of what happens but also differ from one individual to another. This chapter provides an overview of physiological and psychosocial changes, with a special emphasis on the psychosocial aspects of aging as they are relevant to respectful interaction. We urge you to study the burgeoning literature of aging further because the questions and clinical issues surrounding care of older patients are complex.

REFLECTIONS

Close your eyes and imagine yourself at age 85.
- What do you imagine you will be like? Look like?
- What roles will you have? How will they differ from your roles today?
- When you tell your life story, what will the highlights be?

The days of the words from sentimental song "over the river and through the woods to grandmother's house we go" have disappeared in large segments of today's society. Rapid societal changes taking place around older people give them greater opportunity for divergent roles than ever before. Indeed, some grandmothers—and grandfathers—may be home bound, but many are actively involved outside of the home as employees, volunteers, or members of community organizations. Today's elders write books, start new businesses, run marathons, travel, attend college, raise grandchildren, and have active social media accounts. The downside is that if they are unable to take advantage of these opportunities, as many are, they may be burdened by a greater feeling of being left out of the action than were their predecessors. One of the authors was saddened by a patient's remark that he had stopped subscribing to a magazine for older adults because it made him too depressed; everyone his age but him looked younger and did more than he could do. Our experience is that health professionals can play an important role in helping each older person make the best of their opportunities so that their potential for a meaningful old age is optimized.

Views of Aging

Aging in its broadest sense refers to the "changes that occur during an organisms' lifespan."[6] It is a multifactorial process, and as we mentioned the rate at which various changes take place is highly individualized. Extensive gerontological research has documented the interaction among genetics, environmental influences, lifestyles, and disease processes.[7]

Aging also intersects with gender and culture, attaching different social meanings, expectations, attitudes, and evaluations.[8] Theories of aging span the fields of biology, psychology, and sociology. These theories, along with experience and the cultural and societal views of aging, influence how health professionals understand the aging process and how they engage in their work with older patients and their families. You will expand your knowledge of aging theories in various areas of coursework that prepare you to work with the older adult population. The text that follows highlights a few of these theories to support your learning in this area.

BIOLOGICAL THEORIES

Biological theories of aging share the concept that "aging results from a decline in the force of natural selection."[9] There is no known way to stop or reverse the aging process. As adults age, their bodies change and progressively lose function. This increases an individual's vulnerability, to both disease and environmental threats. There are two main types of biological aging theories, genetic (programmed theories) and stochastic (damage theories). Genetic theories propose that "aging is genetically determined and organisms have an internal clock that programs longevity".[9] Stochastic or damage theories propose that "chance error and the accumulation of damage over time cause aging. Stochastic theories include wear and tear, error catastrophe, free radical theory, DNA damage hypothesis, loss of adaptive cellular mechanism, and the mitochondrial theory."[9]

SOCIAL THEORIES OF AGING

We interact with older adults in the context of societies, cultures, and communities. What people see or read in the media or hear from adults plays a critical role in shaping their perceptions of older people.[10] Thus it is important to promote representations of older adults in the full range of their activities and health states. Think for a moment about an older adult you know, perhaps a grandparent. Is this individual active and engaged or immobile and frail? Is the person perhaps pleasant and modern? Or irritable and old fashioned? Or pleasant and old fashioned? Our individual and societal experiences with older adults contribute to our views, which is why it is essential to learn as much as we can regarding healthy aging. Doing so prevents ageism in health care.

Ageism is a type of discrimination and demeaning behavior expressed toward older adults. "Most people, including health care professionals, are more familiar with pathological aging than with healthy aging and tend to generalize and project expectation of pathology. Ageism is thus the composite of stereotypical beliefs and attitudes held about a group of people based on their advanced age."[11]

The *life course approach* is a common societal perspective on aging. This theory "recognizes the social, cultural, and structural contexts of a person's lifelong development."[12] Key principles guiding the life course perspective include historical time and place, timing of events in a person's life, and human agency to make decisions. Appreciating how life events have affected the patient, such as an adverse childhood experience or service in the military during war time, will help you understand how to best support and promote health in this older adult patient. According to societal theory, it is also essential to recognize the contribution of agency to health. *Agency* refers to an individual's "capacity to influence her or his own life and exert control over their actions and outcomes."[12] Agency is linked to physical, cognitive, and mental health. Adults who hold positive views of aging recover from disability at higher rates and are more likely to engage in behaviors that promote successful aging.[7] How an individual adapts to age-related change is important. The life course approach is just one of several social theories focused on aging. Common elements include social engagement later in life and adaptation to age-related changes.

PSYCHOLOGICAL THEORIES OF AGING

Psychological theories of aging refer to both psychological changes as a result of aging and adaptive psychological mechanisms (or lack thereof) to counteract the losses associated with functional decline that results from aging.[13] Psychological theories include staged human development theories that support the individual's lifelong ability to learn and adapt to new challenges. Essential to these theories are the cognitive, emotional, and behavioral skills that support development, and in turn aging, over time. Cognitive plasticity, intelligence, emotional self-regulation, and behavioral regulation are vital skills that allow the older adult to cope and learn to adopt new health behaviors, roles, and routines to support healthy aging.

One of the most positive views of aging is to see people who have lived a long time as a source of wisdom and experience. Recent interest in obtaining oral histories from elders who have witnessed great and mundane historical events is evidence of this insight. The experience of older adults is of value to younger generations and fits well with Erikson's theory of development, introduced in earlier chapters.

REFLECTIONS

Historic events in our society and culture greatly influence our lives. You often hear older adults reminisce about these events. For example, they may say, "I remember exactly where I was the day JFK was shot" or "it was a historic day when man landed on the moon."
Name a historic event that influenced you and/or your family.
- How did it affect you and how you participated in your life roles?
- How did your family talk about this event?
- How has its meaning for your life and society changed over time, if at all?
- When you recount this event to the next generation, what will you say?

NEEDS: RESPECT AND INTEGRITY

Several basic psychological and social processes are evident in the widely divergent lifestyles of today's older adult. Erikson proposes that the success with which an older person can make psychological and social adjustments will depend on his or her ability to meet the most basic psychosocial developmental challenge of old age—that of integrity. In this last stage of human development, the person "understands, accepts, and loves the life he [or she] has led."[14] The person "possesses wisdom" and is willing to share this wisdom with the younger generation.[14] The little girl and older man in Fig. 14.1 perfectly illustrate this sharing of expertise across generations.

Health professionals are delighted, and sometimes awed, by an older person who expresses the breadth and depth of acceptance described by Erikson. These older adults readily accept the psychological and social adjustments that confront them. However, some older persons despair of being old, the psychological and social adjustments of old age overwhelm them, and they find little from their past to support them in their present situation. Key psychological and social processes assist or deter older persons from achieving a sense of wholeness and integrity in old age.

Studies of aging have given rise to the notion and understanding of healthy aging as a lifelong process of optimizing opportunities to preserve and improve health and physical, social, and mental wellness; maintain independence; enjoy a high quality of life; and experience enhancing successful life-course transitions.[15] This includes optimizing physical, cognitive, and mental health and facilitating social engagement.[4] The definition of healthy aging provides avenues to overcome natural losses that occur with age. It is a model of health promotion, injury prevention, and effective disease self-management. Community health programming such as exercise programs, fall prevention, and

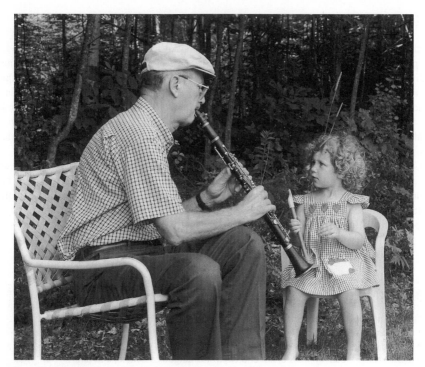

Fig. 14.1   Shared expertise across generations. (© *1995 Joan Beard, from Family: a Celebration, edited by Margaret Campbell, Peterson's.*)

yoga for the older adult all support the healthy aging model. Regardless of what clinical research or health care may define as "successful aging," many older adults have simply defined it as having the physical, mental, and financial means to go and do something worthwhile.[16]

REFLECTIONS

- What theory best describes the attitudes of older adult patients you have treated or observed regarding relationships, gains or losses, health, etc.?
- How might your idea of healthy aging differ from that of such a patient and what might be a barrier to expressing genuine respect to this person?
- Can you think of some problems that could occur clinically if you and a colleague differed in your definitions of "a good old age"?

Friendship and Family Ties

The amount of contact older people maintain with their families and friends varies greatly. Many persons lose a valuable source of natural physical contact and companionship with the diminution of friendship and family ties, whereas others remain actively integrated into family and community circles. When you are treating older patients and take time to assess how many needs for social contact are still being met by friends and family, you will understand a lot about their conduct during their time with you. It is not unusual for people to transfer their needs to health professionals once they have lost other relationships.

Friendships. Until the present ultra-mobile way of life in the United States, the acquisition of a single set of friends continued throughout early life and tapered off when one settled down in a community. One's job seldom changed during the entire period of employment, and as a result the community (and the friends therein) remained the same up through old age. In one sense, this is a secure mode of existence, but reliance on lifelong friendship carries with it the risk that, if these friends all die, the person will be left alone. Many people who have depended on lifelong friendships find it difficult to make new acquaintances at 70 or 80 years of age. An older person whose friendships centered on his or her occupational relationships may find that after retirement the friend is very much alive, but their friendship is dead. Conversely, a distant friendship may thrive after retirement because energy directed elsewhere can now be devoted to the friend. In this sense, the basis of a friendship is an important determinant of its longevity. For older adults, events such as illness, new living arrangements, and mobility problems may make maintaining friendships difficult.[17]

Even though the number of close friends decreases with age, older adults who are active in their communities report more friends than those who are unable to be socially involved or opt not to be.[18] Friendships have been demonstrated to influence a person's psychological well-being and health outcomes.[19] In working with patients, you can understand some important things by exploring who the person's friends are and how friendships are generated and sustained. It is also helpful to keep in mind that low income, poor health, lack of transportation, and infrequent information access are linked to social isolation in the aging adult population.[20] Supporting older adults in social engagement improves health and quality of life.

Family. As we discussed in Chapter 8, the family structure is changing. Participation in families is one of the most lasting and significant roles a person assumes.

In married relationships or other long-term couple relationships, couples usually have an opportunity to spend time alone together. When children become a part of the relationship, attention is transferred to them, and, in many families, much of the communication for years to come takes place in the presence of at least one child. Frequently in these older adults, only after the children have left home or the working years end is the couple alone again. Some couples find this to be an opportunity to engage in activities together that they put off in their younger years.

In the present oldest old population (those 85 years and older) there are many married or formerly married people. Older men are more likely to be married than older women. You may work with elderly women who are not prepared to cope with financial and other home management business affairs because in their youth it was considered improper for women to be thus involved. You may work with elderly men who have never had to prepare a meal or wash clothes because it was considered improper for a man to do "woman's work." Generally, there is a balance of tasks that most married couples and longtime intimate partners develop. In the examples given earlier, the husband did the bills and the wife cooked. When a spouse can no longer perform an essential role because of illness or injury, the partner may become overwhelmed by the need to complete additional tasks. The death of a spouse or partner can be extremely difficult not only emotionally but also because of the disruption to the surviving older adult's patterns, roles, and routines. Some turn to children, nieces, or nephews for help. Older adults often turn to siblings when they find themselves alone. A sibling has the added benefit of a shared history, as is evident in the following poem:

Homecoming

I

after 45 years
of writing letters
& calling, Estelle sent word
to find a contractor—
she wants a home

built next to her sister
the house, brick & modern
is an oddity—
sits prominently among shotgun houses,
cows, chickens, fish ponds, bait shops
& trailer homes
Celeste walks the clay red road
to her Oakland-California-sister—
they have forty-five years to catch up on

II
Estelle & Celeste talk of the other two sisters
who died in their early 70s—
bring out boxes of black & white worn photos
Estelle rakes arthritic fingers
through Celeste's hair
conjuring memory
she parts the white/yellow-stained strands—
braids her sister's hair.

ANDREA M. WREN[21]

A discussion of aging and family relationships must include an assessment of who is most likely to provide support for older people in times of illness. Social support systems for people who are partially or totally dependent include both family caregivers and informal ones (friends, neighbors, or members of a religious or other type of community). As we discussed in Chapter 8, families provide the majority of care for older relatives. Many families struggle to provide this care, as is evident in the following example.

> *Dad may be desperately ill, demanding constant attention and unable to join the family and guests at dinner. Mom may be afflicted with Alzheimer's and can't follow a conversation. Grandma may be bedfast. And in as many cases as not, the woman of the house does the caretaking even though she is poor, busy with a job to stay above subsistence level, preoccupied with her own children, and untrained. In such circumstances—God forbid—there is no extra room for the ill or aged, and little patience or reason for hope. Caring in the home is still the great overlooked medical-social problem among all classes in the United States.[22]*

High levels of caregiver stress can sometimes lead to elder abuse. *Elder abuse* is defined as "physical, sexual or psychological abuse, as well as neglect, abandonment and financial exploitation of an older person by another person or entity."[23] It can occur in any setting an older person engages in and can be engaged in a relationship in which the older adult is trusting of another person or identity. Alternatively, the older adult can be targeted based on his or her age or disability. Elder abuse can take several forms[24,25]:

1. *Rights violations:* Denial of basic rights to adequate medical care, nourishment, or adequate housing
2. *Material abuse/exploitation:* Monetary or material theft, fraud, or undue influence to gain control over an older person's money or property
3. *Physical abuse:* Covers a variety of practices from omission (e.g., leaving a nonambulatory person in bed for long periods) to commission (e.g., beating or injuring the person)
4. *Psychological/emotional abuse:* The person is debased and intimidated verbally, threatened, isolated, or belittled

5. *Sexual abuse:* Sexual contact is forced, tricked, threatened, or otherwise coerced upon a vulnerable elder (including one who is unable to grant consent)

6. *Neglect/abandonment:* Failure or refusal to provide adequately for a vulnerable elder's safety, physical needs, or emotional needs; the desertion of a vulnerable elder by anyone with a duty of care

Elder abuse often is not reported or is underreported because the older person (or others) fear retaliation or believe that nothing will be done to change the situation. Just as with a child whom you suspect is being abused or neglected, you are legally responsible in all 50 states to report suspected elder abuse. Unfortunately, elder abuse is not isolated to the home setting. It occurs in institutional settings as well, such as group homes, nursing homes, adult day care, or even hospitals.

WHERE "HOME" IS

A major challenge for older people is to decide where to make their homes. Aging brings an increased risk for disability, isolation, and financial stress that affect housing decisions.[26] Key components of independent living for older adults include physical health, cognitive health, functional ability, and social ability (including driving and access to the larger community).[27] Security, accessibility to services, transportation, and physical considerations are key variables in elder housing decisions. Reduced income and the desire to be near friends or relatives also often weigh heavily for people who have a choice of location. The preference of many older adults is to age in place. Aging in place is defined by the Centers for Disease Control and Prevention as "the ability to live in one's own home and community safely, independently, and comfortably, regardless of age, income, or ability level."[28] Through the support of formal and informal caregivers, environmental adaptations, and supportive technology, many older adults can achieve this goal, with recent data suggesting that more than three-quarters of individuals over age 80 live in their own homes.[4,29]

Senior apartment communities, intentional retirement communities, and other age-friendly communities are housing alternatives for persons who do not remain in their own homes (or move in with or near relatives) but that allow them to age in place.[30,31] With the dramatic rise in the number of baby boomers who are reaching old age, a burgeoning new industry of "continuing care centers" is expanding. They may be for-profit or not-for-profit sponsored and provide the opportunity for older people to move into an independent living apartment or townhome, graduate to partial assistance, and eventually have full medical and other supports of nursing home arrangements.

For older persons with functional disabilities or those who need more assistance with daily living activities than can be provided at home by family or professional caregivers, an assisted living or nursing home may become their last place of residence. The most common reason for admission to a nursing home is inability to perform activities of daily living. The primary medical conditions associated with nursing home admission are dementia and stroke.[32] About 90% of nursing home residents are older than 65, in fact almost half are 85 years or older, but only 3.1% of the total 65+ population (approximately 1.3 million people) live in a skilled nursing facility.[3] Of this population, most (72%) are women.[33] Not all admissions to skilled nursing facilities are for the rest of a patient's life. Some older adults are admitted only for short-term rehabilitation so that they can regain strength and function to return to independent or partial assisted living.

REFLECTIONS

Imagine you are seriously injured and told that you must live in a nursing home for a minimum of 1 year.
- What would you miss most about your current living situation? Why?
- What about the move would be hardest for you to cope with?
- What supports would make such a move easier for you?

You will benefit from bearing in mind that these challenges may have already occurred for the older person simply because he or she is old rather than because of illness or injury. In many Western societies, the loss of a long-established place of residence, of consequence to anyone, is felt deeply by the older person because self-respect and the power to command the respect of others depend in part on remaining independent. Although many patients experience the loss of independence as temporary, older people usually realize that each loss can be a one-way street to more dependence. Moving out of one's home permanently symbolizes dependence with a capital D.

Each move of residence may have greater significance for older adults than for those of any other age group. For example, a woman who has been forced to move into her daughter's home and who then requires admission to the hospital for elective surgery that results in placement in a nursing home for rehabilitation certainly has grounds for feeling completely "undone" by the number of moves she has had to make in a short period. Thoughtful health professionals take these factors into consideration and are patient in helping the older person adapt accordingly. In fact, a key to respectful interaction with an older person is to promote as much stability in the place of residence as possible.

Challenges of Changes With Aging

Aging brings with it both opportunities and challenges. In the following section, some of the major challenges that present to many older adults are discussed.

CHALLENGE TO FORMER SELF-IMAGE

The discussion so far in this chapter offers ample evidence that humans have the potential to continue to develop throughout the life span, and self-esteem can remain high or even grow stronger in the older years. Some recognize talents they never knew they had or refocus their energies on other hobbies or projects. Consider the following poem and the various transformations of the older adult.

The Layers
I have walked through many lives,
some of them my own,
and I am not who I was,
though some principle of being
abides, from which I struggle
not to stray.
When I look behind,
as I am compelled to look
before I can gather strength
to proceed on my journey,
I see the milestones dwindling
toward the horizon
and the slow fires trailing
from the abandoned camp-sites,
over which scavenger angels
wheel on heavy wings.
Oh, I have made myself a tribe
out of my true affections,
and my tribe is scattered!
How shall the heart be reconciled
to its feast of losses?

In a rising wind
the manic dust of my friends,
those who fell along the way,
bitterly stings my face.
Yet I turn, I turn,
exulting somewhat,
with my will intact to go
wherever I need to go,
and every stone on the road
precious to me.
In my darkest night,
when the moon was covered
and I roamed through wreckage,
a nimbus-clouded voice
directed me:
"Live in the layers,
not on the litter."
Though I lack the art
to decipher it,
no doubt the next chapter
in my book of transformations
is already written.
I am not done with my changes.

STANLEY KUNITZ[34]

REFLECTIONS

- What is this poet saying about adulthood?
- What is the significance of the poem's title—"The Layers"?
- What transitions are highlighted in the verses?
- How would you characterize the poet's view of aging?

Some persons do not even notice changes in how they look, seeing only what they want to see in the mirror (Fig. 14.2). Unfortunately, other people cling to a former visual image and begin to reject the changes brought about by aging. They see themselves as has-beens who are no longer valuable to society and angry or depressed that they cannot perform as they did in the past.

Retirement from a long-held job or career focus often poses a threat to self-image (and, subsequently, to self-esteem) in many older men and women. With almost all adults employed in the workforce at some time in their lives, more people than ever before will face the challenge of retirement. However, many predict that the baby-boomer cohort, which is steadily moving into older adulthood, may not retire at the traditional age of 65 because of concerns about funding shortfalls in Social Security and Medicare, possible cuts in government programs for older people, and cuts in traditional benefit pension plans that previously provided a fixed income in old age. For most, retirement not only involves a substantial reduction in income but also signals a change in daily activity.

As the person looks forward in time to retirement, a central issue becomes replacing time spent in work with other productive activities. Although work is only one part of the person's whole landscape of activities, for many it is a large part. The disappearance of work potentially leaves much of the older adult's landscape unfilled. At a minimum, retirement precipitates change in the person's regular activity pattern.[35] Four basic tasks seem to comprise essential post-job satisfaction: social activity, play, creativity, and lifelong learning.[36]

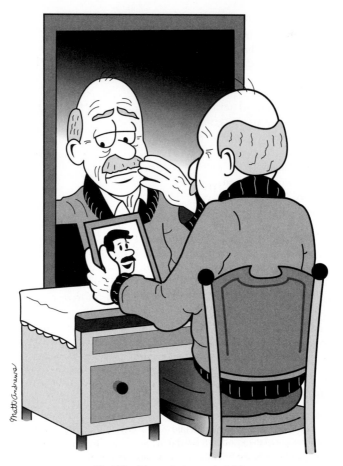

Fig. 14.2   "I haven't changed a bit."

To maintain their self-imposed status as useful members of society, almost all older adults need to be engaged in ongoing activity. This may be a job, a hobby, a volunteer service, or a club. In fact, most volunteer hours are contributed by Americans beginning in midlife and continuing into old age in many areas that US social policy fails to address adequately, such as the provision of basic human services.[37] Regardless of the activity chosen, they do need to have something to look forward to and to know they are needed in a certain place at a certain time. Research suggests that involvement in volunteer activities may significantly improve the health and well-being of older people themselves through lower rates of depression, increased life satisfaction, retention of functional abilities, improved physical activity, and cognitive activity.[38-40] However, not all older people are able to be involved in such activities, and there are some good reasons why:

- They may be shy about meeting new people, particularly if they have maintained one set of friends and acquaintances for many years.
- They may possess too many physical, cognitive, or mental health impairments to participate in ongoing activities.

- They may have no way to get to them.
- They may not be able to afford to go.
- They may be afraid to go out alone or at night.

One or more of these reasons also may prevent them from seeking ongoing health care.

Fortunately, the narrative of the aging adult is changing, and older adults are achieving major milestones later and later in life. As the average age of our society grows, older people will become involved in continuous activities. For example, politics is one area in which the population older than 65 has gained a powerful voice. Political involvement facilitates progress in legislation regarding personal interests and provides a broader perspective for legislation regarding society.

PHYSICAL CHANGES OF AGING

A higher percentage of older adults are remaining in good health longer than ever before; however, as addressed earlier in this chapter, all adults experience physical changes over the life span. Their three most common functional limitations are brought about by reduced strength and endurance, joint problems, and increased risk for falls and greater incidence of household accidents. These functional problems are often associated with both physiologic and cognitive changes. Examples of physiologic age-related changes include bone loss, cartilage thinning, decreased cardiac reserve capacity, loss of muscle mass, sensory changes, and changes in touch, temperature, and pain perception.

Examples of cognitive changes include neuroanatomic changes in the brain that lead to decreased memory, attention, and a general decline in fluid intelligence (the ability to process novel information). With aging, the pattern of intelligence changes. The older adult demonstrates improvements in his or her crystallized intelligence (the ability to apply knowledge gained over time), and thus balance the loss in fluid intelligence, which aids the elder in deciding how to respond to certain situations.[13] Visual changes include declines in acuity, speed of focusing, and accommodation in vision. With aging, adaptation to darkness usually declines, too. Hearing losses are greatest in the high-frequency range. There is a steady loss in perception of body movement, or kinesthesia. The older person may "adjust" to the losses gracefully. An example is an exchange that one of the authors had with her 92-year-old neighbor. As she walked into his living room, where the television announcer was blaring the Boston Red Sox's latest home run, she was surprised to see Tom planted in front of a blank screen. "Tom!" she shouted above the clamor, "There's no picture!"

"Picture went about a month ago!" he shouted back. "Can't see the screen anyway!" Tom, despite his good humor, would probably concede that the savings on the television repair was not worth the price of his failing eyesight. For people with serious sensory impairment, the start of each day must seem like, as Shakespeare put it, the "Last scene of all / That ends this strange eventful history . . . / Sans teeth, sans eyes, sans taste, sans everything" (*As You Like It,* II, vii, 139). Your sensitivity to a patient's feelings about these losses can have profound effects on the extent to which the patient feels respected by you. Understandably, your attention to and authentic care regarding a patient's sensitivity about such matters are critical components of showing respect.

We will not discuss musculoskeletal or neurological changes in the aging process in further detail because many health professionals learn this elsewhere. Posture, balance, strength, endurance, and other physical expressions of aging will vary, but overall wear and tear on the body will affect all adults in their later years. Your role as a health professional is to recognize normal aging and be able to contrast it with signs of pathology. An older adult or family member may mistake a clinical condition for normal aging and think "oh, I am just getting older," when there may be a treatable condition that can be managed clinically to help the patient avoid disease and disability. For example, depression is often underidentified in the older adult. It is commonly mistaken for apathy related to age.

Multiple studies demonstrate that exercise has a positive impact on human beings of almost any age. Regular activity can reverse the decreased mobility that contributes to disease and disability in old age.[41] Furthermore, exercise has been shown to promote modest positive changes in cognitive functioning in this phase of the life span.[42] Given demonstrated improvements in so many areas, a prescription for activity seems indicated for most elderly patients. *Self-efficacy* (conviction to organize and implement effective strategies to deal with potential stressors) is also a positive predictor for aging well. Self-efficacy when linked with activity helps maintain cognitive function and social engagement.[43,44]

One way of dealing with all the physical changes that are a normal part of aging, as well as those that accompany chronic and acute illness and injury, is to share experiences with others who understand what the person is going through.

Your sensitivity to changes, offering the person opportunities to talk about illness and loss and especially what changes mean for his or her feeling of well-being, is an avenue to respectful interaction, too.

MENTAL CHANGES OF AGING

A few minor differences in mental capacity and functioning among all who are older are noteworthy. If attended to, they can enhance the health professional's success in working with older people.

All patients benefit from the security of a set schedule, and this may be especially true for many older persons. The security arises from the knowledge that, at least in this one small area, he or she is in control of the environment. Some older people continue to exercise complete control over the details of their existence, whereas others gradually lose this opportunity. Even if this control extends no further than the patient telling the taxi or ride share service driver to hurry because they are scheduled to be in speech therapy in 15 minutes, that person's self-respect will have been bolstered by exercising this type of agency.

Being able to count on an established schedule is also a way for an older adult to maintain a proper orientation to the environment. Some hospitalized elders become confused about the time of day and the date because they have few clues to orient them compared with the person who works 5 days a week or a peer who has more ongoing routine activity.

An older person's sense of security, control, and orientation can be further enhanced if, in addition to being treated at the same time each day, the routine of a treatment or test is kept reasonably stable from one day to the next. If the treatment or testing situation varies significantly every day, the patient may feel that nothing about it is familiar; it may be an anxiety-producing experience every time the person reports to the health professional. Anxiety can greatly decrease the person's performance and have a detrimental effect on both the relationship with you and the patient's progress.

The ideal situation is to create a balance between the patient's need for stability and his or her continuing interest in life and need for stimulation.

Caring for Older Adults With Cognitive Impairments

Cognitive impairment in the aged person can take many forms, and it is important that you study them in more depth than is appropriate to address in this book. However, impairment in one particular aspect of an elderly person's life, instrumental activities of daily living (IADLs), has been shown to be correlated with the presence of dementia and may be one of the early signs of cognitive changes.[45,46] If there is impairment in one of the following four IADLs, a thorough mental status evaluation should be performed: (1) medication/health management, (2) money/financial management, (3) telephone management/communication device use, and (4) transportation management. We engage you in a general discussion about cognitive impairment and provide some general guidelines for respectful interaction with people with neuropathology that directly affects thought and speech processes.

Acute confusion or disorientation can be caused by a variety of factors, such as an infection, a fluid or electrolyte imbalance, or a cerebral vascular accident. It is important to determine the cause of confusion in an elderly patient and not just ascribe it to "being old." The following case illustrates how critical it is to understand the genesis of a change in mental status in an older patient.

Case Study

Family members brought an 81-year-old man, Abraham Steinman, who was in an acutely agitated and confused state, to the emergency department. The family stated that Mr. Steinman had gradually become more confused over the past few weeks and became violently disturbed earlier in the evening. He was admitted to the adult psychiatric unit because he was physically violent to the staff in the emergency department. The distraught family said he had never had an emotional outburst in his life and could not understand his behavior. The next day a careful physical examination revealed that Mr. Steinman had bilateral pneumonia and some signs of kidney failure. His confusion and agitation had only been symptoms of his physical illness.

REFLECTIONS

- What action might have prevented the admission to psychiatry?
- Would the assessment and treatment have been the same if Mr. Steinman were 40 years old? If he were 20 years old?
- How would you feel if this was your father?
- What can the interprofessional care team treating Mr. Steinman learn from his case to improve the care of future patients?

For such patients, acute confusion can be continual and may be increasingly profound, although you can help diminish the patient's suffering from disorientation at any given moment. Often, a useful approach is to not support the older person's constantly confused ideas, unless correcting them causes him or her to become violent, further disoriented, or deeply agitated. If an old man thinks he is in a hotel, you should try to correct him using a gentle reassuring voice and manner.

If he confuses you with someone else, his mistake can be corrected by showing him your name badge and repeating your name. Chances are that he will be less frightened if the people around him are willing to help him clear up his mind, if only for a few minutes. It is a good general rule of respectful interaction to correct the person. However, you should also remember to listen with interest and politeness to the patient. Listening will help you determine the depth of the confusion, ascertain the wisdom of trying to correct it, and, in some cases, discern that the patient is making sense within a context not immediately evident.

Respect requires that the confused person should always be treated kindly. Spoken correction or redirection should never be condescending but rather should reflect the gentle authority that gives the patient a sense of security.

If the confusion is the result of a disease such as Alzheimer's disease or another form of dementia, many of the same principles apply. Some additional strategies for communicating with patients with dementia are as follows: use broad opening statements or questions, try to establish commonalities, speak to them as equals, speak at a normal rate and without exaggerated intonation, eliminate distractions, repeat when necessary and according to whether the listener misunderstood versus forgot what was said, and try to recognize themes in what the patient is trying to share with you.[47]

Sometimes medication can help an agitated patient relax or in other ways be more comfortable, although with elderly patients it is best to be cautious with the use of medications. Goals must be adapted according to what patients can comprehend. Some patients may be unable to remember the simplest tasks from one testing or treatment period to the next and may never grasp the most elementary verbal instructions. Others, however, will be able to follow astonishingly complex procedures. It is your responsibility and opportunity in such situations to approach each person as an individual and to not take for granted that all confused utterances are signs of organic brain changes. In some cases, the confusion will increase no matter what is done. However, none of these complications should deter you from first attempting, in a kind way, to correct inaccuracies. With a great number of patients, this humane act is the key to respectful interaction.

Assessing a Patient's Value System

The mechanics of adjusting a hearing aid, setting a schedule, or correcting a confused-sounding statement must all be done in a way that supports the older person's value system. Otherwise, the person is reduced to nothing more than an object to be efficiently manipulated. Chapter 1 listed some of the primary societal, cultural, and personal values cherished by people in this society. Older people as a group can be expected to hold the same range and variety of values; no value can be ruled out automatically based on age. However, the topics treated in this chapter can help you understand why so many older adults adhere to some values more than others.

For instance, the primary good of self-respect will often be a more consciously prized value for older people because they perceive, correctly, that they are subject to loss of self-respect in an ageist society. Security, both financial and physical, also may be highly prized by older adults because, again, for many of them the hold on it is more tenuous. Further, continued independent functioning is valued dearly when transition to a nursing home is a threat or when activities that can be performed alone become increasingly limited. Listening for which values the older patient expresses as his or her most precious and then trying to set treatment goals accordingly will greatly enhance your success. This will also help you understand the patient's (and family member's) experience and expectations and build partnerships for shared decision-making. In working with older people, the most important challenge confronting you is resisting the tendency to stereotype them. Society's expectations of its elders, many of which are inaccurate and outdated, are propagated through literature, television, and other popular media.

REFLECTIONS

Some states have instituted mandatory age-based testing for older drivers. This testing varies from state to state but ranges from vision examinations to on-road assessments.

Your patient is seeing you today for his well visit and states, "I am 75 in a few weeks, so I will have to pass the registry test to keep my license. It's not fair. Not only is that policy ridiculous, it is completely ageist! No one asks those tweeting, cell-phone wielding 20-year-olds to retake their test."
- What do you say?
- How do you feel about the issue of age-related mandates?

In thinking about this topic, consider the link between driving and independence in American society.
- How do limitations in this instrumental activity of daily living support or restrict participation for the older adult?

You can learn to appreciate individual differences among aged persons by increasing your contact with people who are older. Programs sponsored by churches, private organizations, and the government offer volunteer opportunities ranging from transportation to recreational activities to providing hot meals for homebound persons. In some cities, senior activity centers, assisted living facilities, and other institutions where older persons live or spend considerable time welcome young people who are interested in volunteering their services or visiting older people. Whether through volunteer services, organizations, or contact as a health professional, your challenge is to develop an acutely discriminating eye for individual differences.

Summary

Care of older adults must be based on a sound understanding of the physiologic and psychosocial aspects of aging. The major developmental tasks of older adulthood are to find integrated meaning and satisfaction with life as it becomes increasingly difficult to keep up with everything that goes on in a quickly changing world. The chief goal of professional care is to maintain and support the patient's self-esteem by affirming his or her strengths and discovering hidden resources. By keeping in mind older patients' emotional and social needs, you can help them retain dignity and self-respect while being mindful not to overlook physical causes for changes in behaviors or attitudes. Overall, the secret to respectful interaction with older adults is to keep their age-related challenges, characteristics, and changes in mind while also supporting and encouraging their abilities, wisdom, and individuality.

See Section 5 Questions for Thought and Discussion on page 265 to apply what you've learned in this section to a variety of case scenarios.

References

1. John Adams as quoted in Wallis CL, ed. *The Treasure Chest: A Heritage Album Containing 1064 Familiar and Inspirational Quotations, Poems, Sentiments, and Prayers From Great Minds of 2500 Years.* New York: Harper and Row Publishers; 1965:12.
2. Schondelmyer E. *Demographics and Living Arrangements: 2013, Household Economic Studies, Current Population Reports.* Washington, DC: U.S. Census Bureau; 2017:1–3.
3. U.S. Census Bureau. *Table 3. Projections of the Population by Sex and Selected Age Groups for the United States: 2015 to 2016 [Data file]*; 2014. Retrieved from https://www.census.gov/data/tables/2014/demo/popproj/2014-summary-tables.html.
4. National Prevention Council. *Healthy Aging in Action.* Washington, DC: U.S. Department of Health and Human Services, Office of the Surgeon General; 2016.
5. Colby SL, Ortman JM. *The Baby Boom Cohort in the United States: 2012 to 2060 Population Estimates and Projections, Current Population Reports*; 2014. Available at https://www.census.gov/prod/2014pubs/p25-1141.pdf.
6. Pinto da Costaa J, Vitorinob R, Silvad GM, et al. A synopsis on aging—theories, mechanisms and future prospects. *Ageing Res Rev.* 2016;29:90–112.
7. Brothers A, Diehl M. Feasibility and efficacy of the aging plus program: changing views on aging to increase physical activity. *J Aging Phys Act [serial online].* 2017;25(3):402–411. Available from MEDLINE Complete, Ipswich, MA.
8. Setterson RA, Hagestad GO. Subjective aging and new complexities of the lifecourse. In: Diehl M, Wahl, HW, eds. Subjective aging: new developments and future directions. Annual Review of Gerontology and Geriatrics, vol. 35. New York: Springer Publishing Company; 2015:29–54.
9. Lipsky M, King M. Biological theories of aging. *Dis Mon.* 2015;61(Issues on Aging):460–466.
10. Wircenski M, Walker M, Allen J, et al. Age as a diversity issue in grades K-12 and in higher education. *Educ Gerontol.* 1999;25:491–500.
11. Rosowsky E. Ageism and professional training in aging: who will be there to help? *Generations.* 2005;29(3):55–58.
12. Hasworth S, Cannon M. Social theories of aging: a review. *Dis Mon [serial online].* 2015;61 (Issues on Aging):475–479.

13. Wernher I, Lipsky M. Psychological theories of aging. *Dis Mon [serial online]*. 2015;61(Issues on Aging):480–488.
14. Erikson EH. *Childhood and Society*. 2nd ed. New York: WW Norton; 1963.
15. Health Canada. Workshop on healthy aging. (website). http://publications.gc.ca/collections/Collection /H39-612-2002-1E.pdf.
16. Bryant LL, Corbett KK, Kutner JS. In their own words: a model of healthy aging. *Soc Sci Med*. 2001;53:927–941.
17. Brossie N, Chop W. Social gerontology. In: Robnett RH, Chop WC, eds. *Gerontology for the health care professional*. 3rd ed. Burlington, MA: Jones & Bartlett Learning; 2015:17–50.
18. Blieszner R, Ogletree AM. We get by with a little help from our friends. *J Am Soc Aging*. 2017;41(2):55–62.
19. Chen Y, Feeley TH. Social support, social strain, loneliness, and well-being among older adults: an analysis of the health and retirement study. *J Soc Pers Relatsh*. 2014;31(2):141–161.
20. Hand C, Retrum J, Ware G, et al. Understanding social isolation among urban aging adults: informing occupation-based approaches. *Occupational Ther J Res*. 2017;37(4):188–198.
21. Wren AM. Homecoming. *Afr Am Rev*. 1993;27(1):157.
22. Marty ME. The "God-forbid" wing. *Park Ridge Center Bull*. 1999;11:15.
23. National Center on Elder Abuse, 2014. *National Center on Elder Abuse: An Introduction to Elder Abuse for Professionals*; 2014. Retrieved from https://ncea.acl.gov/resources/docs/Intro-EA-Pro-Overview-2014.pdf.
24. Benton D, Marshall C. Elder abuse. *Clin Geriatr Med*. 1991;7(4):831–845.
25. National Center on Elder Abuse: Why should I care about elder abuse? Fact Sheet. Available at: https://ncea.acl.gov/faq/index.html.
26. Housing America's Older Adults: Meeting the Needs of An Aging Population. Joint Center for Housing Studies of Harvard University, 2014, President and Fellows of Harvard College. Available at: https://www.nado.org/wp-content/uploads/2014/09/Harvard-Housing-Americas-Older-Adults-2014.pdf.
27. Baker MW. Creation of a model of independence for community-dwelling elders in the United States. *Nursing Res*. 2005;54(5):288–295.
28. Centers for Disease Control and Prevention: Healthy Places Terminology. Available at https://www.cdc.gov/healthyplaces/terminology.htm.
29. Lien L, Steggell C, Iwarsson S. Adaptive strategies and person-environment fit among functionally limited older adults aging in place: a mixed methods approach. *Int J Environ Res Public Health [serial online]*. 2015;12(9):11954–11974.
30. Peek S, Luijkx K, Wouters E, et al. Older adults' reasons for using technology while aging in place. *Gerontology [serial online]*. 2016;62(2):226–237.
31. Jeste D, Blazer I, Feather J, et al. Age-friendly communities initiative: public health approach to promoting successful aging. *Am J Geriatr Psychiatry [serial online]*. 2016;24:1158–1170.
32. Van Rensbergen G, Nawrot T. Medical conditions of nursing home admissions. *BMC Geriatr*. 2010;10:46.
33. Healthy in Aging. Aging & Health A to Z. *Nursing Homes, Basic Facts & Information*. 2017. Available at http://www.healthinaging.org/aging-and-health-a-to-z/topic:nursing-homes/.
34. Kunitz S. *The Collected Poems*. New York: WW Norton Company; 2001.
35. Jonsson H, Kielhofner G, Borell L. Anticipating retirement: the formation of narrative concerning an occupational transition. *Am J Occup Ther*. 1997;51(1):49–56.
36. Vaillant GE. *Aging Well: Surprising Guideposts to a Happier Life From the Landmark Harvard Study of Adult Development*. Boston: Little, Brown; 2002.
37. U.S. Department of Labor, Bureau of Statistics: Table 1. Volunteers by selected characteristics, 2015. Available at https://www.bls.gov/news.release/volun.t01.htm.
38. Moen P. Reconstructing retirement: careers, couples, and social capital. *Contemp Gerontol J Rev Crit Discuss*. 1998;4(4):123–125.
39. Fried LP, Carlson MC, Freedman M, et al. A social model for health promotion for an aging population: initial evidence on the experience corps model. *J Urban Health*. 2004;81(1):64–78.
40. Yuen HK, Huang P, Burik JK, et al. Impact of participating in volunteer activities for residents living in long-term-care facilities. *Am J Occup Ther*. 2008;62:71–76.
41. Gill TH, Guralnik JM, Pahor M, et al. Effect of structured physical activity on overall burden and transitions between states of major mobility disability in older persons. *Ann Internal Med*. 2016;165:833–840.

42. Chu D, Fox KR, Chen L, et al. Components of late-life exercise and cognitive function: an 8-year longitudinal study. *Prevent Sci.* 2015;16(4):568–577.
43. Robnett RH, Chop WC. *Gerontology for the Health Care Professional.* 2nd ed. Burlington, MA: Jones & Barlett Learning; 2009.
44. Schepens S, Sen A, Painter JA, et al. Relationship between fall-related efficacy and activity engagement in community-dwelling older adults: a meta-analytic review. *Am J Occup Ther.* 2012;66:137–148.
45. Cornelis E, Gorus E, Beyer I, et al. Early diagnosis of mild cognitive impairment and mild dementia through basic and instrumental activities of daily living: development of a new evaluation tool. *PLOS Med.* 2017;14(3):1–22.
46. Marshall GA, Rentz DM, Frey MT, et al. Executive function and instrumental activities of daily living in MCI and AD. *Alzheimer's & Dementia: J Alzheimer's Assoc.* 2011;7(3):300–308.
47. Small J, Perry JA. Training family care partners to communicate effectively with persons with Alzheimer's disease: The TRACED program. *Can J Speech-Language Pathol Audiol.* 2012;36(4):332–350.

Some Special Challenges: Creating a Context of Respect

In this section of the book we explore two types of special challenges we think warrant your attention. Chapter 15 addresses relevant considerations you will want to bear in mind while working with patients who are dying and with their loved ones. Patients and their families almost always show evidence of the disruption life-limiting illness has on their present lives and future dreams. The news also may bring challenges, unleash new hopes, and expose unexercised strengths during this time. You have an opportunity to examine these issues and how they affect patients and their families. You will learn about priorities that you as a health professional can set for such patients and their families to show them respect.

In Chapter 16, we examine some situations that health professionals sometimes identify as difficult. In this chapter, our goal is for you to think expansively about your potential for respectful interaction when you encounter complex patients and situations. Example situations include caring for patients with a history of violent behavior and supporting members of the interprofessional care team who make errors in care delivery. Regardless of the situation, effective communication is essential to health care delivery; therefore we summarize 10 evidence-based guidelines that will help you show respect in difficult conversations. Our hope is that these will serve as guideposts throughout your career, providing an opportunity to both optimize patient care outcomes and cope with the emotions that result from difficult conversations.

CHAPTER 15

Respectful Interaction

When the Patient Is Dying

The reader will be able to:

- Recognize the process of dying and death as both a normative and nonnormative part of the life trajectory
- Discuss denial and its effects on respectful interaction
- List several factors that have a bearing on a patient's response upon learning he or she has a life-limiting illness
- Explain several areas of consideration in setting treatment priorities when a patient is dying, including the involvement of the palliative care team or hospice
- Discuss ways to help maintain hope when a patient's condition is irreversible and will result in death
- Identify some important changes in focus health professionals should seek when a patient is near death

Prelude

The newspaper near his chair has a photo of a Boston baseball player who is smiling after pitching a shutout. Of all the diseases, I think to myself, Morrie gets one named after an athlete.

You remember Lou Gehrig, I ask?

"I remember him in the stadium, saying good-bye."

So you remember the famous line.

"Which one?"

Come on. Lou Gehrig. "Pride of the Yankees?" The speech that echoes over the loudspeakers?

"Remind me," Morrie says. "Do the speech."

Through the open window, I hear the sound of a garbage truck. Although it is hot, Morrie is wearing long sleeves, with a blanket over his legs, his skin pale. The disease owns him.

I raise my voice and do the Gehrig imitation, where the words bounce off the stadium walls: "Too-dayyy . . . I feeel like . . . the luckiest maaaan . . . on the face of the earth . . . ."

Morrie closes his eyes and nods slowly.

"Yeah. Well. I didn't say that."

M. ALBOM[1]

This excerpt, from a book titled *Tuesdays with Morrie*, chronicles the last months of a man's dying as it is recorded through the pen of his friend and former student. Here you catch them in one of their many exchanges, the young man trying to make conversation and the dying man bringing the narrative back to the heart of the matter—his own unique experience of dying. Of all the challenges you will face, your work with people with life-limiting illness will provide some of the greatest opportunities to use your skills of communication and collaboration in health care delivery.

One of the challenges of care and treatment for those who are dying is confusing terminology. Even with the simplest of terms, such as the word "dying," there can be different understandings. Thus it is helpful to start with clarification of some commonly used terms when referring to patients with a life-limiting illness or injury. *Terminally ill* is a term that is commonly seen in the literature to describe people who are dying. Like all labels, it allows people in this group to be identified easily according to their needs. At the same time, we refrain from using it in this chapter. One difficulty with the term is its generality. Persons such as Morrie, who suffered from amyotrophic lateral sclerosis (commonly known as *Lou Gehrig's disease*), may live for many months or years. Another person with a different condition may die within days or weeks. Still, both are labeled terminally ill. One of the authors remembers a friend who lived for more than 10 years with a diagnosis of malignant lymphoma. He went into the hospital for his periodic blood test. A health professional who had come back to work after a 5-year hiatus greeted him cheerfully, "Are *you* still around?"

She was apparently astonished that this "terminally ill" patient had not died long ago! The patient recalled that although he knew her intentions were good, her greeting led to the most severe depression of his entire illness. Thus we use the term *life-limiting illness* to indicate that the patient has good reason to believe that the present illness or injury will limit his or her life, leaving the time frame open to the various trajectories of dying.

The reverse problem—that is, not recognizing the trajectory of an illness—is also true. Some diagnoses resist the label of a terminal or life-limiting illness such as Alzheimer's disease in its later stages. Many health professionals, patients, and family members view Alzheimer's disease as a chronic, degenerative illness that progresses over many years, which in fact is generally the case. However, by not recognizing the life-limiting aspects of later stages of Alzheimer's disease, patients and families are far less likely to reap the benefits of care afforded to the dying. As with all types of patients, the key is to look for the distinguishing factors that make this person's situation unique and respond respectfully to the needs that arise out of that individual person's experience. Toward achieving that goal, a first step toward any health professional's understanding of a patient's situation is to gain some general idea of how the dying process and death are viewed within the larger society.

Dying and Death in Contemporary Society

Dying is first and foremost a personal experience. All persons share some awareness that the end of the dying process is the death event. What does this mean to a person? In the minds of some patients or their families, a known diagnosis and somewhat predictable range of symptoms make them feel robbed of the "natural" flow of life. The dying process feels unnatural, an imposition.

A life-limiting condition generates new fears and concerns. Fortunately, for others it is also an opportunity to conduct long-neglected business, put one's affairs in order, or pursue a postponed adventure. Anticipation of the death event, too, creates its own concerns, fears, and hopes. For most people, death remains perhaps the ultimate mystery.

DYING AS A PROCESS

How do we gain an understanding of the relationship of the process of dying to the end point of death? In almost all cultures, stories passed down from generation to generation onward in fairy tales or, in some cultures, the mythic stories deeply inform our understanding of death. Note how in the following popular Western fairy tales death is something that happens to the bad characters, and a notable goal is to help bring it about:

Down climbed Jack as fast as he could, and down climbed the giant after him, but he couldn't catch him. Jack reached the bottom first and shouted out to his mother, who was at the cottage door. "Mother! Mother! Bring me an axe! Make haste, Mother!" For he knew there was not a moment to spare. However, he was just in time. Jack seized the hatchet and chopped through the beanstalk close to the root; the giant fell headlong into the garden and was killed on the spot.

So all ended well. . . .[2]

Then Grethel gave her a push, so that she fell right in, and then shutting the iron door she bolted it. Oh, how horribly she howled! But Grethel ran away, and left the ungodly witch to burn to ashes. Now she ran to Hansel, and opening his door, called out, "Hansel, we are saved; the old witch is dead!"[3]

Many Western childhood portrayals show no connection between the process of dying and the final death event. Both the health professional and patient may share beliefs about the "unnaturalness" of death. Of course, not all cultures have the same understanding of life and death. How might your relationship with a patient be different if, say, he or she grew up with the deep memory of this childhood story recounted by Mitch Albom, the author of *Tuesdays with Morrie* (whose conversations with his dying friend led him to read about how different cultures view death)?

There is a tribe in the North American Arctic, for example, who believe that all things on earth have a soul that exists in a miniature form of the body that holds it—so that a deer has a tiny deer inside it, and a man has a tiny man inside him. When the large being dies, that tiny form lives on. It can slide into something being born nearby, or it can go to a temporary resting place in the sky, in the belly of a great feminine spirit, where it waits until the moon can send it back to earth.

Sometimes, they say, the moon is so busy with the new soul of the world that it disappears from the sky. That is why we have moonless nights. But in the end, the moon always returns. As do we all. . . .[1]

In today's rich diversity of patients an essential step in creating a therapeutic relationship based on care is to try to gain some understanding of dying as a process to be viewed apart from death itself. This provides a starting place for further deliberation about how to respect what a patient or family says, how they behave, and what their attitudes are toward various aspects of their interaction with you and others during the dying process. In addition to paying attention to cultural and social understandings of the dying process and death, it is important to realize that there is also confusion about what it means for a patient to be dead because of different definitions of death. The following is the clinical definition of death in a patient that is most widely accepted in state statutes in the United States. A person who is dead is: "An individual who has sustained either (1) irreversible cessation of circulatory and respiratory functions or (2) irreversible cessation of all functions of the entire brain, including the brain stem, is dead. A determination of death must be made in accordance with accepted medical standards."[4]

Laypeople may not appreciate the distinction between the two definitions of death, but what is important is that those patients who have completely lost the integrating functions of their brain can be considered dead and thus possible donors for vital organs needed in transplantation.

DENIAL

It is often said that Western societies are death denying. What can that possibly mean when all around us people are dying every day from illness, accidents, violence, old age, war, and other causes? Probably the best explanation is that although there is evidence everywhere of our mortality, we do our best to hold the inevitable at arm's length.

In many parts of Western culture, treatment of the dead body is one expression of a need to deny death its power. The dead body is painted and dressed to make it appear alive, although a sign of life, such as a sigh or fluttering eyelash, would cause most people to rush screaming from the room. For the most part, however, denial has simply become subtler. For example, a subtle denial that death is the end of the dying process is manifested in the incredible scenes of violence and killing viewed in films and on television in dramas, cartoons, and the news. The highly popular novels, television shows, and films about the "undead"—that is, vampires and zombies— is another indication of the fascination mainstream American culture holds with death and its denial. Distancing that keeps death at arm's length for as long as possible even during one's dying process is another method of denying the finality of death. This attempt to stave off the inevitable is also experienced by loved ones and poignantly is conveyed in the following quote from a 51-year-old woman who learned that her best friend was dying of cancer:

Before one enters this spectrum of sorrow, which changes even the color of trees, there is a blind and daringly wrong assumption that probably allows us to blunder through the days. There is a way one thinks that the show will never end—or the loss, when it comes, will be toward the end of the road, not in its middle . . . . I meant that I might somehow sidestep the cruelty of an intolerable loss, one rendered without the willful or natural exit signs of drug overdose, suicide, or old age.[5]

At the same time, the health care team can be helpful in assisting both patients and loved ones not to become stuck in prolonged denial, such as happened in the following:

My husband, John, age 55, was handed his diagnosis of liver cancer by a newly graduated doctor— John's own had just retired. "As I'm sure you know," the young man had blushingly begun, and John said simply, "Yes." We walked out of the office holding hands and cold to the marrow.

   Near the end, I started looking for signs that the inevitable would not be inevitable. I watched a few leaves that refused to give up their green to the season. I took comfort in the way the sun shone brightly on a day they predicted rain—not a cloud in the sky! I even tried to formulate messages of hope in arrangements of coins on the dresser top—look how they had landed all heads up . . . what were the odds? I prayed, too, in a way that agnostics do at such times. Sorry I doubted you "dear God, help us now." I stood shivering on our back patio in the early morning with my mug of coffee and told whatever might help us that now would be the time . . . but my dreams betrayed me: John, shrunk to the size of a thumb, fell from my purse where I'd been carrying him and was stepped on. In another dream, I took a walk around the block, and when I came back, my house was gone.[6]

REFLECTIONS

- What, if anything, do you think the doctor could have done at the outset to help set this bereaving wife on a different course?
- Think back to Chapter 7. How would better appreciation of the couple's story helped the health care professionals involved care for them?

Denial mechanisms are so widespread in almost all Western societies that we gave special attention to it here, but, obviously, there are other considerations and responses to dying and death that we turn your attention to now.

Responses to Dying and Death

Individual responses to a life-limiting diagnosis are influenced by a variety of factors, including age, life experiences, religion, culture, etc. Death may be a commonplace occurrence to one person who lives in a neighborhood with high levels of violent crime and sudden deaths. For other people, death might be such a rare occurrence that they do not experience a death until their young adulthood. Even with a wide range of experience with death, most people generally dread the thought of gradual and certain loss. The news of a life-limiting diagnosis, for oneself or a loved one, is almost always disquieting. In this chapter, you have an opportunity to think about what your own and your patients' possible responses to dying and loss are and the challenges to which this inevitable part of life gives rise.

COMMON STRESSES AND CHALLENGES DEMANDING RESPONSE

What would be your biggest challenges if you learned that you were dying? Most people can vaguely imagine and project what they would dread most; once the diagnosis is made, however, the reality of their specific situation intrudes. Then a patient's previous notions about a disease or injury and the known experiences of others who have had it combine to create a vivid picture of what the patient believes to be ahead. The following are some of the most commonly expressed concerns about death and dying.

Anticipation of Future Isolation

As you learned in Chapter 8, separation from the routine and regularity of life and familiar faces can have a disorienting effect on many people. Often a prolonged dying process involves gradual loss of habits, acceptance by others, and familial, social, and societal roles.

The fear of separation from the familiarity of home and routine as a way of ordering one's life becomes a reality for many. At the heart for most is a deeper fear of abandonment by loved ones and caregivers. Anxiety about this may be expressed in comments such as "They are starting to ignore me"; "My family is busy with other things"; "The nurses skipped my medication this morning, so they are probably giving up on me"; and "They spend more time with the woman in the next bed, but of course they know I'm dying." Many persons are aware of the practice of being admitted to the hospital to die or of having to spend the final period of their lives in a care facility, and some contribute to their isolation by rejecting visitors.

You can "treat" (allay) the patient's fears of isolation by your own presence. You cannot always ensure patients that their loved ones will not "jump ship" when the going gets rough, because sometimes families or friends do withdraw from the person. Observing this tapering from supportive relationships is often trying for you, let alone the patient. Relationships are bound to be altered during this time; some friends and relatives disappear because of indifference, despair, or exhaustion, and those who do not become more cherished.

Prospect of Pain

Those who have known others who experienced a painful end to life cannot be sure that their own dying will not be equally distressful or worse. Fortunately, assessment of physical, emotional, and spiritual pain has advanced in modern health care delivery. Pain was declared the fifth vital sign along with temperature, pulse, respirations, and blood pressure measurements.[7] Thus there is a great deal more attention paid to the quality of assessing and managing pain whether chronic or acute. Modern modes of health care intervention for pain today have the potential to nearly obliterate the physical pain of dying, though it is still a challenge in some settings to get positive pain relief.[8] Anxiety and depression can have a heightened effect on pain, whereas distraction and feelings of security tend to diminish the suffering associated with pain. These patterns of response, first characterized by Kübler-Ross several decades ago, have since been shown to better being understood as the range of responses that come and go from time to time.[9] Therefore the patient's suffering may be decreased by your reassurance, presence, compassion, and caring, as discussed in Chapter 10 and elsewhere.

Resistance to Becoming Dependent

Real or feared loss of independence during illness or injury is often a challenge. The extensive literature in end-of-life care supports that patients fear loss of autonomy and loss of dignity. They are concerned about pain management, inability to control bodily functions, and worry about placing undue burden on family or caregivers. Continued independence within whatever sphere of decision-making a person can exercise when in the dying process usually remains a high priority. Proof that they have thought about this is shown in their expressions of astonishment at having reached a point in their symptoms they had previously believed would be totally unbearable. Indeed, everyone has ideas beforehand of what he or she believes to be the "outer limits" of what one could bear: loss of bowel and bladder control; sexual impotence; inability to feed oneself, to communicate verbally, or to think straight; unconsciousness; or other loss. Often (though not always) patients' acceptance changes after a period of fighting and grieving the specific loss. In other words, patients adapt to the "new normal" in the dying process.

Patients' experiences of real or imagined isolation, pain, and increasing dependence are basic, but there are other concerns as well, such as the dread of suffocation and the fear that one's loved ones will not be adequately provided for. A person who dies suddenly in a car accident or plane crash or from a myocardial infarction may have long harbored these fears but did not have a period of prolonged illness during which these concerns surfaced. Those who have time to anticipate their death must find a way of dealing with these fears and concerns. For instance, a man who has had trouble openly expressing affection to his wife may be able to do so by sharing his sorrow that he fears she will not be adequately provided for. An indirect means of communication, such as writing a letter or telling a friend how wonderful she is, serves a similar purpose. You can be instrumental in making suggestions to help such a patient carry out his or her wishes if you get a hint that the patient desires to do so.

In summary, during their dying process, people must rely on their own best inner resources and the support of family, friends, and health professionals to sustain them as they face their challenges. Any hesitance, embarrassment, or disdain you show when a person expresses a concern, even one that seems unfounded to you, will exacerbate the suffering associated with it.

RECKONING WITH WHAT DEATH MIGHT MEAN

Different cultures and individuals treat the moment of transition from alive to dead differently, but for many it is not something to relish. What is the range of expressions about what will happen when death comes?

Many people believe that after this life there is something else. The varieties of religious or philosophical beliefs are many, regarding the relationship of this life to the next.[10] Predominant beliefs in many religions, especially but by no means only those associated with Eastern religions such as Hinduism, propose that "death" is a process of birth and rebirth (e.g., reincarnation). The last step is not extinction but perfection, at which time one is absorbed into a "place" or into a "being" in which complete unity of all beings is realized. Depending on the religion, the type of being one will become after physical death, and the opportunity for the final step into ultimate unity may or may not depend on the type of life one lived on earth during an embodied human lifetime. In Islam, one may be transported through several levels of paradise depending on the type of life one has lived.

Some people believe in the resurrection of souls only, whereas others believe that the actual human body will be restored, usually in an improved form. There is one version of a literal, sudden bodily resurrection (sometimes referred to as the "rapture") in which those—both dead and still living—who have lived holy lives will be immediately transported to heaven, whereas others will be left behind forever to suffer the consequences of their sins. Other Christians have different versions of what it means to be "resurrected," although all share this basic belief.

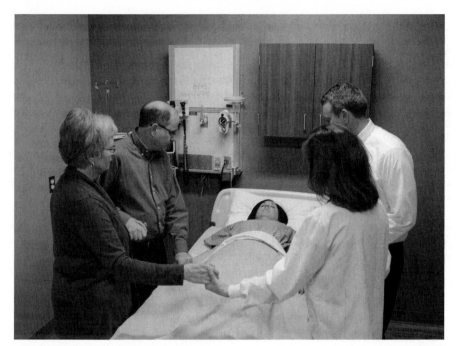

Fig. 15.1 Patients and families often engage in rituals during the dying process. (*Courtesy Maren Haddad.*)

You will meet individuals who talk with anticipation about "going to meet the Lord," whereas others are sure their lives will not meet the standards of acceptability and they will be consigned to suffering of some kind. Knowing that any of these beliefs about immortality may influence the way an individual interprets the impact and meaning of his or her own impending death, you can be better prepared for comments from patients or for rituals a patient and family engage in during the dying process (Fig. 15.1). However, a significant number of people today do not view death as a precursor of immortality in any form. You must be prepared to interact in a respectful way with patients and family members (who may not hold the same beliefs as the patient) who have very different ideas about what happens, if anything, after death.

REFLECTIONS

Before proceeding, think about conversations you may have had with patients or others who hold these positions about what happens after death from a faith-based perspective.
- Which beliefs do you hold, if any?
- How might your beliefs influence your approach to patients who are dying?
- Try to construct a conversation you might have with a patient or family who does not believe in immortality. What kinds of comments might such a person make?
- How would you respond to the person in ways that would be affirming or comforting?

These concepts about death can help you understand patients and their families when they share their feelings and ideas about death and how to prepare for it. When you can enter such conversations with equanimity and express genuine interest in what the person wants or needs to say about death, you will be showing respect for that person.

COPING RESPONSES BY PATIENTS

Although denial is initially a common coping response, the concerns associated with dying and the death event usually become more sharply focused over time, and you can anticipate other emotional-psychological responses as well. For many, the first response is acute shock or disbelief. Coping also may take many other forms, such as periods of depression, anger, and hostility, bargaining behavior, or acceptance.[11] Patients who undergo a long process of dying are likely to feel all of them from time to time and many times over. On one day, a woman denies her impending death; on another, she makes secret bargains with God about how long she will live; on the following days, she feels the relief of acceptance followed by a deep depression, and so on. Although the danger with any such framework is that you or your colleagues may tend to pigeonhole a patient according to the categories provided, we have found them to be a useful general set of benchmarks for thinking about what a patient is experiencing.

The patient's basic personality structure is an important factor in determining which kinds of responses will predominate, too. How each person deals with stress and copes is different. "Most people rely more heavily on one or two things. No style is right or wrong, however some coping styles may be more or less effective in particular life situations."[12]

To further prepare yourself for working with such patients, we suggest you pause here to engage in a reflection on your own life.

REFLECTIONS

Try to think about how you respond to stressful situations in your life.
- Can you imagine what you might be like as a patient or family member faced with the challenge of a dying loved one?
- If you have, in fact, had to face it, try to recall your major types of responses.

Narrative reflection is a resource many use to process the dying experience and cope with end of life. As mentioned in Chapter 7, the writings of novelists, poets, essayists, and others can be a useful tool for patients and families. Many have recorded their experiences in this powerful period of life, and it is to your advantage to avail yourself of these narrative accounts in preparation for your professional encounters with people who are dying.

COPING RESPONSES BY THE PATIENT'S FAMILY

The best and worst aspects of family relationships are exposed when a family member is gravely ill or dying. You will witness a range of behaviors from the most intimate, loving characteristics of family relationships to complicated, lifelong destructive patterns. Regardless of the familial response, the interprofessional care team must recognize the family as essential participants in the death and dying process. Although each families' situation is unique, the great majority of families are brought closer together by an end-of-life experience, and their mutual support during this time is touching to observe. If the patient has not been told of the life-limiting nature of the condition, family members may whisper to you in doorways, trying to involve you in elaborate schemes to ensure continued deception. At times, you may feel torn as to who needs your expertise and support more, the patient or the family member. At the busiest time of day, they may stop you to tell you something, only to burst into tears. You may wonder, why is it important for them to be there? One reason could be that it allows them to cope more effectively with their own stresses and make sense of what is happening in their lives.

Families cope with their stress and anxiety when caring for a person with a life-limiting illness in various ways as well. Some family members pull back and try to get some distance. Others want to get closer to the patient and more involved. Some family members try to maintain control by planning.

Still others become overly optimistic.[12] We include these examples of different coping styles here to help you to understand your own coping mechanisms and those of the people under your care.

Family members also can react to the threat of losing a loved one by experiencing *anticipatory grief* that parallels the symptoms usually seen in the acute grief that follows a death. Symptoms of acute grief may take the forms of a tendency to sigh, complaints of chronic weakness or exhaustion, and loss of appetite or nausea. In addition, a family member may be preoccupied with what a person looks like, express guilt or hostility, and change his or her usual patterns of conduct.[13] Except in extreme situations, family members are so integral to the ongoing life and preferences of the patient that the patient feels lost without this support. They can be an essential element of communication for and about the loved one.

In many instances, patients and families will need the expertise of key members of the interprofessional care team such as social workers, counselors, and chaplains to help them make important decisions in this unique moment of their lives. Your willingness to access and collaborate effectively with these colleagues can extend your own effectiveness considerably.

Setting Priorities in Respectful Interaction

In addition to your role as one who respects the patient and family through listening and responding caringly to them, two additional priorities are appropriate when a patient is dying. They include information sharing and helping patients maintain hope.

INFORMATION SHARING: WHAT, WHEN, AND HOW?

What types of information do patients and families need to know? Start with the patient's diagnosis. The key is for the entire interprofessional care team to be attentive and ready to communicate those things they each have a right to, and are ready to, know. For the most part, in the United States, Canada, and many European countries, medical policies and practices support the position that a patient has a right to information about his or her health status. There is also a conviction that the duty not to harm is best realized by disclosure—the truth "sets free." Thus there is emphasis on involving the patient and those he or she deems appropriate into the shared planning of goals, which is especially important in the dying process.

This trend toward openness is by no means shared universally or even by many of the cultures within the changing US, Canadian, and Western European populations. At the very least, you can be attentive to clues you are receiving from the patient and family as to whether directly sharing this information with the patient is a culturally informed way for members of the health care team to proceed. Do patients figure it out? Probably some do and some do not.

Whatever combination of considerations make up the interprofessional care team's decisions, most are now telling patients with life-limiting conditions their diagnoses, usually in direct terms with emphasis on keeping communication channels open after the initial discussion.[14] In the end, there is no substitute for personalized, sensitive communication by all members of the interprofessional care team, initially and throughout the patient's course of interaction with them.

REFLECTIONS

- Do you think you would want to be told the news that you have a life-limiting condition that the physicians have just discovered? If yes, try to imagine the physical setting, people you would hope were (or were not) present, and key points you would want to know in this initial exchange.
- What would you like to have happen over the course of your dying that would most help you feel that you were being treated with respect from the start of your ordeal?
- What (if any) role would health professionals play in this process?

Seldom will it be within the boundaries of your role to personally shoulder the sole responsibility of a life-limiting diagnosis. Typically, the interprofessional care team will discuss and plan for the time to speak to a patient about the diagnosis, prognosis, and goals of care. As part of that team, you should listen to the patient's story with focused attentiveness. Your attention to patient and family questions will provide some relief to their anxieties because it will show that you care and respect even their most unusual concerns. It also conveys your willingness to keep communication channels open.

Using language and words the patient really understands is imperative. Without this translation from medical/clinical terminology to everyday language, nothing will make sense in the conversation.

For example, in *Endings and Beginnings,* a young woman's account of her husband's terminal diagnosis and eventual death, the author recalls that after exploratory surgery the doctor tried to be reassuring by saying they had found a "lymphatic tumor" but did not go on to tell them that it was an aggressive, life-limiting malignancy. In fact, that evening her husband reassured her that, because it was "lymphatic," at least it was not cancer. Their reassurance was short lived:

> *That evening, as I left the hospital elevator I was startled to have the head resident under Dr. C. (the surgeon) turn to me and say, "Try not to worry; we'll do everything we can." It was clear there was much more going on than any of us was admitting.*[15]

Following her encounter, the young couple spent many days trying to verify the truth that the husband had something serious. In reflecting on the whole course of his dying, the author remembers that period of unclarity as one of the most painful for both.

Talking with a patient and family about a life-limiting prognosis has its own challenges because almost always the prognosis is not known with absolute certainty. Today physicians often talk about probability: "You have a 50% chance of a 5-year survival." This approach allows certain information to be transmitted to the patient and may permit the patient to learn what usually happens to people in similar situations. At the same time, probabilistic information does not answer the key question of "what, exactly, does this mean for me?"

HELPING PATIENTS MAINTAIN HOPE

In the first part of the chapter we emphasized the importance of recognizing and understanding patients' challenges during this unique period of their life. Many life-limiting conditions are accompanied by a gradual or quick diminution of strength, endurance, control of movement, or sensory acuity. Helping the person and family adjust to each of the gradual losses in function, or "little deaths" as they are experienced, is a continuing challenge. Your respectful caring requires being attuned to the losses while affirming the patient's remaining strengths.

When a patient is dying, the focus of hope will change over time, from a hope for cure to a hope for meaningful activities in the remaining life left to this person. Hope may be directed toward events such as seeing a loved one or pet another time, visiting a favorite place, or hearing a familiar piece of music played.

Some hopes are less tangible: that one will be able to keep a positive spirit or sense of irony to the end, that one will be remembered and missed, or that a tradition will be carried on in one's absence. Previously sought long-term goals are put into perspective, and the patient focuses his or her hopes on the most important ones, knowing that some will no longer be attainable.[16]

Families also adjust their hopes for what is possible given the new circumstances. As one husband wrote when he learned that his wife was not going to recover from her early bouts of ovarian cancer:

There is a transition between the certainty of living and the acceptance of dying. When there is such acceptance, there is a kind of emotional purgatory. The cartoon character stands still in space beyond the edge of a cliff and awaits the fatal fall. That is where things were for us in early October. There were choices, however, even in this purgatory. They remained a moment to live in . . . if only a moment. After that we will go on with our lives. Before it was over and before I began my desperate search for a new life, there would be a time for us as a family that was like none other. Most important was that we manage the pain. The first priority was comfort. The second priority was to get Lezlie back home not so much so that she could die there as that she could live there before she left.[17]

How can you show respect in terms of supporting hope? Hope itself depends significantly on the attitudes of health professionals, as well as on those of family and friends when the patient dares to disclose a hope. We have witnessed tender scenes between family or friends and the patient when one dares to say, "I was hoping . . . ." Your listening for clues can help maintain the person's feeling of worth and provide a human context into which hopes may be more freely expressed. Health professionals also often can play a significant role in helping the patient realize some specific hopes by making a few important telephone calls to the right people, by mentioning the patient's wishes to the family and others, or by other similar means.

Most people faced with dying hope that they will be treated kindly, that everything clinically reasonable will be done for them, and that meaningful human interaction will not disappear. You can do your best in your role to support those general hopes.

The Right Care, in the Right Place, at the Right Time

The site, timing, and focus of caring interventions have been the source of much discussion and policy in health care. An important factor is considerations arising from an improved understanding of physiological and other responses to pain or other disturbing symptoms associated with many life-limiting conditions, and where the interventions can best be delivered. Most people still die in the hospital, though the actual figures will vary according to the number of hospital beds and general demographics of the area's population. This is usually the appropriate site for interventions that require complex technologies and specialties available in the hospital setting. The second most likely setting for death in the United States is a skilled nursing facility. However, where people die is not always the place they want to die. About 80% of Americans report they would prefer to die at home, but only 20% of them do[18] (Fig. 15.2). There are many barriers to dying at home that include the emphasis on cure regardless of prognosis, lack of understanding about what palliative care or hospice can offer to patients with a life-limiting illness, and fear and anxiety on the part of family as to their roles and responsibilities for a dying loved one. Regardless of the actual setting of care delivery, palliative care and hospice are of importance to patients with a serious or life-limiting illness or injury.

PALLIATIVE CARE

Palliative care traditionally was thought of as what health professionals can offer when cure no longer is possible. In other words, it becomes appropriate when all else has failed. From Hippocrates' time onward the suggestion was that if cure was no longer possible, the disease had gone beyond the "art of medicine" and should not be interfered with by the doctor. So, all too often palliation meant that dying patients received little medical intervention. At the same time, you can understand that the idea of palliative care is important because, applied appropriately, it allows you to have better insight into how to respond well to patients' fears of abandonment, pain, and other distress associated with the dying process.

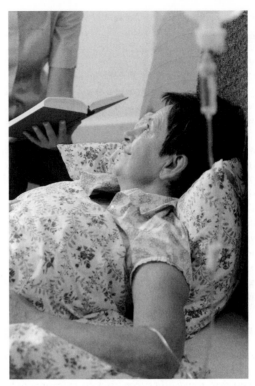

Fig. 15.2 Most Americans would prefer to die at home in familiar surroundings although most do not. (© *KatarzynaBialasiewicz/iStock/Thinkstock.com.*)

Today the growing focus on appropriate end-of-life care has shed new light on what palliative care entails. Palliative care goes well beyond the traditional "hand-holding at the bedside" so often portrayed in the pictures before modern medicine could offer so much. Comfort can be achieved for patients through many varieties of intervention, such as medications, respiratory therapies, surgical procedures, and psychological and spiritual counseling, to name some. Contemporary palliative care and the medical sub-specialty of palliative medicine are defined as:

> *[S]pecialized medical care for people living with serious illness. It focuses on providing relief from the symptoms and stress of a serious illness. The goal is to improve quality of life for both the patient and the family. Palliative care is provided by a team of palliative care doctors, nurses, social workers and others who work together with a patient's other doctors to provide an extra layer of support. It is appropriate at any age and at any stage in a serious illness and can be provided along with curative treatment.*[19]

Palliative care is growing and expanded in the United States and other countries. "Over 1700 hospitals with more than 50 beds have a palliative care team today."[19] Along with this heightened consciousness and technology focus, there also has been a rethinking about the traditional assumption of a progression from "treatment" to "palliation" as the patient's dying ensues as is suggested by the inclusion of "at any stage" of a serious illness in the Center to Advance Palliative Care definition given previously. Using cancer as a model, the National Academy of Medicine (formerly the Institute of Medicine) in the United States proposes that treatment geared to cure

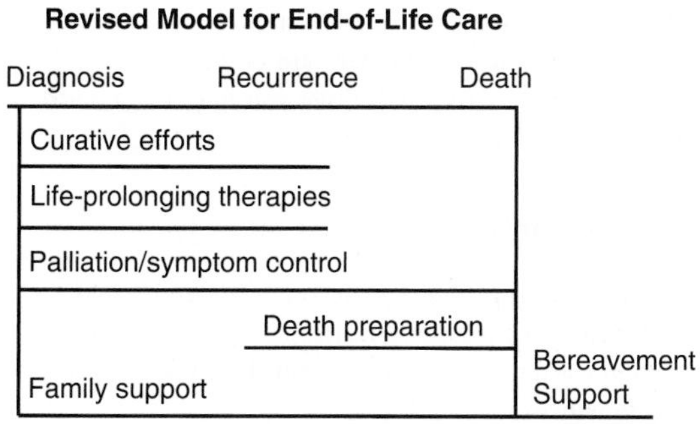

Revised Model for End-of-Life Care

Fig. 15.3   A revised model for end-of-life care. (*From Field MJ, Cassel CK, eds. Approaching Death: Improving Care at the End of Life. Washington, DC: Committee on Care at the End of Life, Institute of Medicine, National Academies Press; 1997.*)

versus treatment geared to palliation does not progress in a tidy, linear way (Fig. 15.3). Different combinations of education about how to prevent deterioration or the appearance of new symptoms, responsiveness to rehabilitative needs, acute care interventions, and comfort measures all may remain appropriate from the beginning to the end of a serious illness or eventually when the patient begins the dying process.[20]

HOSPICE

The modern hospice, which began in England and has spread to Canada, the United States, and many other countries, provides treatment and care expressly designed to meet the needs of patients who are expected to die within 6 months. Hospice is holistic in its approach to caring for patients, family members, and their friends. Hospice services are available for all types of patients with life-limiting conditions such as end-stage cardiac or renal disease, Alzheimer's disease, progressively deteriorating neurological conditions, cancer, and chronic obstructive pulmonary disease.

Hospice focuses on comfort measures when cure or remission is no longer possible. The hospice setting is characterized by interprofessional care team approaches. When there is a family, it (and not the patient alone) is the unit of care. Family perspectives on end-of-life care for elders with advanced-stage cancer in different settings showed significantly more favorable experiences of their loved ones dying outside of the hospital setting with hospice services than those whose loved ones died in hospitals. The authors concluded that this setting is far better equipped to provide symptom relief, communication with health professionals, emotional support, and less aggressive treatment.[21]

Hospice services are "without walls"; that is, they are designed to provide care within the home with devices such as hotlines, care networks, and respite programs for caregivers or a designated hospice care facility or a skilled nursing facility. Churches and other organizations sometimes become involved in filling the gaps not covered by hospice staff or the family members who are expected to provide a significant amount of the direct care the patient requires. Families and informal caregivers are often shocked when they learn there is no full-time personal care coverage for dying patients under the Medicare hospice benefit or other insurance plans. The responsibilities that families are expected to assume are often overwhelming, especially when they cannot afford to pay out of pocket for additional help. You and your patients will benefit if you take time to acquaint yourself further with the functions and structure of each of these settings in the communities where you work. This will prepare you to inform patients of their options when it becomes appropriate and to be active in their information-gathering process. You may even find yourself drawn to these aspects of health care and be one of the growing numbers of health care providers working in hospice. Other alternative care delivery models that are fine-tuned to patients' and families' real needs are also being developed. You are entering the health professions at a time when the attention devoted to these issues will assist you in doing a better job than your forbears did in providing care for dying patients.

When Death Is Imminent

At some point during a life-limiting illness it becomes apparent that the person will die soon. Persons who do not suffer from a prolonged illness as such also face the moment of imminent death: the accident victim, the attempted suicide or murder victim, and the young person seriously injured in battle or other violence.

INDIVIDUALIZED CARE

The patient whose death is imminent should not be barraged with routine requests and procedures that no longer matter. As one woman sitting by her dying father's bedside asked dismayingly, "Does it matter, really, if his bowels haven't moved on the last day he will probably be alive?"

Attempts to relieve pain by medication, massage, and other therapeutic means may have been started long before, and these should be continued unless the patient asks that they be withdrawn. Some people, knowing that they are experiencing the final days of their lives, find the stupor induced by heavy medication more troublesome than uncomfortable symptoms.

However, maximizing comfort goes beyond alleviating pain. It involves the relief of real or potential suffering. Suffering is a far more inclusive, personalized concept than pain, and your assistance in helping patients and their families have a final time together as free of pain and suffering as possible is a laudable goal. Families do many things to try to provide a meaningful and peaceful transition. We have seen families who read to their loved ones, bathe them, sing songs they loved, or fill the room with flowers. A friend of one of the authors sneaked her 2-month-old daughter up to the hospital room so that her husband could witness his wife nursing their child for one last time. A religious leader may be called in for instruction or rituals. The patient who has been nourished only intravenously for days or weeks may request that all medications and intravenous lines be removed. Specific activities will vary from person to person influenced by personal preference and cultural, ethnic, religious, or other beliefs. When they exist, respect requires you to alter your treatment procedures to honor them.

Caregivers in the health care environment can be facilitators by allowing the family and friends their final day or days together, remaining "on standby" if needed. This might mean breaking hospital rules and readjusting one's schedule. It also means knowing whom should be called if the patient's condition worsens and death appears near.

SAYING GOOD-BYE

Many people find it difficult to say good-bye to a friend or other loved one who is going away. It is often more difficult still when the person is dying—so much so that good-byes are seldom said, especially by the health professional to the patient and the patient's family. This is, however, something that you can do to show respect for the people and their situation when many other forms of interaction have been suspended. One psychiatrist offers this suggestion:

What should be said is, I want you to know the relationship was meaningful, I'll miss this about you, or . . . it won't be the same, I'll miss the bluntness that you had in helping me sort out some things, or I'll just miss the old bull sessions, or something like that. Because those are things you value. Now what does that do for the other person? The other person learns that although it's painful to separate it's far more meaningful to have known the person and to have separated than never to have known him at all. He also learns what it is in himself that is valued and treasured by [you]. And some of those underlying, corrosive feelings of low self-esteem that plague people are shored up.[22]

This encounter also allows the patient and his or her family to express similar feelings. There is often a real sense of closeness and gratitude felt toward the health professional, and to be able to show it is a great relief. In addition to what the exchange does for the patient and family, it is important to realize how much it can help in your own grieving. Giving patients and families an opportunity to express gratitude to you may sound odd, but it is one way in which some patients and families can be assisted in their own grieving. When they observe that the health professional receives his or her thanks humbly, they will appreciate this show of human caring.

However, you should also prepare for the patient and family to reject your attempts to show respectful caring during this intense period of their lives. Sometimes when a person is close to dying, he or she shuts out many people. Such a patient may not want to have anything more to do with you. There are many possible reasons for this:

- Many have great difficulty saying good-bye under any circumstance.
- The person has accepted his or her death and no longer needs any people around, except the closest few of whom you are not one.
- The patient and his or her family may direct their anger about the death toward you and other members of the team.
- You are inextricably linked to the whole setting in which suffering and the dying process have taken place. So much anguish may be associated with you and your professional environment that it is painful for the patient to be in your presence.

In short, when your final efforts and good intentions are neither wanted nor welcomed, you may feel hurt by these sudden or unexpected rebuffs and can do little more than forgive the person responsible for them. At times when hurt is present, support from your professional colleagues may become vital. Sharing feelings of failure, rejection, or bewilderment with an understanding colleague can lend insights into the reasons listed earlier.

Summary

This chapter considers some key factors that can be helpful to you in your attempts to show respect in the extreme life situation in which death is approaching for a patient in your care. The patient needs your professional skills, compassion, and wisdom in this situation. At the same time, you are confronted with your own uncertainties and fears about dying and death along with the irony that, no matter what you do, the result for this patient will be death. Your part in making the remainder of life for a dying patient as rich and worthwhile as possible may be the motivation you will need to sustain that person and his or her loved ones.

References

1. Albom M. *Tuesdays with Morrie*. New York: Doubleday; 1997.
2. Jack and the beanstalk (a traditional English fairy tale). *The Arthur Rackham Fairy Book*. Philadelphia: Lippincott; 1950.
3. Hansel and Grethel (a Grimm's fairy tale). *The Arthur Rackham Fairy Book*. Philadelphia: Lippincott; 1950.
4. Annual Report, 12/15/1980, Domestic Policy Staff – James Mongan's and Joseph Onek's Subject Files, "Report of the President's Commission for the Study of Ethical Problems in Medicine and Biomedical and Behavioral Research," Box 3, Jimmy Carter Library.
5. Caldwell G. *Let's Take the Long Way Home*. New York: Random House; 2010.
6. Berg E. *The Year of Pleasures*. New York: Random House; 2005.
7. Pasero C, McCaffrey M. Pain ratings: the fifth vital sign. *Am J Nursing*. 1997;97(2):15.

8. Brennan F, Carr DB, Cousins M. Pain management: a fundamental human right. *Pain Med 105*. 2007;105(1):205–221.

9. Kübler-Ross E. *On Death and Dying*. New York: Macmillan; 1969.

10. Burt RA. *Death Is That Man Taking Names: Intersections of American Medicine, Law, and Culture*. Berkeley: University of California Press; 2002.

11. Balber PG. Stories of the living dying: the Hermes listener. In: Corless I, Germino BB, Pittman MA, eds. *Dying, Death, and Bereavement: A Challenge for Living*. 2nd ed. New York: Springer Publishing; 2003.

12. Purtilo R, Robinson E. *Maintaining Compassionate Care: A Companion for Families Experiencing the Uncertainty of a Serious and Prolonged Illness*. Boston, MA: MGH Institute of Health Professions, Inc.; 2007:34.

13. Hodgson H, Krahn L. *Smiling Through Your Tears: Anticipatory Grief*. North Charleston, SC: Booksurge LLC; 2005. www.booksurge.com.

14. Brighton IJ, Bristowe K. Communication in palliative care: talking about end of life, before end of life. *Postgrad Med J*. 2016;92:466–470.

15. Albertson SH. *Endings and Beginnings*. New York: Random House; 1980.

16. Purtilo RB. Attention to caregivers and hope: overlooked aspects of ethics consultation. *J Clin Ethic*. 2006;17(4):358–363.

17. Surman O. *After Eden: A Love Story*. New York: iUniverse; 2005.

18. Institute of Medicine. *Dying in America: Improving Quality and Honoring Individual Preferences Near the End-of-Life*. Washington, DC; 2014.

19. Center to Advance Palliative Care: www.capc.org/about/palliative-care.

20. Field MJ, Cassel C, eds. *Approaching Death: Improving Care at the End of Life*, National Academy of Medicine Report. Washington, DC: National Academies Press; 1997.

21. Wright AA, Keating NL, Ayanian JZ, et al. Family perspectives on aggressive cancer care near the end of life. *JAMA*. 2016;315(3):284–292.

22. Cassem NH. The caretakers. In: Langone J, ed. *Vital Signs: The Way We Die in America*. Boston: Little, Brown; 1974.

CHAPTER 16

Respectful Interaction in Complex Situations

The reader will be able to:

- Identify three potential sources of difficulties that create barriers to respectful health professional and patient interaction
- Discuss how disparities in power within the health care context can lead to anger and frustration for all involved
- Identify attributes and behaviors of patients, such as manipulative, sexually provocative, or aggressive behaviors, that may challenge the health professional's ideal of respectful care in all its forms
- Recognize patients with "high need," and understand how the interprofessional care team can collaborate to effectively meet the care demands of this population
- Describe strategies to cope with the emotions that result from difficult conversations
- Reflect on personal expectations of what it means to be a "good" health professional and how this affects interactions with patients
- Describe environmental factors that may contribute to difficulties in health professional and patient interaction
- List and evaluate guidelines for managing and, when possible, preventing difficult interactions to optimize health professional and patient relationships and health care outcomes
- Identify 10 strategies for effectively managing difficult conversations in health care

Prelude

She asks for help and I have given it to her. She has been on various medications but nothing seems to work. She is a sad case really, and her anxiety seems to stem from a poor home environment. She gets anxious and then gets anxious about being anxious. I prescribe, but I know she will be back again in a short time. It would not be so bad if she tried to help herself.

I. SHAW[1]

Difficult conversations are part of everyday life in health care. Patients and families present for care when they are most vulnerable, and the interprofessional care team is often responsible for communications that bring both joy and sorrow. There are patient care situations in which you will come away with a sense of satisfaction and others that may elicit profound frustration. As a health professional, you must be prepared for all types. This chapter focuses on difficulties inherent in the health professional and patient interaction that have not specifically been addressed elsewhere in this book or that bear reemphasizing. We suggest that you refer to Chapters 2 and 3 to review the content on establishing relatedness, recognizing boundaries, and creating professional closeness. You will need to use these insights and skills in your work with patients who challenge your conceptions of what it means to be a "good" health professional. Moreover, you will have an opportunity to think about other factors that can create great tension in the health professional and patient interaction, such as disparities in power and role expectations or an unsafe working environment that can cause harm to the health professional or patient. We devote this chapter to some summary statements about how to work more effectively with complex patients and families and offer ways to effect change in "difficult" settings and situations.

Sources of Difficulties

Generally, when you enter a relationship with a patient, you have good reason to expect that things will go well, or if there are problems, you expect that they can be resolved. However, there are situations in which even your best efforts cannot make things right. When this happens, a common response is to look for a place to lay the blame. For example, you might wonder what else you could have done for the patient, or you might reason that the patient was not ready for treatment, or you might become defensive and decide that the patient was disruptive, maladjusted, or any number of other negative labels. Refer to the quote that opened the chapter regarding a patient who does not seem to be meeting the health professional's expectations for improvement. Especially note the last sentence, indicating that the patient is at least partly to blame for the situation. Difficulty relating to a patient may originate in the health professional, in the interaction itself, or within the setting where the interaction takes place.

SOURCES WITHIN THE HEALTH PROFESSIONAL

As emphasized throughout this book, you bring a wealth of experiences, education, biases, and values to your interaction with patients and their families. These factors can affect how you react to a particular patient. For example, recall the discussion on transference and countertransference in Chapter 2. A patient may remind you of your third-grade teacher, whom you particularly feared and disliked. This experience can arouse intense emotional reactions in the present relationship. In addition, your personality and how you deal with stress will play a large part in how you manage patient care situations that are interpersonally difficult.[2] In fact, your personality, more than your professional or demographic background, may explain why you react negatively to some patients and certain situations and have little difficulty with others.

For the health professional, the most reliable indicator of a negative emotional response is an unfavorable gut response or sense of discomfort in encounters with a patient.[3] If you are attuned to monitoring your feelings, you can try to assess how much anger, fear, or guilt you bring to the interaction and try to manage those feelings before trying to manage the patient. After you identify the emotions you are experiencing, two questions often follow: "Why is this happening?" and "Where is this emotion coming from?"

Although it is a widely held belief, which has certainly been emphasized in this book, that health professionals should be nonjudgmental in their relationships with patients, it is a fact that health professionals often find some patients more difficult than others.

In general, patients who do not affirm the health professional's identity (i.e., accept and appreciate professional assistance) can be considered "bad patients." The patient's rejection of the health professional's help can be easily misread as rejection of the health professional. This rejection can take many forms, ranging from complaints to incessant demands, manipulative behavior, ingratitude, or basic unwillingness to follow advice or treatment. The literature categorizes "difficult patients" as patients who are needy, demanding, help-rejecting, and self-destructive.[4] Patients with these characteristics may evoke strong negative feelings (including guilt, hostility, and aversion). They may attempt to intimidate, devaluate, and ignore recommendations. They also may become aggressive and frighten or sometimes even threaten or physically harm health professionals. Still others may make unacceptable sexually explicit or racist remarks that undermine the relationship or challenge the safety or comfort of health professionals or others in the health care environment.

During your program of study to become a health professional, the ideal that is reinforced is that you should be able to function effectively in all patient situations and you are solely responsible for the success or failure of these interactions. This may not be what your instructors and mentors or we want to convey, but it is often what health professionals think. Thus long before you have a full complement of skills and a breadth of experience with which to deal with difficult situations, you may blame yourself for failing to meet the needs of a challenging patient encounter. In fact, we have found that new situations can raise old doubts or uncertainties at any period in one's career.

SOURCES WITHIN INTERACTIONS WITH PATIENTS

What makes a patient "difficult"? Patients who are overly demanding or who do not adhere to treatment generally are labeled as problematic, as this family physician notes:

> *Let's be blunt. It's hard to care for difficult patients. It's sometimes impossible to actually like them. This species of sick individuals tends to strain time, patience, and resources. They often generate a cascade of phone calls. They sometimes demand a heap of medically unnecessary tests. They occasionally refuse recommended treatment. Many have unreasonable expectations. Some whine and gripe incessantly. A few threaten to sue.[5]*

Other types of behaviors that commonly elicit a negative response from health professionals are violence, anger, or self-harm behaviors such as in the case of substance use disorders. Kelly and May[6] proposed a theoretical framework for the way health professionals conceptualize "good" and "bad" patients using an interactionist perspective. According to this view, patients come to be regarded as good or bad, not because of anything inherent about them or in their behavior but because of the interactions between health professionals and patients. Patients are not passive recipients of care but active agents in the interaction process. Kelly and May explain that patients have the power to "influence, shape and reject professionals' attempts to impose a definition on their situation, with profound consequences for nurse-patient relations and the professional task."[6] Even though Kelly and May focus on the nurse and patient interaction, their framework appears applicable to all health professionals and their reaction when patients withhold affirmation for the health professionals' roles.

As you can see, the focus of the dislike can easily move from dislike for the consequences of inappropriate or unacceptable attitudes or behavior to dislike for the person who is a patient. For example, patients with illnesses that are socially unacceptable are often labeled as difficult even if their behavior is a model of adherence. People with substance use disorders such as alcohol or drug use are often viewed as "bad" patients. Even if a health professional views alcoholism as a disease rather than a behavior a patient should be able to control, the patient who has a problem with substance use can be rejected by health professionals. In a recent study of facilitators and barriers in substance use treatment, a health professional commented that "the terminology seems to be more punitive and judgmental towards this population when they are cycling in and out. I mean it's not enjoyable to be dealing with that, but I think the judgmental aspect actually gets in the way."[7]

Patients who are judged to be responsible in some way for their illness or injury, such as people who are obese or addicted to tobacco or other substances, are often also labeled as less worthy of respect than patients who are "blameless" for their present health condition. These patients have one thing in common: Either because of the nature of their health problems or the way they respond to the health professionals involved in their care and treatment, they withhold the legitimacy that makes health professionals feel good about who they are and what they do.

Thus a large part of the label a patient receives depends on our role expectations of patients in general and of patients with specific characteristics. One of the most basic expectations of patients is adherence with agreed-on treatment. *Adherence* is defined as the extent to which a person's behavior—taking medication, following a diet, and/or executing lifestyle changes—corresponds with agreed recommendations from a health care provider.[8] Adherence is affected by multiple factors, including the patient, the social context, the health system, and the health professional. *Nonadherence* is largely viewed in health care literature as a problem to be resolved: we assume patients are not following professional advice because they do not understand or have some misconception that prevents them from understanding. Major efforts, then, are directed toward getting patients to understand so they will adhere to treatment. This often includes attending to the social circumstances in which patients live their lives.[9] If health professionals approach the problem of nonadherence by trying to understand the factors in patients' lives that mediate their cooperation, efforts can be made to change factors that are amenable to change or adjust treatment to meet the reality of a patient's life.

HIGH-NEED PATIENTS

As you recall from Chapters 13 and 14, about 12 million adult patients in the United States are living with three or more chronic conditions. These patients, as well as others with complex needs, have recently been the focus of attention in the study of health care delivery and expenditure. The literature suggests that the top 1% of patients who use health care resources account for more than 20% of health care expenditures, and the top 5% account for nearly half of US spending on health care.[10] *High-need patients* have been defined as those with "complex conditions and circumstances requiring multiple services that, for the most part, are not currently delivered easily or effectively by the health care system."[11] Many high-need patients are adults over the age of 65 with multiple chronic conditions or advanced illness, but young adults with disabilities, individuals with chronic mental health conditions, and/or those with substance use disorders also fall into this category.[12]

Because of the functional difficulties many of these patients experience with activities of daily living and navigating the health care system, they warrant collaborative and integrated interprofessional care. Multidimensional care models that attend to the medical, functional, behavioral, and social needs of patients with high needs can help improve the cost and quality of care delivery.[13]

SOURCES IN THE ENVIRONMENT

The health professional and patient interaction takes place in a particular context. At times, the context can be the source of difficulty in an interaction. For example, if the environment is strange and frightening, the patient or health professional may react in a fearful or angry manner. Fig. 16.1 illustrates that for many patients, a health care facility can be an extremely threatening place. Taken in this context, even a simple activity such as bathing can be viewed as menacing. Rader[14] noted that for a person with apraxia (inability to execute purposeful, learned motor acts despite the physical ability and willingness to do so), agnosia (inability to recognize a tactile or visible stimulus despite being able to recognize the elemental sensation), and aphasia (loss of language function either in comprehension or expression of words)—symptoms often found in patients who have had a cerebral vascular accident—the standard nursing home bathing experience may be perceived as horrific. Consider the following limitations and place yourself in the patient's position.

A person the resident does not recognize comes into her room, wakens her, says something she does not understand, drags her out of bed, and takes off her clothes. Then the resident is moved down a public corridor on something that resembles a toilet seat, covered only with a thin sheet so that her private parts are exposed to the breeze. Calls for help are ignored or greeted with, "Good morning." Then she is taken to a strange, cold room that looks like a car wash, the sheet is ripped off, and she is sprayed in

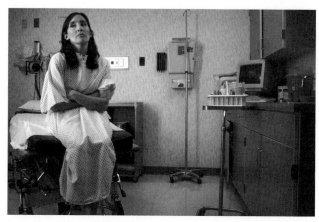

Fig. 16.1 Patients often feel overwhelmed and out of place in health care settings. (© *Photodisc/Photodisc/Thinkstock.com.*)

the face with cold and then scalding water. Continued calls for help go unheeded. Her most private parts are touched by a stranger. In another context this would be assault.[14]

An environment can be equally strange and intolerable to the health professional. For example, we have noted in other chapters that, in community health practice, health professionals may go into the unknown realm of the patient's living environment. One of us recalls a home visit to a small, run-down house literally butted up against the back fence of the holding pens for cattle at the stock market. The smell of manure was overwhelming both outside and inside the house. The elderly woman who lived there (and the subject of the home visit for management of diabetes) seemed oblivious to the odor. In fact, she had just finished hanging a load of clean sheets on the line to dry in her tiny backyard!

Other environmental factors that make care difficult include the aesthetics of a space, crowding, noise, and climate. Similar stresses can arise in a hectic and crisis-ridden environment. Patients who are kept waiting in an overcrowded emergency department or office are more likely to be frustrated and hostile to health professionals when they are finally seen. Understaffing often leaves health professionals feeling frustrated and dissatisfied as they attempt to meet the needs of too many patients with too little time and too few resources. Overworked staff worry about the effect of stretching themselves too thin and the impact this can have on patient care. Physical and psychological exhaustion resulting from excessive professional demands that can drain you have been aptly dubbed compassion fatigue. Introduced in Chapter 3, compassion fatigue is "the convergence of secondary traumatic stress and cumulative burnout, a state of physical and mental exhaustion caused by a depleted ability to cope with one's everyday environment."[15] Creating a repertoire of strategies for attending to the emotions that may arise from difficult patient encounters is one way to prevent compassion fatigue and realize more success in these interactions. Luff and colleagues[16] identified several common strategies that experienced health professionals use to assist them in problem-solving through difficult conversations. They include self-care, development of preparatory and relational skills, empathic presence, use of a team approach, and reliance on one's professional identity. These strategies are summarized in Table 16.1.

Disparities of Power

We have noted several times in this book that patients are placed in a position of diminished power upon entering the health care environment. The numerous losses that patients face

TABLE 16.1 ■ Strategies Used by Health Professionals to Manage Emotions Related to Difficult Conversations

Category	Strategies
Self-care	Identify personal emotions before conversation Breathe deeply Take breaks or use self-calming techniques Find an outlet to decompress (exercise, writing) Talk about experience with others Acknowledge individual and system-level limitations
Preparatory and relational skills	Anticipate family's needs Consider how patient/family would most prefer to hear the news Rehearse conversations ahead of time Speak slowly; allow silence Adapt approach based on patient/family responses/emotional cues
Empathic presence	Put yourself in patient's/family's shoes Imagine the context of the patient/family health care journey Remember primary role to support patient/family
Team approach	Include other team members in conversation to broaden expertise offered to patient/family Consult with more experienced peers and mentors before conversation Debrief with other team members after conversation
Professional identity	Lead with compassion Separate emotion from responsibility Leave professional problems at the workplace

From Luff D. Martin EB, Mills K, Mazzola NM, Bell SK, Meyer EC. Clinicians' strategies for managing their emotions during difficult healthcare conversations. Patient Education and Counseling 99, 1461–1466. 2016.

because of illness or trauma include independence, social status, ability to fulfill responsibilities, and other expressions of identity. Often these expressions of identity are taken away precipitously when people enter a health care institution. These factors contribute to feelings of powerlessness. A common reaction to powerlessness is anger, and a common target of anger is the most accessible and least-threatening health professional involved with the patient.[17] Thus students are often the target for a torrent of rage from a patient that has little to do with the student or his or her abilities. Few studies have explored patients' perceptions of this inequity in power, but in one study of mental health workers and patients, both groups reported an awareness of the struggle to gain or retain power and control. Patients noted that when health professionals demonstrated respect, took time with them, and were willing to give them some control and choice in their own care, feelings of anger were reduced.[18]

Role Expectations

Because we are socialized not to use negative terms such as "bad," we substitute euphemisms to describe patients with the attributes listed earlier. They are described as disruptive, unmotivated, maladaptive, and manipulative. Patients who are perceived to be difficult to treat evoke intense negative affective responses in the health professional that can work against establishing a positive, constructive relationship.[19] Furthermore, there is also a strong possibility that the professional's language exerts a powerful impact on thought and, consequently, action. Negative words lead to negative thoughts and actions regarding difficult patients. An example from rehabilitation medicine highlights the impact of language.

Most rehabilitation staff members have encountered patients who resist their best efforts to engage them in therapeutic activities. These patients seem to not want to be in rehabilitation.

They may view therapies as trivial, irrelevant, uninteresting, or too demanding, and they must be constantly coaxed to attend therapy sessions; if they do attend, they do not participate. Staff members become quickly frustrated with patients who do not share the "rehabilitation perspective" that places a high premium on attaining optimal independent functioning within constraints imposed by the patient's condition.

Any patient behavior that is inconsistent with expected patient role behavior (read "good patient behavior") could negatively influence the care of the patient. Not only might you be tempted to diminish your efforts in the care of a nonadhering patient, but you might also resort to distancing yourself from the patient. Unfortunately, avoidance and distancing may result in the reinforcement of deviant behavior as a patient response to nonsupportive care. In extreme cases, health professionals have been known to respond to difficult patients with their own version of negative behavior. In a national study of transplant coordinators, a full 62% revealed a belief that a hostile or antagonistic patient should not receive an organ transplantation.[20] The irony and tragedy in such findings are that expressions of anger and frustration (behavior that can be labeled as *hostile*) may be a natural response by patients to chronic illness.

Most health professionals can control these kinds of strong emotional reactions and continue, at least marginally, to meet their obligations to the patient. The result is a sort of "grudging attention" (i.e., the patient gets the minimal care that he or she needs and nothing more). Grudging attention occurs because of a combination of factors. Once a negative label is attached to a patient, it is difficult for health professionals to look past it and process other data about the patient. Negative labels often get "passed on" until a patient develops a bad reputation.[21] It is as if we see only one aspect of the patient. Couple these stereotypes about the difficult patient with idealistic role expectations of health professionals as caring, nonjudgmental, and capable of reaching every patient, and the result is an interaction devoid of everything but going through the motions.

Although it is important to work toward the goals of acceptance and constructive problem-solving, sometimes the only solution is to do what you must for the patient and then leave. This is exactly what happened in the case of a sexually aggressive patient who made lewd propositions and repeatedly exposed himself to his caregivers. The health professionals in the below case responded with grudging attention.

Case Study

Mr. Leland was getting only the absolute necessities—no extras. After all, who wants to sit down and chat with someone who talks about nothing but his sex life—or yours? Once our professional responsibilities were met, we avoided Mr. Leland. He could not fail to notice this, and as a result his demands for attention become angrier and more disruptive.[22]

REFLECTIONS

- If you were assigned to care for Mr. Leland and he continued to talk explicitly about sex after you asked him not to, what would be your next step?
- What are some possible negative outcomes of "grudging attention" for the patient or the health professional staff?

Going through the minimal motions of care is a temporary and ineffective solution to a much larger problem. Often it results in guilt on the part of the health professional and can result, as in the case of Mr. Leland, in an escalation of the behavior that led to avoidance in the first place. Although the following quote refers to nurses, the same can be applied to all health professions: "If patients interpret a nurse's manner as uninterested, or if they overhear pejorative comments, they fear that they will not be cared for adequately. It is as valuable to examine staff's behaviors as it is to understand a patient's motivations."[23]

Difficult Health Professional and Patient Relationships

In this section, we introduce you to two patients who share some of the attributes that have been identified as difficult by most health professionals. As you examine some of the character traits and behaviors of the two patients and the nature of the relationships with health professionals, perhaps you will gain insight into your own values and attitudes and reflect on how you will respond.

Working With Patients Who Are Self-Destructive

Sometimes the most difficult patient is not the one who commits actions that are outrageous or inappropriate but who shrinks from constructive action and resorts to self-harm behavior such as that encountered in the case of Violet Mercer and Tina Kramolisch.

Case Study

Tina Kramolisch worked evenings and weekends in a busy urban emergency department (ED) as a technician while she finished her last year of professional preparation. Tina often commented to classmates that you really do not have a taste for what it is like in practice without the experiences you find in an ED. In fact, Tina felt as if she had seen it all and was quite proud of her ability to work with different types of patients in various levels of distress. However, after taking care of Violet Mercer, Tina wondered if she was ready to care for all types of patients.

Tina entered the holding area where Violet lay still on the examination table under a sheet. When Tina said Violet's name, there was no response, so Tina gently touched the woman's arm. Violet flinched so violently at the touch that it startled Tina as well and she jumped back from the cart. Tina was even more shocked at how Violet looked. Violet murmured, "You scared me." The words were somewhat difficult to understand as Violet's lips were swollen and split in one corner. Violet had lacerations, contusions, and swelling all over her face. Tina had never seen anyone so badly beaten. Tina noticed old bruises and injuries all over Violet's body as she conducted her intake assessment. Tina knew the physician would have to confirm her observation, but she was almost certain that several of Violet's ribs were fractured.

Because Tina had been trained to work with women who had been abused, she knew the right questions to ask and did so. Violet admitted, cautiously, that her husband, Donnie, had lost his temper and done this to her. Tina reported her findings to the nurse and physician, and they set into motion the services and protection the health care and criminal justice systems can offer battered women. In fact, Donnie was being treated down the hall for a scalp laceration that Violet had inflicted as she tried to defend herself. The police who brought the Mercers into the ED were waiting outside Donnie's room to see if Violet would press charges. Tina was holding Violet's hand as the rib binder was put into place when the nurse entered the room and said, "The social worker can take you to the women's shelter after you talk to the police." Violet did not look up as she said in a flat voice, "I've changed my mind. I don't want to press charges. I'm going with Donnie." Tina was speechless as she watched every effort to change Violet's mind fail. Tina felt hot tears of frustration and anger run down her cheeks as she watched Violet and Donnie leave the ED arm-in-arm.

REFLECTIONS

- Why do you think Tina felt a combination of frustration and anger with Violet?
- What would your reaction be?

In this case, Violet adheres to Tina's professional interventions, willing to accept them—to a point. In Violet's case, the perception of difficulty rests to some extent on the invalidating effects of Violet's behavior on Tina and the other health professionals caring for her. In the eyes of the professionals, intervention in Violet's case should include more than merely suturing her cuts and bandaging her broken ribs; it should also include offering her a way out of an abusive, potentially life-threatening situation. When Violet fails to accept the help that is offered to her, the primary treatment goal is thwarted and the health professional's role as a therapeutic agent can feel invalidated.

Working With Patients With a History of Violent Behavior

Many health professionals feel inadequately prepared to deal with patients who have a complex medical condition that is complicated further by a history that involves violent behavior. The case on Darrin Block and Austin Greder involves a seriously ill patient and behavior that is generally unacceptable in an acute care institution.

Case Study

Darrin Block was a nurse on the step-down unit at an urban medical center. Because of the medical center's location in a large city, the intensive care unit got more than its fair share of victims of gunshot wounds. Most of these patients were male, young, unemployed, and knew their assailants. Many were members of gangs and had to be admitted under aliases for their own protection. Austin Greder fit this description exactly. He was a 21-year-old high school dropout who had been shot by a rival gang member. Although he lacked formal education, Austin was bright. His major sources of support were his mother and a girlfriend. He was admitted to the surgical intensive care unit in serious condition but had begun to recover, so he was moved to a medical/surgical step-down unit. His wound was not healing as well as the treatment team expected. Since his admission to the step-down unit, the staff had referred to Austin and his numerous visitors as "nothing but trouble." Large numbers of visitors moved in a steady stream in and out of Austin's room, even though the staff had told them about the restrictions on visitors in the unit. Austin's girlfriend, Alicia, had practically taken up residence in Austin's room. One time, Darrin walked into Austin's room and found him and Alicia involved in what appeared to be sexual activity. Darrin left in confused embarrassment but was somewhat angry, too. He did not expect to walk in on a sexual encounter and did not think he should have to apologize. After this incident, Darrin asked Alicia to leave whenever he entered the room to provide care. In response, Austin became angry and dismissive to Darrin, refusing to let him perform wound care and asking for one of the other nurses to care for him. To make matters worse, Austin revealed his alias to a friend even though this undermined maintenance of security on the unit. Darrin thought the right thing to do was set limits on Austin's behavior because things were clearly getting out of control. However, he was fearful of retaliation by Austin's friends outside of the safety of the hospital. He had heard more than one other member of the interprofessional care team talk about being confronted in the parking garage by one of "these gang members."

REFLECTIONS

- Put yourself in Darrin Block's position. What would you do the next time the patient refused wound care?
- What resources might there be in the hospital to assist Darrin and the interprofessional care team in working with Mr. Greder to "set limits"?

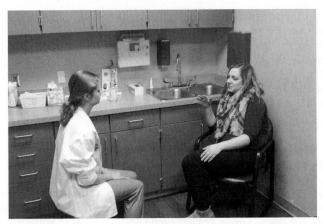

Fig. 16.2 Patients and health professionals sometimes must engage in difficult discussions. (*Courtesy Maren Haddad.*)

These patients challenge the notion of what it means to be a "good" health professional. They make us realize that, although we are generally able to effectively help patients, sometimes we fall far short even with our best efforts. In the following section, we offer various techniques that may help you in working with difficult patients of all types. We also share some ideas about changing a difficult working environment.

Showing Respect in Difficult Situations

When patients are uncooperative, manipulative, angry, or they reject help, this is not a license to show disrespect toward them as persons (Fig. 16.2). You will have to be responsive to your own feelings of disgust, fear, anger, and so forth, as well as manage patients' unacceptable behavior.

Reframing. An appropriate place to start is to show respect by initially refusing to believe that you are dealing with a person whose character is flawed. Reframing the interaction is important to recognize that the patient has complex health and social needs. The behaviors and attitudes may be the result of a treatable or modifiable factor. For example, one of your first determinations is to make certain that the patient has received a thorough, understandable explanation of the treatment or therapy in question. The patient may also be unmotivated or uncooperative if he or she has not been shown the respect of participation in establishing personally meaningful goals. After these more obvious problem areas are explored and resolved and problems persist, you can turn to the following types of behaviors that have been found to be effective in working with difficult patients.

Structuring and Consistency. As a rule, for all types of difficult situations, structure and consistency in communication in every aspect of patient care are important.[24] A key component of a deliberate, consistent approach is setting limits. Setting firm limits is a part of setting boundaries with all patients but with additional safeguards given the extremity of the situation. By setting forth clear, consistent expectations in a nondefensive manner, you can help strengthen the patient's inner control. Be open to negotiation. Listen for opportunities to find out what is important to the patient.

When you are involved in setting limits, respect for the patient must govern the interaction. You should ask yourself whether the limits you are setting are arbitrary—that is, do they stem from your need to be in control or punish the patient—or whether the patient' welfare would indeed be best served by establishing external limits. Any plan to set limits should be agreed on by all members of the interprofessional care team to avoid the potential for a patient to "split" the staff (i.e., divide staff into all good or all bad). Good communication lines among all members of the team are essential. For example, the patient may use charm and flattery to manipulate some staff members but make disparaging and critical comments about their co-workers.[25]

Focus on Behaviors. It is also helpful to focus on a patient's unacceptable behaviors rather than on the patient himself or herself. This allows for open communication and avoids negative labeling that tends to stick to patients and obscure the real problem. One way to avoid negative labeling of patients is to be honest with them and tell them exactly how you feel. Again, your honest comments should be directed at the patient's behavior and not at the patient. This way you can share your reactions and still not humiliate the patient. Look for opportunities to give plenty of positive feedback for desired behaviors. Also, focus on the here and now rather than long-term aspects of behavior. If all else fails, a behavioral contract can be developed to focus on specific actions. A contract, sometimes called a *patient care agreement,* "outlines the expectations, plans, and responsibilities of the patient and the consequences for noncompliance."[24]

Contribute to a Respectful Environment. On a broader basis, you can encourage the development of an environment that is respectful of everyone. Such a setting encourages patients to ask questions and challenge the system's rules and practices. If just a single member of the health care team prompts the patient legitimately to question his or her care, the rest of the team could come to see the patient as "difficult." Having patients ask about the care they receive and make decisions about their care must be considered the normal, desired state. The safety of health professionals also should be encouraged in a respectful environment. There must be practices and policies in place to give staff members basic protection from harassment, abuse, and other threats. You may find yourself in an environment that is amenable to change through education and support for staff. In fact, the support of supervisory staff in the form of validation and insight is an essential component of an environment that fosters positive health professional and patient interactions.

DIFFICULT CONVERSATIONS

Communication is the most common procedure in health care. It is so central to a respectful relationship that Chapters 7 and 9 are devoted directly to aspects of it. Unlike other procedures, there are no easy checklists or algorithms for executing communication because each conversation involves different individuals, topics, and contexts. However, studies show that health professionals who practice difficult conversations improve the quality and outcomes of their communications. The text that follows summarizes 10 evidence-based guidelines for showing respect toward patients and families in difficult conversations[17,22,26–34]:

1. *Timeliness matters.* Many people avoid difficult conversations because the topic may be hard to discuss, or those involved may have difficult behaviors. Do not avoid or wait too long. Most individuals appreciate information that is timely, clear, and direct.
2. *The setting matters.* One would think this might go without saying; however, in busy health care environments, health professionals are more likely to have hallway conversations and forget that patients and families need the proper space and place to hear important messages. Aim to always talk at the bedside or in a private space.
3. *Establish goals for the conversation and practice in advance.* If you are on an interprofessional care team, make sure all members of the team understand the goals before the meeting. Ask yourselves "what is the one message we want the patient or family member to take away from this conversation." As part of planning, expect, rather than avoid uncertainty and complexity.
4. *Start the conversation by communicating the big picture and why all involved should care.* Respectfully acknowledge the emotions in the room with candor. Commit to seek shared decision-making and mutual purpose.

5. *Remember that the caring function is as important as other interventions.* Make an empathetic statement such as, "I know you must be frustrated or disappointed." This kind of response tells the patient that you understand. In the words of Brene Brown "empathy is a strange and powerful thing. There is no script. There is no right or wrong way to do it. It is simply listening, holding space, withholding judgment, emotionally connecting, and communicating that incredibly healing message of you are not alone."[33]

6. *Talk less and listen more.* Generally, if you are talking more than half of the time, you are talking too much. Ask open-ended questions such as "What is your understanding of the situation?" or "What are your fears?" and "What are your hopes?" This helps you understand the patient or family perspective. Next share your point of view. Avoid trying to persuade; rather, work together to solve problems and achieve shared decision-making.

7. *State facts and observations to remain as objective as possible.* Avoid the use of derogatory labels as a means of reducing your frustration or anger. Label the encounter, not the patient. It is also helpful to use "I" statements versus "you" statements. For example, instead of saying "Your mental health is not good, you cannot think clearly" say "Given the care team's observations of your disorganized thinking, I am concerned about your mental health."

8. *Set realistic expectations.* Your own power as a health professional to achieve treatment adherence must be based on realistic expectations. Do not expect to change aspects of the patient's situation beyond your control. Instead, try to help change the underlying social and institutional conditions or attitudes that lead to nonadherence in high-need populations.

9. *Ensure safety.* When interacting with an aggressive patient or family, always ensure personal safety for yourself, members of the interprofessional care team, and the patient. Monitor body language and tone of voice that can quickly escalate to a threatening stance. If a patient or family member is hostile, diffuse the situation by allowing him or her to vent uninterrupted. Then strive to understand the problem, affirm what can be done, and follow through. Bring in additional resources such as ethics consultants and security personnel as needed. Affirm policies and practices (e.g., the patient rights and responsibilities statement) that are in place in your institution to encourage mutual respect.

10. *Conclude by clarifying expectations and summarizing the conversation.* Document the plan so that all members of the interprofessional care team know the direction of care and any emotional support that the patient, family, or team may require.

Although all your efforts as a health professional should be directed at acknowledging negative biases and keeping them in check, you may find that you cannot operate in the best interest of a given patient, no matter how much you try. If it comes to letting a patient go, be certain that you are referring him or her to a capable professional and not abandoning the person. Respect includes everybody, but as humans we come in all shapes and forms, so the wise health professional recognizes that unresolvable difficulties with patients and situations will arise.

PROFESSIONALS' MISTAKES AND MAKING APOLOGY

An additional difficult situation that is unfortunately all too common in health care is dealing with errors in patient care, whether they are the result of individual mistakes or generated by system-level problems. All errors include challenges between the individual health professional and patient involved, as well as within the broader system in which the error occurred.

In recent years, significant literature in the health professions has emerged on the topic of the response of health professionals to a patient when a mistake related to the patient's care is made by individual professionals or as a result of a systems error in the health care institution. Communication breakdowns, diagnostic errors, poor judgment, and inadequate skill have all been found to result in patient harm and death.[35] The number of deaths and serious injuries that occur in the United States each year alone is staggering. Recent literature estimates an incidence range of 210,000 to 400,000 deaths per year associated with medical errors and preventable adverse events in hospitalized patients.[36] When compared to the Centers for Disease Control and Prevention rankings, this suggests that if medical error was categorized as a disease, it would be the third most common cause of death in the United States.[35] Errors that have serious negative consequences for the patient must be disclosed to the patient or his or her family, and appropriate restitution must be made. However, disclosure of an error is generally difficult for health professionals.

There are numerous reasons why disclosure of errors to a patient and his or her family is so difficult for health professionals. One is that health professionals often think they are immune to error, so they find it difficult to admit that an error has occurred. The second reason is that it is experienced as a sign of failure. Third, until recently there have been few mechanisms in place for health professionals to talk freely with peers about the circumstances surrounding an error because of shame and irrational legal fears. Finally, disclosing an error to a patient and following the disclosure by apologizing requires a great deal of humility and skill on the part of the health professional. The case of Melanie Lieberman and Laura Keenan deals with the various facets of disclosure of an error that resulted in harm to the patient.

Case Study

It was an exceptionally busy night on the medical/surgical floor where Melanie Lieberman worked. To make matters worse, one of the nurses called in sick at the last moment and the supervisor was unable to get a replacement for the first 4 hours of the 7 p.m. to 7 a.m. shift. Melanie had responsibility for twice the number of patients that she usually would during the beginning of the shift, the busiest time during the 12 hours she would be on duty. One of the patients under Melanie's care was Laura Keenan, who returned to the unit in the early evening from surgery for a mastectomy and breast reconstruction. Melanie was able to manage a full assessment of Laura at the beginning of the shift, but after that she was on a dead run with medications, dressing changes, pages, and phone calls from physicians for new orders on a transfer from the emergency department, etc. When Melanie sped past Laura's room, she did look in once or twice to affirm that the patient was resting quietly but she did not have time to complete a more thorough assessment. When the replacement nurse finally arrived at 11 p.m., Melanie offered up a quick report to her colleague on the patients he would assume responsibility for the rest of the shift and then went straight to Laura's room. Melanie realized after taking Laura's blood pressure and pulse that something was wrong. A quick look at the dressings covering the reconstruction indicated that Laura was bleeding and likely suffering from hypovolemic shock. Melanie knew that the most common postoperative problem for breast reconstruction patients was bleeding and she had not checked for the most obvious signs of this complication. After summoning additional assistance to monitor Laura, Melanie rushed to contact the surgeon and supervisor and upon returning learned that in her brief absence Laura's vital signs indicated worsening shock. Melanie increased the rate of the intravenous fluid and reinforced the dressing, all the while mentally berating herself for missing such an obvious problem. She knew she was overstretched but thought she could handle the workload. Now her lack of monitoring for a predictable problem was going to require another trip to the operating room for Laura and perhaps life-threatening consequences if the surgical team did not get the bleeding stopped fast enough. As if things were not bad enough, Melanie knew that she would have to talk to Laura's family and explain what happened. She dreaded this more than anything. Nothing like this had ever happened to Melanie before.

REFLECTIONS

- Review the case and indicate where you think the error of lack of monitoring could have been prevented. In other words, would you have handled the situation differently from the way Melanie did given the same set of circumstances?
- What are the system-level problems that contributed to the error?
- What are the individual-level issues that contributed to the error?

The type of error in the case of Melanie Lieberman and Laura Keenan is a combination of the failure of the individual, in this case the nurse, to meet basic standards of postoperative care and system-level problems, including staffing issues. To prevent errors from occurring in the future, health professionals must view errors as a learning opportunity that is different from the "shame-and-blame culture that focuses only on individual responsibility or culpability."[37]

Melanie's error is not uncommon. Neither is her reaction to the expectations of negotiating the rough terrain of owning up to her share of the responsibility and disclosing what happened in a manner that is meaningful to the patient and her family. She knows that this will mean taking accountability and communicating a genuine apology. The right apology, at the right time, in the right context can do wonders for reestablishing trust, allowing patient, family, and health professional to move forward. The science of safety, including root cause analysis and the development of safety culture tools and systems, helps support the health professional when an error occurs. They serve to break the silence surrounding such events in clinical practice. Institutional supports are in place for health professionals to report, resolve, and reflect on errors. These supports begin with members of the interprofessional care team and extend to supervisors and employee assistance programs. Many organizations have offices of quality and safety who will provide on-call support, including incident debriefing. These supports are key to ensuring efficient, effective, and high-quality patient outcomes, while at the same time ensuring that both individual health professionals and systems learn from mistakes.

Summary

This chapter makes suggestions about respectful interaction with types of patients whom many health professionals find difficult to treat without negative feelings or behaviors intruding on the relationship. Sources may be the patient's personality and behavior, societal stereotypes, the professional's own countertransference and learned behaviors, or the opinions of peers. The environment in which the relationship takes place also can cause difficulties and add to frustration, anger, and other negative responses by both parties. The environment often plays a significant role in one of the most difficult health professional and patient situations, the occurrence of an error and its aftermath. Despite such challenges, your responsibility to show respect for the patient as a person remains and can be expressed through attempts to use strategies that provide an opportunity to minimize the negative aspects of the relationship and optimize care outcomes.

See Section 6 Questions for Thought and Discussion on page 266 to apply what you've learned in this section to a variety of case scenarios.

References

1. Shaw I. Doctors, "dirty work" patients, and "revolving doors." *Qual Health Res*. 2004;14(8):1032–1045.
2. Santamaria N. The relationship between nurses' personality and stress levels reported when caring for interpersonally difficult patients. *Aust J Adv Nurs*. 2000;18(2):20–26.
3. Herbert CP, Seifert MH. When the patient is the problem. *Patient Care*. 1990;24(1):59.
4. Hawking M, Curlin FA, Yoon JD. Courage and compassion: virtues in caring for so-called "difficult" patients. *AMA J Ethics*. 2017;19(4):357–363.
5. Miksanek T. On caring for "difficult" patients. *Health Affairs*. 2008;27(5):1422–1428.
6. Kelly MP, May D. Good and bad patients: a review of the literature and a theoretical critique. *J Adv Nurs*. 1982;7:147–156.
7. Timko C, Schultz NR, Britt J, et al. Regular article: transitioning from detoxification to substance use disorder treatment: facilitators and barriers. *J Subst Abuse Treat*. 2016;7064–7072.
8. World Health Organization. *Adherence to Long-term Therapies: Evidence for Action.* Geneva: Switzerland; 2003.
9. Lofland P. *Adherence to Treatment in Clinical Practice*. New York: Nova Science Publishers, Inc.; 2014.

10. Cohen DJ, Davis MM, Hall JD, et al. *A Guidebook of Professional Practices for Behavioral Health and Primary Care Integration: Observations From Exemplary Sites.* Rockville, MD: Agency for Healthcare Research and Quality; 2015.

11. Salzberg CA, Hayes SL, McCarthy D, et al. *Health System Performance for the High-Need Patient: A Look at Access to Care and Patient Care Experiences.* New York: The Commonwealth Fund; 2016.

12. Zodet M. *Characteristics of Persons with High Health Care Expenditures in the U.S. Civilian Noninstitutionalized Population.* Agency for Healthcare Research and Quality; 2014.

13. Long PM, Abrams A, Milstein G, et al., eds. *Effective Care for High-Need Patients: Opportunities for Improving Outcomes, Value, and Health.* Washington, DC: National Academy of Medicine; 2017.

14. Rader J. To bathe or not to bathe: that is the question. *J Gerontol Nurs.* 1994;20(9):53.

15. Cocker F, Joss N. Compassion fatigue among healthcare, emergency and community service works: a systematic review. *Int J Environ Res Public Health.* 2016;13:1–18.

16. Luff D, Martin EB, Mills K, et al. Clinicians' strategies for managing their emotions during difficult healthcare conversations. *Patient Educ Couns.* 2016;99:1461–1466.

17. Mittal D, Ounpraseuth ST, Reaves C, et al. Providers' personal and professional contact with persons with mental illness: relationship to clinical expectations. *Psychiatr Serv.* 2016;67(1):55–61.

18. Breeze JA, Repper J. Struggling for control: the care experiences of "difficult" patients in mental health services. *J Adv Nurs.* 1998;28(6):1301–1311.

19. Gallop R, Lancee W, Shugar G. Residents' and nurses' perceptions of difficult-to-treat short-stay patients. *Hosp Comm Psychiatry.* 1993;44(4):352.

20. Neil JA, Corley MC. Hostility toward caregivers as a selection criterion for transplantation. *Prog Transplant.* 2000;10(3):177–181.

21. Juliana CA, Orehowsky S, Smith-Regojo P, et al. Interventions by staff nurses to manage "difficult" patients. *Holist Nurs Pract.* 1997;11(4):1–26.

22. Wasan AD, Wootton J, Jamison RN. Dealing with difficult patients in your pain practice. *Reg Anesth Pain Med.* 2005;30(2):184–192.

23. Nield-Anderson L, Minarik PA, Dilworth JM, et al. Responding to the "difficult" patient: manipulation, sexual provocation, aggression—how can you manage such behaviors? *Am J Nurs.* 1999;99(12):26–34.

24. Morrison EF, Ramsey A, Synder B. Managing the care of complex, difficult patients in the medical-surgical setting. *Medsurg Nursing.* 2000;9(1):21–26.

25. Daum AL. The disruptive antisocial patient: management strategies. *Nurs Manage.* 1994;25(8):49.

26. Browning DM, Solomon MZ. The initiative for pediatric palliative care: an interdisciplinary educational approach for health care professionals. *J Pediatr Nurs.* 2005;20:326–334.

27. Farrell M. Difficulty conversations. *J Libr Adm.* 2015;55:302–311.

28. Hinkle LJ, Fettig LP, Carlos WG, et al. Twelve tips for just in time teaching of communication skills for difficult conversations in the clinical setting. *Med Teach.* 2017;39(9):920–925.

29. Cline C. Why some conflicts involving "difficult patients" should remain outside the province of the ethics consultation service. *Am J Bioethics.* 2012;12(5):16–18.

30. Hinkle LJ, Fettig LP, Carlos WG, et al. Twelve tips for just in time teaching of communication skills for difficult conversations in the clinical setting. *Med Teach.* 2017;39(9):920–925.

31. American Association for the Advancement of Science. *Communication Fundamentals;* 2017. https://www.aaas.org/page/communication-fundamentals-0.

32. Gawande A. *Being Mortal: Medicine and What Matters in the End.* New York: Metropolitan Books; 2014.

33. Brown B. *Daring Greatly: How the Courage to be Vulnerable Transforms the Way We Live, Love, Parent, and Lead.* New York: Avery Publishers; 2015:125.

34. Stone D, Patton B, Heen S. *Difficult Conversations: How to Discuss What Matters Most.* New York: Penguin Books; 2010.

35. Makary MD, Daniel M. Medical error—third leading cause of death in the US. *BMJ.* 2016;353:1–5. https://phstwlp2.partners.org:3267/10.1136/bmj.i2139.

36. James JTA. A new, evidence-based estimate of patient harms associated with hospital care. *J Patient Safety.* 2013;9:122–128.

37. Woods A, Doan-Johnson S. Executive summary: toward a taxonomy of nursing practice errors. *Nurs Manage.* 2002;32(10):45.

Section Questions for Thought and Discussion

Section 1

1. What important ways is your education—designed for a career in the health professions—similar to and different from other types of formal education? From what you have read so far, do you think the emphasis on respect is more compelling for persons practicing in the professions than other lines of work (e.g., business, home construction, the performing arts)? Discuss why or why not.

2. As you have learned, professional respect requires you to adapt to the challenges of everyday situations. One such example is that everyone who treats patients sometimes gets into a time bind for one reason or another. Cecilia has been caught short today because so many patients on her schedule needed a little extra time with her for her to feel she has given them their fair share of professional attention. As the afternoon progresses, she is becoming increasingly further behind and is aware that three patients are in the waiting area and she needs a solution to fit three into a time frame usually reserved for two before the unit closes. None of them knows the time when the others were scheduled to be seen.

   For her to show due respect for each person, what should she do? Discuss why each of the options offered here is or is not acceptable. You can combine some of the choices or add others of your own.
   a. Continue to take them in the order they were originally scheduled, cutting the time for each one, and explain the situation to each one privately.
   b. Tell all of them together what the situation is and let them decide among themselves the order in which they will be seen.
   c. Make an independent decision about who is most in need of care, and take them in that order, telling all three of them what you are doing and apologizing for what has happened.

3. You have become good friends with Colin, a professional colleague who works closely with you and now has come to you for advice. He tells you that he is planning to take a weekend trip with Tony, a male patient who was discharged from your institution 2 weeks ago. Everyone thought this patient had progressed sufficiently to be discharged, but already it is apparent he will benefit from further treatment in the ambulatory care clinic. Neither of you works in that part of the institution. You both were part of Tony's interprofessional care team, and so he is aware you know what a fine person Tony seems to be. Colin asks you, "Do you think there is any reason I shouldn't go with him? I suppose he could become my patient again. But I like him, and, obviously, the attraction was mutual. Between you and me, he asked me out when we first started working together. I told him hooking up in the institution wasn't much fun, and we both laughed. I thought it had cooled down, but he called 2 days after discharge with his offer."

   As a co-worker and friend, how will you respond to your colleague Colin's question? Discuss the factors you will consider that support your decision to respond in this way.

Section 2

1. You have been asked by colleagues to run for office in the state organization of your profession. You are already busy with work and your personal commitments, and still you are tempted and honored to be recognized by your peers. List your most important priorities, and decide what would be compromised the most by taking on this new position should you be elected. What values will determine whether you will choose to run for this office?

2. You are the supervisor of an ambulatory clinic. You recognize an increase in the number of Mayan immigrants in your patient population. You are also surprised to learn that English is their third language. The Mayans speak Spanish as a second language and commonly do not read Spanish. Where should you start in preparing yourself and peers to care for these patients?

3. An 8-year-old girl presents at the emergency department with her mother. Both are recent immigrants from Afghanistan. The child has several unusual neurological symptoms, but when the physician recommends a lumbar puncture to rule out encephalitis, the child's mother refuses. When asked why, she explains that a "djinn" (a spirit in Islamic folk belief) is involved and the lumbar puncture will upset the djinn and her daughter will become more ill.[1] As a health professional involved in her care, how should you proceed?

4. Obtain an organizational chart from a clinical site, and identify the various administrators such as the Chief Executive Officer and the lines of communication that link various departments and employees. Notice if the organizational chart includes such areas as quality assurance, risk management, compliance, and human resources and any information about reporting mechanisms. What does the organizational chart tell you about the organization? Are the lines of reporting and responsibilities clear and understandable?

Reference

1. Seelman C, Suuromond J, Stronks K. Cultural competence: a conceptual framework for teaching and learning. *Med Educ*. 2009;434:229–237.

Section 3

1. Find a standard "case study" in a professional journal. Rewrite it from the patient's perspective. Now, rewrite it from the family's perspective.

2. In groups of four, have one student act as a patient with an injury such as a fall from a ladder; have the second act as the interviewer trying to find out how the patient was injured and what sort of pain or other symptoms that patient is experiencing; have a third student act as the patient's family member who heard the fall and arrived to find the loved one on the ground; and have the fourth student observe and then critique the interview process. Change roles four times so that all get to play the patient, health professional, family member, and observer/critic. What do you discover about the patient's story with the different interview techniques? What works well, and what does not? What did you learn about how to best interact with the family member as a member of the team supporting the patient's care?

3. A patient asks you if she can bring her friend to treatment with her. You know that this patient has been asking a lot of questions and seems to be anxious. When the friend comes, she starts asking you some of the same questions that the patient asked you previously. Some are what you would take as private matters. You want to honor the patient's privacy and so are hesitant to respond. The friend states, "You know how anxious she gets. I just want to be able to reassure her, and I can't do that without knowing what is going on."

   You ask the patient what she would like you to share, and she just shrugs her shoulders. You really cannot tell whether the shrug is a passive resignation or what else. Not feeling completely comfortable with your answer, you say to them that you are not free to share information with anyone unless the patient is more positive that it is OK. At that she shrugs her shoulders again.

What steps can you take to show this patient and her friend respect in spite of your concerns about the patient's privacy? What specific questions might you ask to better understand the role of this friend in supporting the patient's recovery?

4. A single woman in her 60s comes to you with symptoms you know are related to the stress of her position as the primary family caregiver for her elderly father who has Alzheimer's disease. You know the best thing for her is to have some respite from the situation. You first ask her about other family members who might share her responsibility, but she claims to have none who are willing or able to help share her burden. Her situation seems perilous to you, and you begin to think of a perfect society where she would not be stuck in this seemingly endless and intense situation. List all the things you can think of to design an environment for her and her father so that both can realize the respect they deserve.

5. You are asked to participate on the planning committee charged with designing the new waiting room for families in the emergency room at your institution. The architects report that they are eager for "front line clinicians" to provide input. What suggestions will you provide to the architects, decorators, and administrators?

Section 4

1. Form interprofessional teams or role-play different members of the interprofessional team in groups of five or six; assign roles such as timekeeper, recorder, and observer. Assume you all work within the same outpatient pediatric clinic. In 45 minutes, establish goals for a standard procedure for communicating with parents about vaccination that incorporates the unique perspectives of each member of the interprofessional team particularly regarding parents who are selective about vaccination or refuse to have their children vaccinated at the clinic where the team works. Who took the leadership position and why? Were all the appropriate members of the team present who would have helpful input and expertise for this planning session? Was everyone given an opportunity to be heard? What did the observer note that members of the team did not?

2. Think of a clinical situation that you participated in or witnessed where interprofessional communication (verbal or nonverbal) was essential to the outcome—for example, a situation that took a turn, for better or worse, because of the quality of the communication? In what ways was communication key to the outcome? If a negative outcome, what barriers were evident that prevented effective communication?

3. Write out instructions for a simple procedure such as using a cane or giving a subcutaneous injection that a patient might carry out at home. Share the instructions with a classmate and see if he or she is unclear about any of the written instructions. Work together to improve the clarity of the written instructions. What do other modes of communication such as email messages, texts, or web-based patient education materials offer that basic written instructions do not? Experiment with delivering the same instructions but in an electronic format. Which works better and why?

4. Dennis is a 24-year-old man who has had surgery to control his epilepsy. Unfortunately, postoperatively he remains somewhat confused and apprehensive about health care settings. His wife brings him to your department, and you can see his anxiety. You must perform some tests on him that will not hurt him but will require his cooperation.
   a. What parts of this setting may be causing his anxiety?
   b. What aspects of your appearance may be causing his anxiety?
   c. What steps will you take to establish communication with him?
   d. How may his wife be helpful in facilitating effective "dialogue" between you and Dennis?

Section 5

1. You are approached by a parent of a child in the elementary school setting where you work. The parent is concerned that her daughter is falling behind in her schoolwork, and she is concerned that "no one appears to be listening to her." Her two older sons have learning disorders, and she is worried that her daughter may be at risk as well. How would you respond to this parent's concern?

2. You are the supervisor of an adolescent unit in a hospital. The patient, a 16-year-old named Sam, is mature for his age, and you have found him to be very thoughtful. Sam has cancer that you know has metastasized. His parents have decided with the surgeon that he should have an amputation, although all agree that the hope of saving him completely from the spread of the disease is negligible. One evening you notice that Sam is withdrawn. He says, "My parents and the doctor are going to cut off my leg, and they haven't even asked me what I think about it. I'd rather die than lose my leg."
   a. What should you do?
   b. To whom should you speak about this conversation? Why?
   c. How can the interprofessional care team best support Sam, and his family, guided by the principles of patient- and family-centered care?

3. You are hurrying down the hospital corridor when you notice an acquaintance of your family, a firefighter in his middle 50s, who is apparently a patient. You express surprise at seeing him there because he has always been the picture of good health. He tells you that he has had a heart attack. Suddenly he begins to pour out a blow-by-blow description of the incident. As he talks, he becomes increasingly agitated and finally bursts into tears, sobbing, "It's all over. I'll never be able to go back to my job or anything. What am I going to do?"
   a. What can you say or do right then to calm this man's immediate anxious state?
   b. Will you report this interaction? To whom and why?
   c. How can the interprofessional care team work together to treat the middle-age person's anxiety about the long-term effects of illness on family, job, and self-esteem?

4. Young adulthood is often referred to as "the healthy years and the hidden hazards." What does this mean? What are the implications for the life span?

5. Given what you know about the theories of aging, which theory do you find aligns best with your chosen health profession? Why? How will it support healthy aging in the patients you will be treating? How do you think the baby boomer generation will change or inform theories of aging over the next decade?

6. An alert 92-year-old patient who has been in your care for several days arrives late for treatment one morning at your ambulatory care clinic. She explains that she missed her usual bus and had to wait in the rain and cold for the next bus to arrive. You begin to converse with her in your usual manner and quickly realize that something is wrong; she does not answer your questions appropriately. Once or twice, she mentions her son (whom you know was killed years ago in the service of his country). Her sentences are disconnected and incomplete.
   a. What possible reasons may there be for her apparent confusion?
   b. Where will you start in your attempt to diagnose her problem?
   c. Who on the interprofessional care team will serve as resources to you as you navigate this change in presentation?

Section 6

1. You are in a patient's room performing a procedure. The patient, who has a type of cancer that is always fatal, has been told of his condition. While you are there, a man visiting a

patient in the next bed begins to describe the horror of his wife's last days before she died of cancer. Your patient becomes increasingly tense and finally begins to sob.

a. What can you do to console or reassure this patient?

b. What could you have done to prevent this situation?

c. What members of the interprofessional care team would you involve in responding to this patient and why?

2. You are working in an outpatient clinic in an economically depressed area of the city. A disheveled woman comes in dragging three young children behind her. One of the children begins to whine that she is hot. You are in the receiving area and see the woman hit the child so hard that the child falls to the floor and begins to scream. The woman looks at you in panic. You are already late for your next appointment. Your next patient is anxiously waiting to be seen and looks with scorn at the woman and you.

a. What feelings does this scene trigger?

b. You probably think there are some things you should do in this situation, but what would you really like to do?

c. What does this teach you about the possible difference between your emotional and "professional" reaction to this extreme situation?

d. What might you say to either the woman who hit the child or the observers of the incident to show respect to all involved? Instead of saying I would say "X," pair up with a partner and actually say the words out loud. Reflect on how you feel hearing yourself talk through difficult messages/conversations.

3. What types of patient care situations make you (or, if you are still a student, do you *think* will make you) the most uncomfortable? Identify two or three concrete interventions you would take to effectively deal with the challenging situations you identified.

INDEX

Note: Page numbers followed by "f" indicate figures, "t" indicate tables, and "b" indicate boxes.